Case Studies in Infectious Diseases

Case Studies in Infectious Diseases

Editor: Nyla Wright

AMERICAN
MEDICAL PUBLISHERS
www.americanmedicalpublishers.com

AMERICAN
MEDICAL PUBLISHERS
www.americanmedicalpublishers.com

Cataloging-in-Publication Data

Case studies in infectious diseases / edited by Nyla Wright.
p. cm.
Includes bibliographical references and index.
ISBN 979-8-88740-606-0
1. Infection. 2. Communicable diseases. 3. Infection--Case studies.
4. Communicable diseases--Case studies. I. Wright, Nyla.
RC111 .I543 2023
616.9--dc23

American Medical Publishers,
41 Flatbush Avenue,
1st Floor, New York,
NY 11217, USA

ISBN 979-8-88740-606-0 (Hardback)

Contents

Preface ... XI

Chapter 1 **Rhino-Orbital-Cerebral Mucormycosis in a Post-COVID-19 Patient from Peru** ... 1
Linda Ponce-Rosas, Jose Gonzales-Zamora, Nelson Diaz-Reyes, Oliver Alarco-Cadillo and Jorge Alave-Rosas

Chapter 2 **Pulmonary Mucormycosis in Chronic Lymphocytic Leukemia and Neutropenia** ... 7
Izza Mir, Sijan Basnet, David Ellsworth and Elan Mohanty

Chapter 3 ***Saccharomyces cerevisiae* Laryngitis and Oral Lesions in a Patient with Laryngeal Carcinoma** ... 11
Jumanah N. Algazaq, Kevan Akrami, Fernando Martinez, Allen McCutchan and Ajay R. Bharti

Chapter 4 **Infection of a Ventricular Septal Defect Patch with *Acremonium* Species** ... 15
Nosheen Nasir, Kauser Jabeen, Joveria Farooqi, Binish Arif Sultan, Afia Zafar, Aamir Hameed Khan, Muneer Amanullah and Farheen Ali

Chapter 5 **Cutaneous Fusariosis in a Patient with Job's (Hyper-IgE) Syndrome** ... 19
Ahmed M. Altibi, Radhika Sheth, Ayman Battisha and Vivek Kak

Chapter 6 ***Fusarium* Infection in a Kidney Transplant Recipient Successfully Treated with Voriconazole** ... 24
Ahmed M. Alkhunaizi, Ali M. Bazzi, Ali A. Rabaan and Elwaleed A. Ahmed

Chapter 7 **Rare Case of Four Osseous Lesions of the Skull in a Patient with Secondary Syphilis** ... 28
Jace Kusler and Supha Arthurs

Chapter 8 ***Cystoisospora belli* Gallbladder Infection in a Liver Transplant Donor** ... 31
Clifford Akateh, Christina A. Arnold, Dathe Benissan-Messan, Anthony Michaels and Sylvester M. Black

Chapter 9 **Unusual Radiographic Presentation of Pneumocystis Pneumonia in a Patient with AIDS** ... 36
Brian L. Block, Tejas Mehta, Gabriel M. Ortiz, Sean P. Ferris, Thienkhai H. Vu, Laurence Huang and Adithya Cattamanchi

Chapter 10 **Primary *Klebsiella pneumoniae* Osteomyelitis with Bacteremia and Sepsis in a Patient with Cirrhosis** ... 42
Akshay Khatri, Naga Sasidhar Kanaparthy, Bright Jebaraj Selvaraj, Eunna Cho and Marc Y. El Khoury

Chapter 11 **A Rare and Potentially Catastrophic Infection: Primary Intestinal Aspergillosis—Case Report in an HIV Patient** ... 46
Cátia Dias, Filipa Duarte-Ribeiro, Sara Pipa and Margarida Mota

Chapter 12 **Cryptococcal Meningitis in a HIV Seronegative Patient: A Rare Complication of Cerebrospinal Fluid Leak Detected with a New Cisternographic Technique** 49
Chukwunonso Chime, Charbel Ishak, Kishore Kumar, Muhammad Kamal, Srinivasan Krishna, Paul Kelly and Sridhar Chilimuri

Chapter 13 **From Bilateral Periorbital Necrotic Wound to Fungal Brain Abscess: A Complicated Case of COVID-19-Associated Mucormycosis** 54
Bahram Eshraghi, Nastaran-Sadat Hosseini, Rasoul Mohammadi, Seyed Hamid Reza Abtahi, Alireza Ramezani-Majd, Roya Azad and Mohsen Pourazizi

Chapter 14 **Disseminated Cryptococcosis in a Non-HIV Patient in Singapore** 59
Jonathan See, Kok Choon Raymond Fong and Humaira Shafi

Chapter 15 ***Candida* Empyema as a Red Flag for Esophageal Rupture: A Case Report and Literature Review** 64
Naureen Ali and Getahun Abate

Chapter 16 **Failed Early Intervention of Pyomyositis in an Immunocompetent Individual** 68
Ranna Al-Dossari and Sana Zekri

Chapter 17 **The Forgotten Disease: A Case of Lemierre's Syndrome with Distal Extremity Involvement** 71
John Gaskill and Michael Aronson

Chapter 18 ***Burkholderia cepacia* Complex Lumbar Spondylodiscitis: A Rare Nosocomial Infection** 75
Rachel Subramanian and Lynn Fitzgibbons

Chapter 19 **A Case of *Fusobacterium necrophorum* without Lemierre's Syndrome Mimicking Acute Leptospirosis** 79
Ryo Yasuhara, Shunichi Shibazaki and Takayoshi Yamanouchi

Chapter 20 **Bilateral Facial Diplegia: A Rare Presenting Symptom of Lyme** 83
John Ashurst and Matthew Perry

Chapter 21 **Prepatellar Bursal Infection Caused by *Mycobacterium tuberculosis* with an In Situ Total Knee Arthroplasty: A Case Report and Comprehensive Literature Review** 86
Abdulrahman D. Algarni

Chapter 22 ***Neisseria meningitidis* Infecting a Prosthetic Knee Joint: A New Case of an Unusual Disease** 90
Berta Becerril Carral, Elvira Alarcón Manoja, Salvador López Cárdenas and Jesús Canueto Quintero

Chapter 23 **Typhoid Fever due to Extended Spectrum β-Lactamase-Producing *Salmonella enterica* Serovar Typhi: A Case Report and Literature Review** 93
Abdul Azeez Ahamed Riyaaz, Vindya Perera, Sabaratnam Sivakumaran and Nelun de Silva

Chapter 24 **All Signs Point to Cancer: A Case of Cryptic Miliary Tuberculosis in the Setting of Concomitant Cancer** 98
Victoria Cress, Sue Min Sophia Kwon and Michael T. Ulrich

Chapter 25 *Streptococcus constellatus* **Causing Empyema and Sepsis, Necessitating Early Surgical Decortication** 101
D. Chrastek, S. Hickman, D. Sitaranjan, I. Vokshi, O. Kakisi, J. Kadlec, W. Bartosik, F. Van Tornout and V. Kouritas

Chapter 26 **A14-Year-Old Male Patient with Kawasaki Disease Presented with Stroke after COVID-19** 105
Nexhmedin Shala, Fisnik Jashari, Dren Boshnjaku, Argjend Shala, Pranvera Ibrahimi, Vera Kukaj and Shemsedin Dreshaj

Chapter 27 **Encephalopathy Associated with Severe Cytomegalovirus Infection in an Immunocompetent Young Woman** 110
Syuichi Tetsuka, Tomohiro Suzuki, Tomoko Ogawa, Ritsuo Hashimoto and Hiroyuki Kato

Chapter 28 **Atypical Manifestation of VZV Infection in a Vaccinated Immunocompetent Adult** 116
Deesha Bhojwani, Mohamed Zakarya and Suha Abu Khalaf

Chapter 29 **Parainfluenza 3 Respiratory Infection Associated with Pericardial Effusion in a Very Low Birthweight Infant** 120
Cristina Aranda Cazón, Luis Arruza Gómez, Gloria Herranz Carrillo, Cristina González Menchén, Zarife Daoud Pérez, José Antonio Martínez-Orgado and José Tomás Ramos Amador

Chapter 30 **Successful Treatment of High-Level Aminoglycoside-Resistant** *Enterococcus faecalis* **Bacteremia in a Preterm Infant with Ampicillin and Cefotaxime** 124
Jennifer Tam, Santina J. Lee, Vibhuti Shah and Shaun K. Morris

Chapter 31 **Coronavirus Disease 2019 and Acute Hemorrhagic Edema of Infancy** 127
Mohsen Jari

Chapter 32 **An Unusual Case of CMV/EBV Ventriculoencephalitis with Evolution to Primary Central Nervous System Lymphoma in HIV-Positive Patient** 130
Gisela Borges, Diana Neves, Inês Pintado Maury, Aida Pereira and Maria de Jesus Silva

Chapter 33 **Non-ST Elevation Myocardial Infarction and Severe Peripheral Artery Disease in a 20-Year-Old with Perinatally Acquired Human Immunodeficiency Virus Infection** 133
Purva Sharma, Mohamad Kabach, Samineh Sehatbakhsh, Rashida Tharpe, Shaun Isaac, Robert Chait and Kleper De Almeida

Chapter 34 **Cerebral Venous Thrombosis as Rare Presentation of Herpes Simplex Virus Encephalitis** 137
José Leite, Ana Ribeiro, Diana Gonçalves, João Sargento-Freitas, Luís Trindade and Victor Duque

Chapter 35 **Acute Brucellosis Presenting with Bleeding Tendency due to Isolated Severe Thrombocytopenia** 142
M. Aon and T. Al-Enezi

Chapter 36 **Acute Cytomegalovirus Illness in an Immunocompetent Adult Causing Intravascular Hemolysis and Suspected Hemophagocytic Lymphohistiocytosis** 145
Ross P. Elliott, Brian P. Freeman, Jeffery L. Meier and Rima El-Herte

Chapter 37 *Streptococcus thoraltensis* **Bacteremia: First Described Case as a Fever of Unknown Origin in Human** ... 152
Nikolaos Petridis, Athanasia Apsemidou, Georgios Kalopitas, Georgios Pilianidis and Iakovos Avramidis

Chapter 38 *Candida krusei* **Empyema Thoracis: A Community-Acquired Infection Requiring a High Index of Suspicion** ... 155
Hazim Bukamur, Waseem Ahmed, Yazan Numan, Ibrahim Shahoub and Fuad Zeid

Chapter 39 **Add-On Therapy with Ertapenem in Infections with Multidrug Resistant Gram-Negative Bacteria: Pediatric Experience** ... 159
Sevgen Tanır Basaranoglu, Yasemin Ozsurekci, Kubra Aykac, Kamile Oktay Arıkan, Ayse Buyukcam, Ali Bulent Cengiz, Mehmet Ceyhan and Ates Kara

Chapter 40 **Massive Haemoptysis due to Obscure Aetiology: Perils and Management Dilemmas** ... 163
A. Shreenivasa, K. A. Vishak, K. Sindhu, Kauslya Sahu and G. V. Chaithra

Chapter 41 **Presentation of Ocular Syphilis in a HIV-Positive Patient with False-Negative Serologic Screening** ... 166
Mahsaw N. Motlagh and Cameron G. Javid

Chapter 42 **Successful Management of Biliary Ascariasis in a High-Endemic Zone and Low-Resource Setting in Ethiopia** ... 171
Yonathan Aliye Asfaw, Girum Tesfaye Asrat, Tesfanew Bekele Uddo, Bethlehem Aliye Asfaw, Ayush Anand, Helen Huang, Eden Demessie Firew and NagaSpurthy Reddy Anugu

Chapter 43 **Emergence of Lassa Fever Disease in Northern Togo: Report of Two Cases in Oti District in 2016** ... 175
Akouda Akessiwe Patassi, Dadja Essoya Landoh, Agballa Mebiny-Essoh Tchalla, Wemboo Afiwa Halatoko, Hamadi Assane, Bayaki Saka, Mouchedou Abdoukarim Naba, Issifou Yaya, Kossi Atsissinta Edou, Tsidi Agbeko Tamekloe, Abiba Kere Banla, Kokou Mawule Davi, Magloire Manga, Yao Kassankogno and Dominique Salmon-Ceron

Chapter 44 **Severe Presentation of Nontypeable** ***Haemophilus influenza*** **(NTHi) Infection in a Previously Healthy Toddler** ... 180
Eiman Al Boloushi, Abdulla Al Amri, Ghassan Ghatasheh and Huda Al Dhanhani

Chapter 45 **A Case of Malaria Predisposing to** ***Salmonella*** **Bacteremia in a Returning Traveler from Nigeria** ... 184
Robert Jakubowski, Lisa L. Steed, Susan E. Dorman and Camelia Marculescu

Chapter 46 *Plasmodium vivax* **Infection in Multiple Family Members in Texas, USA** ... 187
Roukaya Al Hammoud, James R. Murphy and Michael L. Chang

Chapter 47 **Herpes Zoster Infection Presenting as Aseptic Meningitis and Dermatomal Rash in Immunocompetent Adult** ... 190
Suyash Dawadi, Sudesh Lamsal and Bhupendra Shah

Chapter 48 **A Case of Bacteremia and Meningitis Associated with Piperacillin-Tazobactam Nonsusceptible, Ceftriaxone Susceptible *Escherichia coli* during *Strongyloides* Hyperinfection in an Immunocompromised Host** 193
Santosh Dahal, Jeffrey Lederman, Jesse Berman, Marius Viseroi and Stephen Jesmajian

Chapter 49 **Invasive *Malassezia pachydermatis* Infection in an 8-Year-Old Child on Lipid Parenteral Nutrition** 197
Zheyi Teoh, Joel Mortensen, and Joshua K. Schaffzin

Permissions

List of Contributors

Index

Preface

The diseases which are caused by pathogenic microorganisms, such as bacteria, viruses, fungi and parasites are known as infectious diseases. These diseases can invade the body and disrupt its normal functioning. Infectious diseases can range from common infections like the flu or a cold to more severe conditions such as tuberculosis, HIV/AIDS, malaria, and hepatitis. The diagnosis of infectious diseases begins with a thorough medical history and physical examination. This includes a study of the patient's symptoms, duration of illness, recent travel history, exposure to sick individuals and any underlying medical conditions. Imaging studies, such as X-rays, computed tomography (CT), and magnetic resonance imaging (MRI) are used to determine the extent and severity of certain infectious diseases, particularly those affecting the lungs, bones, or central nervous system. This book includes some of the vital pieces of work being conducted across the world, on various topics related to infectious diseases. It will provide comprehensive knowledge to the readers.

This book unites the global concepts and researches in an organized manner for a comprehensive understanding of the subject. It is a ripe text for all researchers, students, scientists or anyone else who is interested in acquiring a better knowledge of this dynamic field.

I extend my sincere thanks to the contributors for such eloquent research chapters. Finally, I thank my family for being a source of support and help.

Editor

1

Rhino-Orbital-Cerebral Mucormycosis in a Post-COVID-19 Patient from Peru

Linda Ponce-Rosas,[1] **Jose Gonzales-Zamora**,[2] **Nelson Diaz-Reyes**,[3,4] **Oliver Alarco-Cadillo**,[5] **and Jorge Alave-Rosas**[3,4]

[1]*Peruvian American Medical Society, Especialistas en Gestion de Salud Ocupacional, Lima, Peru*
[2]*Department of Medicine, Division of Infectious Diseases, University of Miami Miller School of Medicine, Miami, FL, USA*
[3]*Peruvian Union University, Lima, Peru*
[4]*Department of Internal Medicine, Good Hope Clinic, Lima, Peru*
[5]*Department of Internal Medicine, Good Hope Clinic, Peruvian University of Applied Sciences, Lima, Peru*

Correspondence should be addressed to Linda Ponce-Rosas; linluzponce@gmail.com

Academic Editor: Mohd Adnan

Mucormycosis has been reported increasingly in patients affected by COVID-19, especially in India where the first cases were described. In Latin America, there is limited information about this association, mainly coming from Brazil, Mexico, and Peru. Herein, we report the case of a 66-year-old female that presented with rhino-orbital-cerebral mucormycosis, diabetic ketoacidosis, and COVID-19. The patient had the compromise of all the sinuses, orbital invasion, and intracranial extension. Isavuconazole was promptly initiated because amphotericin B was not available. She had a single open surgical debridement of necrotic tissues at the beginning of the diagnosis then multiple manual sessions to clear the residual or recurrent disease during approximately 5 months. Isavuconazole was effective and well-tolerated for 10 months without side effects. We highlight the importance of considering mucormycosis in post-COVID-19 patients with uncontrolled diabetes. The report emphasizes the favorable outcome of isavuconazole as an alternative therapy.

1. Introduction

Coronavirus disease 2019 (COVID-19) is a disease caused by the novel coronavirus SARS-CoV-2 first documented in China and subsequently causing a lethal pandemic.

According to the World Health Organization (WHO), the pandemic has so far produced more than 318 million confirmed cases and more than 5.5 million deaths throughout the world [1]. COVID-19 has unevenly affected Latin American countries. The Johns Hopkins University database reported that Peru has the highest fatality rate (8.4%) and about 625 people per 100,000 residents have lost their lives to COVID-19 [2].

COVID-19 infection in patients with multiple risk factors such as diabetes mellitus, hypoxemia, and steroid use may increase the susceptibility of opportunistic fungal infections such as mucormycosis (MCR), a disease that can be potentially fatal [3]. Recently, several cases of MCR in people with COVID-19 have been reported worldwide. India, Iran, and Egypt were the most affected countries with hundreds of cases [4–6]. Invasive MCR has been described in patients with severe COVID-19 infection who received corticosteroid and/or tocilizumab as part of their treatment. It has also been associated with mechanical ventilation, supplemental oxygen therapy, and healing rituals with cattle manure. In the majority of patients, diabetes mellitus (DM) was a predisposing condition [4–9]. Similarly, there are increasing numbers of cases reported in Brazil, Mexico, and Peru [7–11]. Here, we report a case of rhino-orbital-cerebral mucormycosis (ROCM) in a patient recovered from COVID-19 infection with uncontrolled DM.

2. Case Report

A 66-year-old woman with a 5-year history of poorly controlled diabetes mellitus was admitted to the hospital with drowsiness. Two weeks earlier, the patient went to her primary care physician (PCP) because her son was diagnosed with COVID-19 infection at work. At that time, she was diagnosed with COVID-19 infection by RT-PCR from nasopharyngeal swap. During the evaluation, she reported approximately ten days of headache, for which she self-medicated with dexamethasone 8 mg PO daily for 10 days (a medication that can be obtained without prescription in Peru). Dexamethasone was stopped immediately by her PCP. She had a mild infection with sore throat, headache, fatigue, muscle aches, decreased appetite, anosmia, and dysgeusia. No dyspnea, cough, or fever was reported by the patient. She received symptomatic treatment at home with no oxygen supplementation. Four days prior to admission, the patient noticed a violaceous palate lesion and started to develop accentuated fatigue and confusion. In the following days, her symptoms got progressively worse. On arrival, her temperature was 37°C (98.6 F), blood pressure was 145/75 mmHg, pulse was 123/min, and respiratory rate was 22/min. Oxygen saturation was 97% on room air. On physical examination, she appeared to be in moderate distress with altered mental status. Her mucous membranes were dry. On ophthalmic examination, the left eye (OS) had no light perception (NLP), and there was chemosis and mild proptosis. The direct and consensual light reflexes were absent OS. Fundoscopic exam revealed a normal retina and macula and was notable for pallor and atrophy of the optic disc OS. Visual acuity in the right eye (OD) was 20/100 with corrective lens, unchanged from the previous examination as well as a normal anterior segment and fundoscopic exam. Nasal examination showed necrotic tissue and erosion of the nasal septum, edema, and necrosis on the mucosa of both nasal turbinates and lateral walls of the nasal cavity. A black eschar in the hard palate was also noticed. Lung auscultation revealed diffuse crackles. Neurological examination revealed a patient arousable to painful stimuli and oriented to person, place, and time. The Glasgow score was 13/15. Cranial nerves II–XII were grossly intact. Strength was 5/5 in all extremities. Sensory deficit was not found. Deep tendon reflexes were normal. Coordination was normal. There were no meningeal signs.

Laboratory studies on admission showed leukocytosis (white blood cell (WBC) count of 28.5 K/uL with 91% neutrophils and 3.4% lymphocytes). Serum chemistry was significant for hyperglycemia (glucose 407 mg/dL); metabolic acidosis (sodium 135 mEq/L, potassium 3.4 mEq/L, chloride 99.2 mEq/L, and bicarbonate 11.2 mEq/L). Arterial blood gases revealed a pH 7.3, pO2 97.1 mmHg, and pCO2 22.6 mmHg. Hemoglobin A1c was 11%. Creatinine was 0.83 mg/dl. The chest radiograph showed bilateral lung opacities predominantly in the left lower zone compatible with viral pneumonia. Computed tomography (CT) scan showed multifocal small areas of consolidation and perilobular opacities associated with some ground-glass areas in the left lower lobe. CT scan of the brain without contrast was unremarkable. CT scan of paranasal sinuses revealed severe mucosal thickening of the bilateral maxillary sinuses as well as frontal, ethmoid, and sphenoid sinuses. There were no intra, periorbital, or brain lesions (Figure 1). A contrast-enhanced magnetic resonance imaging (MRI) of the brain was not available on admission.

Due to the development of diabetic ketoacidosis (DKA), the patient was started on intravenous fluids, sodium bicarbonate, and insulin drip. Vancomycin and piperacillin-tazobactam were initiated for suspected bacterial pansinusitis. Isavuconazole (200 mg IV as a loading dose, then 200 mg VO daily) was added for treatment of presumptive invasive fungal infection. Amphotericin B was not available. Maxillofacial surgery was consulted, and the patient was taken to the operating room for an open surgical debridement. Intraoperatively, nasal septum resection was performed, ethmoid sinus antrostomy, and maxillectomy. Left orbital exenteration was indicated but it was not performed due to patient's own choice. Palatal necrosis was managed with palatectomy according to the extension of the invasion. Sinus cultures were positive for multidrug resistant *Pseudomonas aeruginosa*. Vancomycin was discontinued, and piperacillin-tazobactam was switched to colistin and meropenem to complete 21 days. Histopathology revealed broad nonseptated hyphae with right-angle branching consistent with mucormycosis (Figure 2). A contrast-enhanced MRI of the brain was obtained after surgical debridement, revealing orbital invasion and central nervous system (CNS) involvement highly consistent with invasive mycosis (Figure 3). In the following days, the patient improved significantly, showing near resolution of neurologic symptoms and minimal necrotic tissue in affected areas. At 3-month follow-up from admission, she was discharged home with antifungal therapy (isavuconazole) and weekly manual drainage, lavage, and debridement of residual or recurrent necrotic tissues. At 5-month follow-up, the ophthalmic examination revealed exotropia and NLP on the left eye, fundoscopic exam was notable for atrophy of the optic nerve OS. Visual acuity and funduscopic exam were unchanged from the initial examination. At 5- month follow-up, a contrast-enhanced MRI of the brain showed reduced hyperintense signal in cortical anterobasal frontal lobes (Figure 4).

The patient received oral treatment with isavuconazole during 10 months without side effects. She only had a single open surgical debridement at the beginning of the diagnosis then multiple sessions of manual lavage, drainage, and debridement of necrotic tissues for approximately 5 months. Currently, the patient is undergoing periodic ambulatory evaluations to ensure eradication of the disease.

3. Discussion

Mucormycosis in patients with COVID-19 infection has been reported worldwide. In a systematic review by Bhattacharyya, the majority of cases (92%) of MCR in patients with COVID-19 reported were from India with 350 cases, followed by 15 cases from Iran, 6 from Egypt, and 11 cases from Turkey [5]. In a cross-sectional study conducted by Pakdel et al. [12], 15 cases from Iran were described. Additionally, Fouad et al. [13] reported 26 cases from Egypt. In

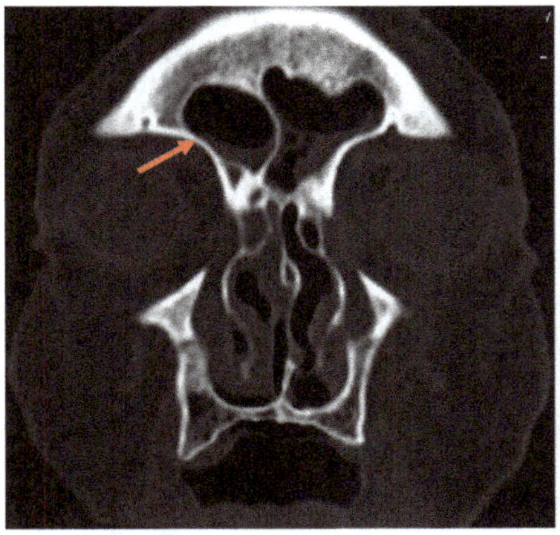

(a)

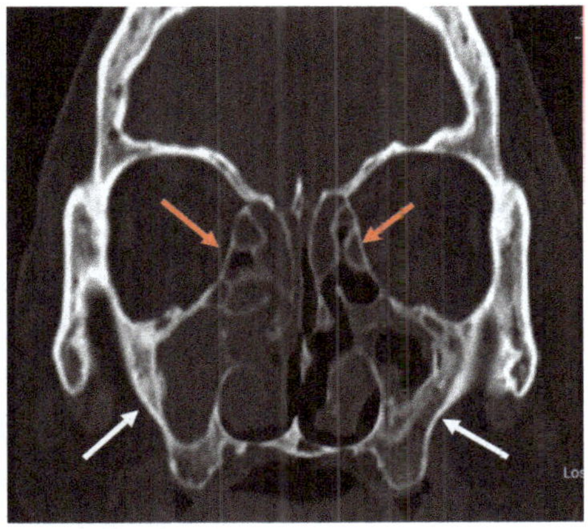

(b)

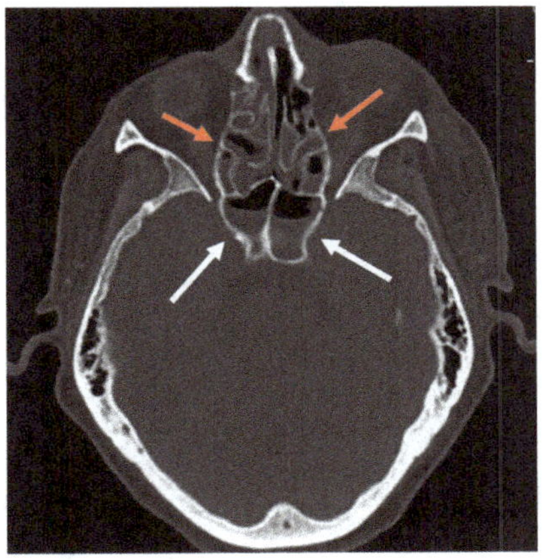

(c)

Figure 1: (a) Paranasal sinuses CT scan showed fluid level of frontal sinuses, (b) mucosal thickening of bilateral maxillary (white arrows) and ethmoid sinuses (red arrows), and (c) mucosal thickening of bilateral ethmoid sinuses (red arrows) and fluid level of bilateral sphenoidal sinuses (white arrows).

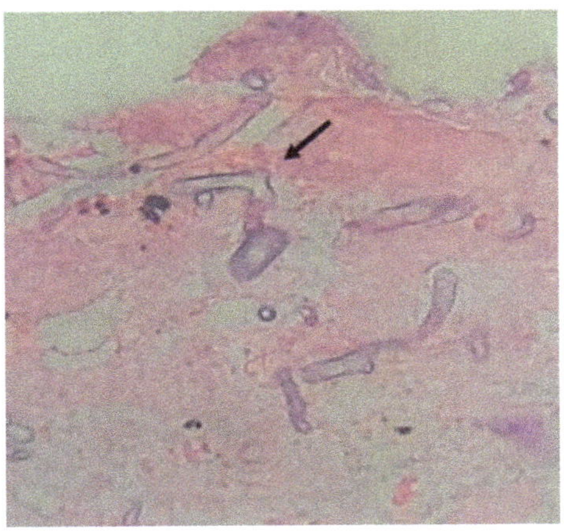

Figure 2: Histopathology showing broad, nonseptate hyphae with 90-degree angle branching (hematoxylin and eosin staining, original magnification ×400).

our region, 2 cases were from Brazil and 1 case was described in Mexico [7, 8, 10]. In Peru, the literature is scarce, with only four cases reported by Elguera-Falcon and Cumpa-Quiróz [11].

COVID-19 infection may cause persistent lymphopenia in 85% of the affected patients, which may potentially result in an increased risk of opportunistic infections [14, 15]. The primary reason that appears to facilitate fungal spores to germinate in people with COVID-19 is an ideal environment of low oxygen, high glucose, acidic environment, high iron levels, and decreased phagocytic activity of WBC due to immunosuppression (SARS-CoV-2-mediated, steroid-mediated or background comorbidities) coupled with several other risk factors including prolonged hospitalization with or without mechanical ventilation [16].

In a systematic review conducted by John et al. [17], 41 confirmed MCR cases in people with COVID-19 were described, and DM was reported in 93% of cases, while 88% were receiving corticosteroids. Similar data were presented by Singh et al. and Bhattacharyya et al. [4, 5]. Collectively, these results suggest a strong relationship of MCR with diabetes and steroid use in COVID-19 patients, which was also seen in our case.

Direct mycological and histological examinations remain the gold standard for diagnosis. The histopathologic identification of mucormycosis (large, broad nonseptated hyphae with right-angle branching) may provide the only

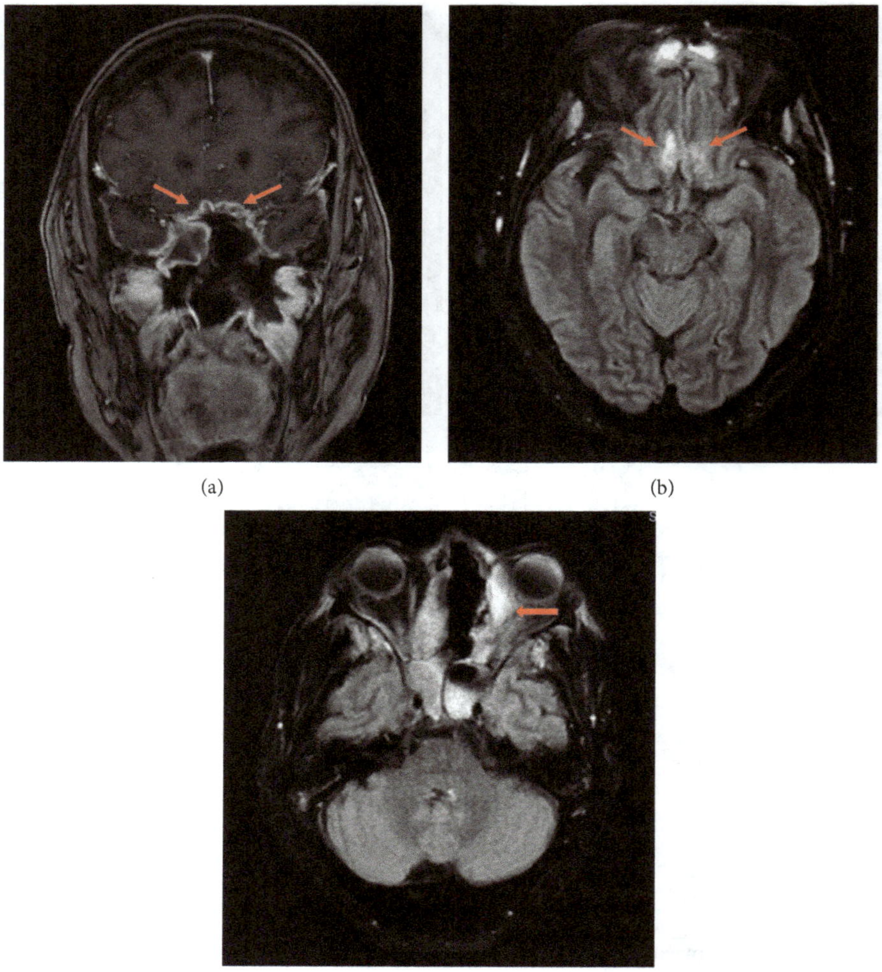

(a) (b) (c)

Figure 3: (a) Coronal T1-weighted contrast-enhanced MRI reported frontal anterobasal dural thickening and strong pachymeningeal enhancement (arrows). (b) Fluid attenuated inversion recovery (FLAIR) sequence showed hyperintense signal in cortical anterobasal frontal lobes (arrows). (c) FLAIR sequence revealed an abscess adjacent to the inferior rectus muscle of the left orbit (red arrow).

evidence of infection because the culture often yields no growth [3, 18]. A CT scan is crucial for the identification of the bony destruction. Contrast-enhanced MRI provides early detection of meningeal or intraparenchymatous spread and intracranial vascular occlusion [3, 18]. In a prospective study conducted by El-Kholy et al. [19], the most affected sinuses were ethmoid (72.2%) and sphenoid (55.6%) sinuses. Sen et al. [6] reported in the orbit, diffuse involvement predominated in 40% (674 of 1731) followed by involvement of the medial orbit in 27% (469). Orbital apex was involved in 21% (371) patients. In the CNS, the cavernous sinus was most commonly involved in 53% (285 of 539). Bilateral CNS involvement was documented in 5% (133 of 2669) cases with the cavernous sinus being the most common route of spread (70%, 299 of 430).

Treatment of MCR consists of a combination of surgical debridement of involved tissues and antifungal therapy [3]. It remains crucial the appropriate treatment of the underlying medical condition, correction of hypoxia, acidosis, hyperglycemia, electrolyte abnormalities, and a judicious evidence-based use of corticosteroids in patients with COVID-19 [4, 5]. Due to the difficulties in establishing a definitive diagnosis, many patients are treated empirically for MCR because they have risk factors for infection and positive cultures and/or compatible clinical syndromes [3]. Intravenous amphotericin B is the drug of choice for initial therapy. Posaconazole or isavuconazole is used as step-down therapy for patients who have responded to amphotericin B. They can also be used as salvage or alternative therapy for patients who do not respond to or cannot tolerate amphotericin B [18, 20, 21]. Our patient received empiric treatment with isavuconazole because amphotericin B was not available on admission. Isavuconazole was effective and well-tolerated by the patient. She did not develop any side effects, such as gastrointestinal symptoms, confusion, decreased appetite, or QT prolongation. Aggressive surgical debridement of involved necrotic tissues should be considered as soon as the diagnosis of any form of MCR is suspected because these areas are unreachable with antifungals. In the case of

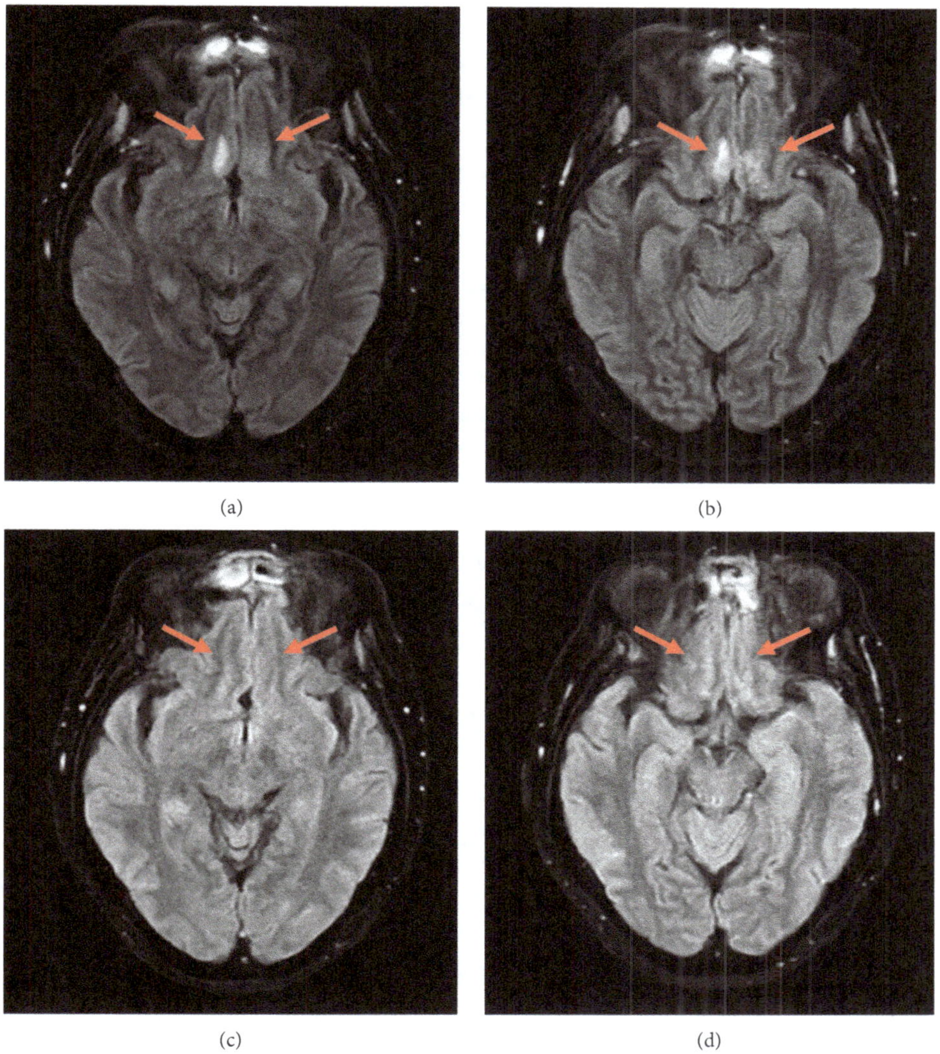

FIGURE 4: (a, b) FLAIR sequence showed hyperintense signal in cortical anterobasal frontal lobes (arrows) at the beginning of the treatment (first week). (c, d) FLAIR sequence showed reduced hyperintense signal in cortical anterobasal frontal lobes (arrows) at 5 months follow-up.

rhino-cerebral infection, debridement to remove all necrotic tissue can often be disfiguring, requiring removal of the palate, nasal cartilage, and the orbit [18]. However, more recent experience shows that endoscopic debridement with limited tissue removal can also be attempted [18, 19].

Despite early diagnosis and aggressive combined surgical and medical therapy, the prognosis for recovery from MCR is poor [22]. The overall mortality was around 38.6% in cases with concomitant MCR and COVID-19 infection [4–6, 17, 19]. We believe our patient had a good outcome due to a prompt diagnosis and management.

4. Conclusion

This case highlights the presentation of ROCM in patients recovered from COVID-19, which is a complication that should be considered in the differential diagnosis for an early detection and appropriate treatment. We advocate a multidisciplinary approach that combines medical management and surgical debridement of necrotic tissues to achieve favorable outcomes. As shown in this report, isavuconazole may be used as an alternative medication for ROCM in places where the administration of intravenous amphotericin is not feasible.

Consent

Patient written consent was obtained. Patient consent for publication was obtained.

Disclosure

All authors meet the International Committee of Medical Journal Editors (ICMJE) criteria for authorship and take responsibility for the integrity of the work. They confirm that this paper will not be published elsewhere in the same form, in English or in any other language, including electronically.

Authors' Contributions

LPR, JGZ, and JAR conceptualized the study, analysed and interpreted the data, and revised the manuscript. LPR drafted the manuscript. JGZ edited the manuscript. NDR, OAC, and JAR performed the management of the patient. JAR collected the data. JGZ, NDR, OAC, and JAR gave final approval of the manuscript. All authors agreed mutually to submit for publication.

Acknowledgments

The authors offer their sincere appreciation to Dr. Katia Villa who helped with the captions of the radiological images. The authors deeply acknowledge Dr. Jaime Caceres who contributed by choosing and describing the histopathological images.

References

[1] WHO, *Global Database of COVID-19 Confirmed Cases and Deaths*World Health Organization (WHO), Geneva, Switzerland, 2022.

[2] Johns Hopkins University & Medicine, *Mortality in the Most Affected Countries*, Johns Hopkins University & Medicine, Baltimore, ML, USA, 2022.

[3] K. Bhatt, A. Agolli, M. H. Patel et al., "High mortality co-infections of COVID-19 patients: mucormycosis and other fungal infections," *Discoveries*, vol. 9, no. 1, p. 126, 2021.

[4] A. K. Singh, R. Singh, S. R. Joshi, and A. Misra, "Mucormycosis in COVID-19: a systematic review of cases reported worldwide and in India," *Diabetes & Metabolic Syndrome: Clinical Research Reviews*, vol. 15, no. 4, Article ID 102146, 2021.

[5] A. Bhattacharyya, P. Sarma, D. J. Sharma et al., "Rhino-orbital-cerebral-mucormycosis in COVID-19: a systematic review," *Indian Journal of Pharmacology*, vol. 53, no. 4, pp. 317–327, 2021.

[6] M. Sen, S. G. Honavar, R. Bansal et al., "Members of the collaborative OPAI-IJO study on mucormycosis in COVID-19 (COSMIC) study group: epidemiology, clinical profile, management, and outcome of COVID-19-associated rhino-orbital-cerebral mucormycosis in 2826 patients in India—collaborative OPAI-IJO study on mucormycosis in COVID-19 (COSMIC), report 1," *Indian Journal of Ophthalmology*, vol. 69, no. 7, pp. 1670–1692, 2021.

[7] E. S. d. Monte Junior, M. E. L. d. Santos, I. B. Ribeiro et al., "Rare and fatal gastrointestinal mucormycosis (zygomycosis) in a COVID-19 patient: a case report," *Clinical Endoscopy*, vol. 53, no. 6, pp. 746–749, 2020 Nov.

[8] P. Bonates, G. A. P. João, K. S. Cruz et al., "Fatal rhino-orbito-cerebral mucormycosis infection associated with diabetic ketoacidosis post-COVID-19," *Revista da Sociedade Brasileira de Medicina Tropical*, vol. 54, Article ID e03582021, 2021.

[9] L. A. B. G. Farias, L. S. Damasceno, S. P. Bandeira, F. K. d. A. Barreto, T. d. M. J. S. Leitão, and L. P. d. G. Cavalcanti, "COVID-19 associated mucormycosis (CAM): should Brazil be on alert?" *Revista da Sociedade Brasileira de Medicina Tropical*, vol. 54, Article ID e04102021, 2021.

[10] S. Waizel-Haiat, J. A. Guerrero-Paz, L. Sanchez-Hurtado, S. Calleja-Alarcon, and L. Romero-Gutierrez, "A case of fatal rhino-orbital mucormycosis associated with new onset diabetic ketoacidosis and COVID-19," *Cureus*, vol. 13, no. 2, Article ID e13163, 2021.

[11] F. Elguera-Falcón and R. Cumpa-Quiróz, "Mucormicosis en pacientes diabéticos post infección por COVID-19," *Revista de la Sociedad Peruana de Medicina Interna*, vol. 33, no. 4, pp. 176–182, 2020.

[12] F. Pakdel, K. Ahmadikia, M. Salehi et al., "Mucormycosis in patients with COVID-19: a cross-sectional descriptive multicentre study from Iran," *Mycoses*, vol. 64, no. 10, pp. 1238–1252, 2021.

[13] Y. A. Fouad, H. M. Bakre, M. A. Nassar, M. O. A. Gad, and A. A. K. Shaat, "Characteristics and outcomes of a series of COVID-associated mucormycosis patients in two different settings in Egypt through the third pandemic wave," *Clinical Ophthalmology*, vol. 15, pp. 4795–4800, 2021.

[14] M. Salehi, K. Ahmadikia, H. Badali, and S. Khodavaisy, "Opportunistic fungal infections in the epidemic area of COVID-19: a clinical and diagnostic perspective from Iran," *Mycopathologia*, vol. 185, no. 4, pp. 607–611, 2020.

[15] J.-P. Gangneux, M.-E. Bougnoux, E. Dannaoui, M. Cornet, and J. R. Zahar, "Invasive fungal diseases during COVID-19: we should be prepared," *Journal de Mycologie Médicale*, vol. 30, no. 2, Article ID 100971, 2020.

[16] P. Nori, K. Cowman, V. Chen et al., "Bacterial and fungal coinfections in COVID-19 patients hospitalized during the New York city pandemic surge," *Infection Control & Hospital Epidemiology*, vol. 42, no. 1, pp. 84–88, 2021.

[17] T. M. John, C. N. Jacob, and D. P. Kontoyiannis, "When uncontrolled diabetes mellitus and severe COVID-19 converge: the perfect storm for mucormycosis," *Journal of Fungi*, vol. 7, no. 4, p. 298, 2021.

[18] O. A. Cornely, A. Alastruey-Izquierdo, D. Arenz et al., "Global guideline for the diagnosis and management of mucormycosis: an initiative of the European confederation of medical mycology in cooperation with the mycoses study group education and research consortium," *The Lancet Infectious Diseases*, vol. 19, no. 12, pp. e405–421, 2019.

[19] N. A. El-Kholy, A. M. A. El-Fattah, and Y. W. Khafagy, "Invasive fungal sinusitis in post COVID-19 patients: a new clinical entity," *The Laryngoscope*, vol. 10, no. 1002, Article ID 29632, 2021.

[20] F. M. Marty, L. Ostrosky-Zeichner, O. A. Cornely et al., "Isavuconazole treatment for mucormycosis: a single-arm open-label trial and case-control analysis," *The Lancet Infectious Diseases*, vol. 16, no. 7, pp. 828–837, 2016.

[21] J. A. van Burik, R. S. Hare, and H. F. Solomon, "Posaconazole is effective as salvage therapy in zygomycosis: a retrospective summary of 91 cases," *Clinical Infectious Diseases*, vol. 42, no. 7, pp. 61–65, 2006.

[22] A. Werthman-Ehrenreich, "Mucormycosis with orbital compartment syndrome in a patient with COVID-19," *The American Journal of Emergency Medicine*, vol. 42, no. 264, p. 264, 2021.

2

Pulmonary Mucormycosis in Chronic Lymphocytic Leukemia and Neutropenia

Izza Mir, Sijan Basnet, David Ellsworth, and Elan Mohanty

Department of Medicine, Reading Health System, 420 S. Fifth Avenue, West Reading, PA 19611, USA

Correspondence should be addressed to Izza Mir; izza.mir@readinghealth.org

Academic Editor: Sinésio Talhari

Pulmonary mucormycosis is a rare life-threatening fungal infection associated with high mortality. We present the case of a 61-year-old man with history of chronic lymphocytic leukemia who presented with fever and cough, eventually diagnosed with pulmonary mucormycosis after right lung video-assisted thoracoscopic surgery. The patient was successfully treated with amphotericin B and right lung pneumonectomy; however, he later died from left lung pneumonia.

1. Introduction

Pulmonary mucormycosis is a rare but life-threatening, rapidly progressive infection that occurs in immunocompromised patients with mortality as high as 76% that is 10–50 times less likely than aspergillus or candida infection [1–3]. Early clinical diagnosis can be delayed in the setting of concomitant infections such as pneumonia and bacteremia. However, prompt diagnosis is critical to initiate early aggressive management. We report the case of a patient with chronic lymphocytic leukemia (CLL) with resultant neutropenia undergoing chemotherapy diagnosed with pulmonary mucormycosis.

2. Case Description

A 61-year-old man with past medical history of sarcoidosis, deep vein thrombosis on rivaroxaban, and CLL treated with bendamustine and rituximab complicated by neutropenia presented to the outpatient office with (four) days of fevers and scant hemoptysis. On physical exam, patient had temperature of 38.4°C, blood pressure of 128/60 mm Hg, respirations of 18 per minute, heart rate of 92 beats per minute, and oxygen saturation of 96% in room air. Lung sounds were diminished bilaterally. His white blood cell count was 88,200/μL with absolute neutrophil count 1900/UI (2.15%), hemoglobin level 7.4 g/dL (decreased from 8.8 g/dL three weeks prior), and platelet count 291,000/μL. Chest radiograph revealed a large mass-like consolidation in the right upper lobe, which was new compared to computerized tomography (CT) imaging two months prior.

The patient was transported to the hospital, admitted for sepsis secondary to community-acquired pneumonia, and initiated on intravenous broad-spectrum antibiotics. CT chest was obtained due to concern for hemorrhage on ibrutinib. It revealed a mass-like consolidation in the right upper lobe along with diffuse nodules and multifocal airspace disease suspicious for invasive aspergillosis (Figure 1). Aspergillus antibody was obtained; however, empiric antifungal therapy was deferred while blood cultures grew *S. pneumoniae*. The patient failed to improve clinically prompting bronchoscopy evaluation, which identified purulent airway secretions. Bronchial aspirate cytology was unrevealing, and specimens were sent for further microbiology testing. The patient continued to decline. CT-guided needle biopsy of the consolidation established presence of scattered Gomori methenamine silver (GMS) and periodic acid-Schiff (PAS) positive structures suggestive of fungal etiology. So, voriconazole was started.

Repeat chest CT demonstrated worsening airspace disease, and the patient underwent video-assisted thoracoscopic surgery (VATS) with right upper and middle lobe wedge resection. VATS revealed severe dense adhesions, thickened and necrotic pleura, and the lung was found to be

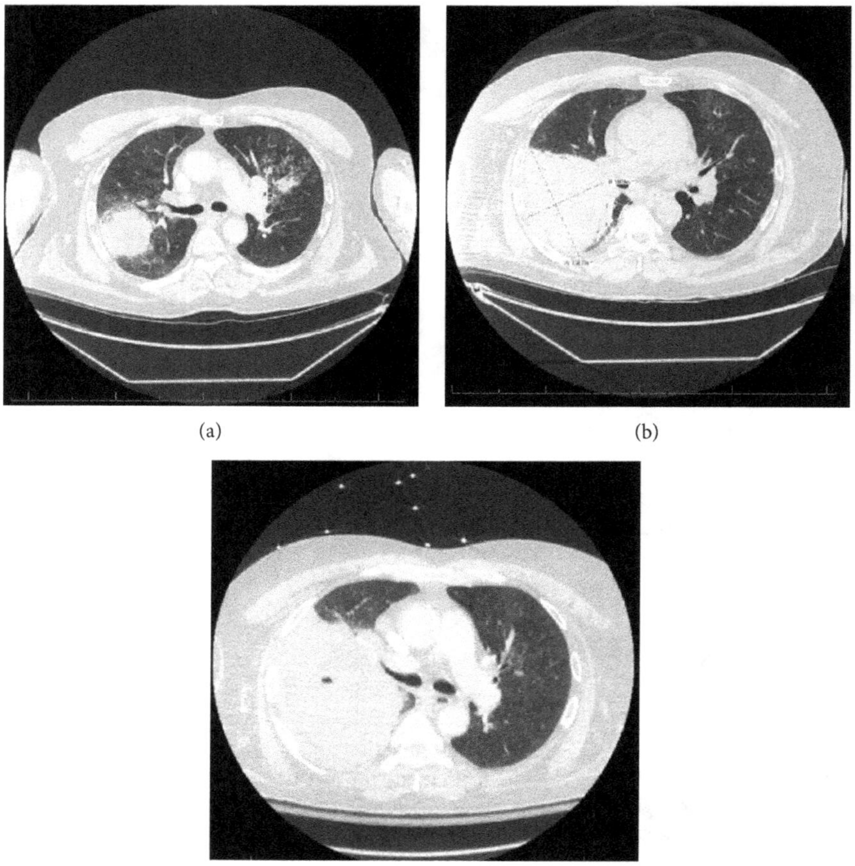

(a) (b) (c)

Figure 1: CT chest from day of admission (a), day of fine needle biopsy (b), and prior to VATS (c).

consolidated, hard, and hepatized with necrosis (Figure 2). Preliminary cultures were negative but eventually grew *Rhizopus* species. Since voriconazole is not effective against *Rhizopus*, it was discontinued and the patient was started on amphotericin B liposomal 5 mg/kg/24 hours. Six days after VATS, histopathologic analysis revealed presence of non-septate fungal hyphae with right-angle branching suggestive of mucormycosis. Patient failed to improve after VATS; thus, patient underwent right pneumonectomy with subsequent clinical improvement. He was initially discharged to rehab eight days after pneumonectomy (43 days after admission) with plan for a 14-day course of amphotericin B after pneumonectomy followed by initiation of posaconazole as recommended per infectious disease specialist. Unfortunately, the patient returned to the hospital eleven days after discharge with complications of wound dehiscence and bronchocutaneous fistula formation that grew *Rhizopus*. Thus, patient's amphotericin B course was prolonged to a total of 46 days after pneumonectomy after which he was transitioned to posaconazole. This gentleman unfortunately suffered from further wound complications, VRE infection, and was unable to return home, and discharged to a nursing facility several months later. Patient returned to the hospital from nursing home with left lung pneumonia positive for rhinovirus-enterovirus and eventually passed away seven months later due to complications during that admission.

3. Discussion

Mucormycosis can take several forms including rhinocerebral, pulmonary, cutaneous, gastrointestinal, and disseminated disease [2]. Risk factors include diabetes mellitus, hematologic malignancy, receiving hematopoietic stem cell transplant, deferoxamine therapy, injection drug use, and trauma or burns [1–4]. Pulmonary infection is most commonly found in patients with hematologic malignancy, as was the case in our patient [1, 2, 5]. Additional risk factors for pulmonary infection include male gender, neutropenia, chronic steroid use, underlying rheumatologic disorders, and voriconazole prophylaxis in patients undergoing chemotherapy [2, 5–7]. Bendamustine and rituximab have been associated with impaired lymphocyte recovery in patients with CLL, and both agents have also been associated with an increased risk of serious opportunistic infections [8, 9]. Thus, in the case of our patient, these chemotherapy agents may also have contributed to the development of mucormycosis.

The symptoms are typically nonspecific even in later stages of infection, and co-infection can further complicate diagnosis. Infection most commonly presents as acute-onset

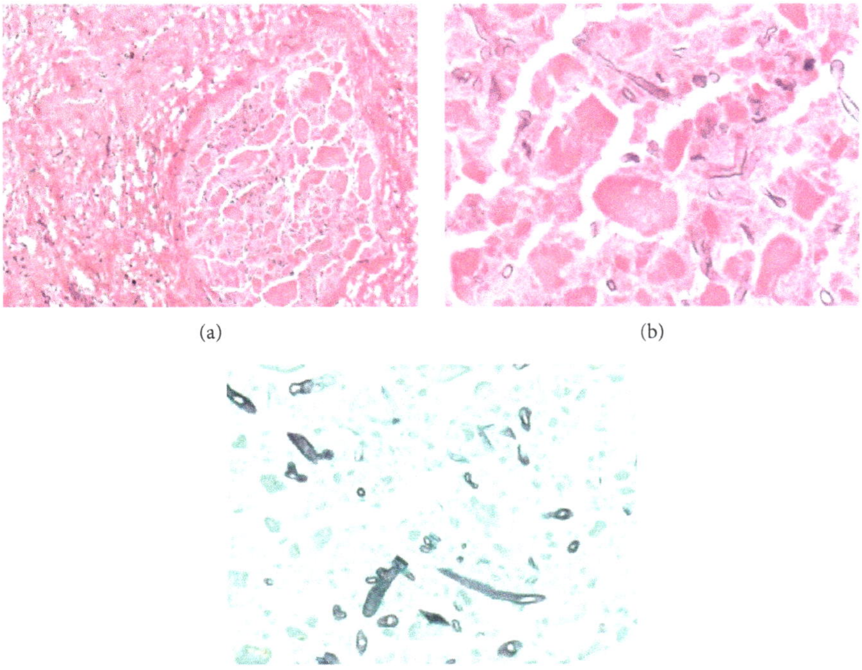

(a) (b) (c)

FIGURE 2: Histologic sections of pulmonary parenchyma showing prominent necrosis and angioinvasion by fungal species. Fungal hyphal forms noted in lumen and wall of pulmonary vessel (a). Intravascular broad and ribbon-like hyphal forms with right-angle branching and absence of septations, morphologically consistent with zygomycetic infection (hematoxylin/eosin stain (b); GMS staining (c)).

high fever with nonproductive cough, dyspnea, or chest pain that is unresponsive to broad-spectrum antibiotics [2, 4, 7].

Radiological manifestations are mostly nonspecific, and disease tends to impact the upper lobes [4]. Findings on imaging that suggest pulmonary mucormycosis are greater than ten nodules, presence of pleural effusion, and a reverse halo sign on CT chest [2, 10, 11]. Bourcier et al. found that the presence of the reverse halo sign is more common in neutropenic patients with pulmonary mucormycosis, enough for them to suggest initiation of mucormycosis antifungal therapy based on the presence of this sign [10]. Sputum secretions and broncheoalveolar lavage cultures are notoriously insensitive for detection of mucormycosis, and even cultures from fine needle aspiration often fail to grow [4, 5]. The sensitivity can be improved by placing tissue sections directly on a culture plate without prior grinding or homogenizing the material, as it can disrupt the fungal structure [4, 5]. Colonies can take three to five days to grow. Diagnosis is achieved by demonstrating hyphae with variable width (from 6 to 25 μm), zero or sparse septations, irregular ribbon-like appearance, and nonpigmented and wide-angle bifurcations including 90-degree angles. PAS and GMS stains must be used to properly visualize the hyphae [5]. Mucorales PCR has been shown to be useful for confirmation of the diagnosis of mucormycosis; however, it requires further investigation as a method of improving detection of mucormycosis in the clinical setting [12].

3.1. Management. Pulmonary mucormycosis has a poor prognosis. Patients who undergo combination of pharmacological and surgical management have been shown to do better compared to either treatment alone [4, 12, 13]. The drug of choice for initial therapy is amphotericin B while posaconazole or isavuconazole can be used for step-down therapy [14, 15]. Correction of underlying predisposing conditions, such as acidosis or neutropenia, and discontinuation of steroids or iron-chelating agents is required. Posaconazole has been reported as an effective salvage therapy in studies [14, 16]. Cornely et al. also showed that posaconazole improved survival and more effectively prevented invasive fungal infections than fluconazole or itraconazole in patients with hematologic malignancy undergoing chemotherapy [17]. Thus, to prevent severe mucor infections, posaconazole could potentially be considered for prophylaxis in patients with hematologic malignancy, especially those undergoing chemotherapy who are at risk for neutropenia.

4. Conclusion

Pulmonary mucormycosis is a rare but potentially fatal fungal infection that occurs in immunocompromised patients, most commonly in those with hematologic malignancy [1, 4]. Early recognition is crucial for prompt initiation of pharmacological and surgical comanagement to improve high rates of associated morbidity and mortality [2, 12]. Due to its nonspecific presentation, diagnosis is often difficult. However, suspicion and early initiation of therapy should be considered in immunosuppressed patients, especially neutropenic patients with hematologic malignancy, who present with fever and cough that is unresponsive to broad-spectrum antibiotics.

Acknowledgments

The authors appreciate the assistance of Dr. Sharon Swierczynski MD, PhD, from the Department of Pathology, for preparation and interpretation of the histology slides.

References

[1] M. M. Roden, T. E. Zaoutis, W. L. Buchanan et al., "Epidemiology and outcome of zygomycosis: a review of 929 reported cases," *Clinical Infectious Diseases*, vol. 41, no. 5, pp. 634–653, 2005.

[2] G. Petrikkos, A. Skiada, O. Lortholary, E. Roilides, T. J. Walsh, and D. P. Kontoyiannis, "Epidemiology and clinical manifestations of mucormycosis," *Clinical Infectious Diseases*, vol. 54, no. 1, pp. S23–S34, 2012.

[3] R. Samarei, N. Gharebaghi, and S. Zayer, "Evaluation of 30 cases of mucormycosis at a university hospital in Iran," *Mycoses*, vol. 60, no. 7, pp. 426–432, 2017.

[4] F. Y. W. Lee, S. B. Mossad, and K. A. Adal, "Pulmonary mucormycosis the last 30 years," *Archives of Internal Medicine*, vol. 159, no. 12, pp. 1301–1309, 1999.

[5] T. J. Walsh, M. N. Gamaletsou, M. R. McGinnis, R. T. Hayden, and D. P. Kontoyiannis, "Early clinical and laboratory diagnosis of invasive pulmonary, extrapulmonary, and disseminated mucormycosis (zygomycosis)," *Clinical Infectious Diseases*, vol. 54, no. 1, pp. S55–S60, 2012.

[6] G. Chamilos, E. M. Marom, R. E. Lewis, M. S. Lionakis, and D. P. Kontoyiannis, "Predictors of pulmonary zygomycosis versus invasive pulmonary aspergillosis in patients with cancer," *Clinical Infectious Diseases*, vol. 41, no. 1, pp. 60–66, 2005.

[7] E. Lin, T. Moua, and A. H. Limper, "Pulmonary mucormycosis: clinical features and outcomes," *Infection*, vol. 45, no. 4, pp. 443–448, 2017.

[8] R. G. Munoz, A. Izquierdo-Gil, A. Munoz, V. Roldan-Galiacho, P. Rabasa, and C. Panizo, "Lymphocyte recovery is impaired in patients with chronic lymphocytic leukemia and indolent non-Hodgkin lymphomas treated with bendamustine plus rituximab," *Annals of Hematology*, vol. 93, no. 11, pp. 1879–1887, 2014.

[9] A. Nosari, "Infectious complications in chronic lymphocytic leukemia," *Mediterranean Journal of Hematology and Infectious Diseases*, vol. 4, no. 1, p. e2012070, 2012.

[10] J. Bourcier, P. M. Heudes, F. Morio et al., "Prevalence of the reversed halo sign in neutropenic patients compared with non-neutropenic patients: data from a single-centre study involving 27 patients with pulmonary mucormycosis (2003–2016)," *Mycoses*, vol. 60, no. 8, pp. 526–533, 2017.

[11] R. A. Murphy and W. T. Miller Jr., "Pulmonary mucormycosis," *Seminars in Roentgenology*, vol. 31, no. 1, pp. 83–87, 1996.

[12] S. P. Hammond, R. Bialek, D. A. Milner, E. M. Petschnigg, L. R. Baden, and F. M. Marty, "Molecular methods to improve diagnosis and indentification of mucormycosis," *Journal of Clinical Microbiology*, vol. 49, no. 6, pp. 2151–2153, 2011.

[13] M. Tedder, J. A. Spratt, M. P. Anstadt, S. S. Hegde, S. D. Tedder, and J. E. Lowe, "Pulmonary mucormycosis: results of medical and surgical therapy," *Annals of Thoracic Surgery*, vol. 57, no. 4, pp. 1044–1050, 1994.

[14] J. A. Van Burik, R. S. Hare, H. F. Solomon, M. L. Corrado, and D. P. Kontoyiannis, "Posaconazole is effective as salvage therapy in zygomycosis: a retrospective summary of 91 cases," *Clinical Infectious Diseases*, vol. 42, no. 7, pp. e61–e65, 2006.

[15] B. Spellberg, A. Ibrahim, E. Roilides et al., "Combination therapy for mucormycosis: why, what, and how?," *Clinical Infectious Diseases*, vol. 54, no. 1, pp. S73–S78, 2012.

[16] G. Chamilos, R. E. Lewis, and D. P. Kontoyiannis, "Delaying amphotericin B-based frontline therapy significantly increases mortality among patients with hematologic malignancy who have zygomycosis," *Clinical Infectious Diseases*, vol. 47, no. 4, pp. 503–509, 2008.

[17] O. A. Cornely, J. Maertens, D. J. Winston et al., "Posaconazole vs. fluconazole or itraconazole prophylaxis in patients with neutropenia," *New England Journal of Medicine*, vol. 354, no. 4, pp. 348–359, 2007.

3

Saccharomyces cerevisiae Laryngitis and Oral Lesions in a Patient with Laryngeal Carcinoma

Jumanah N. Algazaq,[1] Kevan Akrami,[2] Fernando Martinez,[3] Allen McCutchan,[2] and Ajay R. Bharti[2]

[1]*Department of Health Sciences International, The University of California, San Diego, CA, USA*
[2]*Division of Infectious Diseases, The University of California, San Diego, CA, USA*
[3]*Division of Pathology, University of Texas MD Anderson Cancer Center, Houston, TX, USA*

Correspondence should be addressed to Ajay R. Bharti; abharti@ucsd.edu

Academic Editor: Gernot Walder

Saccharomyces cerevisiae is increasingly being promoted as a nutritional supplement by health food enthusiasts and is also recommended as prophylaxis against antibiotic-associated diarrhea. However, severe opportunistic infections due to *S. cerevisiae* have been reported in patients with chronic disease, cancer, and immunosuppression. Fungemia, endocarditis, pneumonia, peritonitis, urinary tract infections, skin infections, and esophagitis have been described. It is important to consider infections due to *S. cerevisiae* in appropriate clinical settings. Here, we describe the first case of *S. cerevisiae* laryngitis in a patient with a history of laryngeal carcinoma who also had oral lesions.

1. Introduction

Saccharomyces species are ubiquitous yeasts that have been used for centuries in baking and the production of beer and wine and are commonly known as baker's or brewer's yeast. *Saccharomyces cerevisiae* is used as a probiotic for prophylaxis of antibiotic-associated diarrhea [1] and is also promoted as a nutritional supplement by health food enthusiasts. It is part of the normal flora of the oral, gastrointestinal, and respiratory tracts and the vaginal mucosa [2]. Severe opportunistic infections due to *S. cerevisiae* have been reported in patients with chronic disease, cancer, and immunosuppression presenting as fungemia, endocarditis, pneumonia, peritonitis, urinary tract infections, skin infections, and esophagitis [3]. Here, we describe the first case of *S. cerevisiae* laryngitis in a patient with a history of laryngeal carcinoma who also had oral lesions.

2. Case Report

A 63-year-old Caucasian female with squamous cell carcinoma of the vocal cords developed a small grayish lesion on the ventral surface of her tongue one month after local external radiation therapy (XRT). It gradually increased in size and the patient noticed 2 new lesions (3×2 cm and 4×2 cm), one on either side of the tongue (Figures 1(a) and 1(b)). The lesions had well-demarcated margins with slightly raised and rolled edges, without bleeding or discharge, and were initially painless, but later became extremely painful. Biopsy did not reveal any malignancy. Symptoms progressed and she developed shortness of breath, stridor, and hoarseness of voice that prompted evaluation by an otolaryngologist. Laryngoscopy revealed grayish exudates on both vocal cords that were similar in appearance to the oral lesions. No oropharyngeal mucositis was seen. Complete blood cell count at the time of presentation did not reveal any abnormalities. Information regarding mucositis or leukopenia immediately following XRT was not available. The patient was started empirically on oral fluconazole 400 mg/day for presumed candidal infection. There was no improvement despite 2 weeks of therapy, and she presented to the emergency room with severe difficulty in breathing. Repeat laryngoscopy revealed worsening of the grayish exudates on the vocal cords, vocal cord edema, and narrowing of the airway that required tracheostomy.

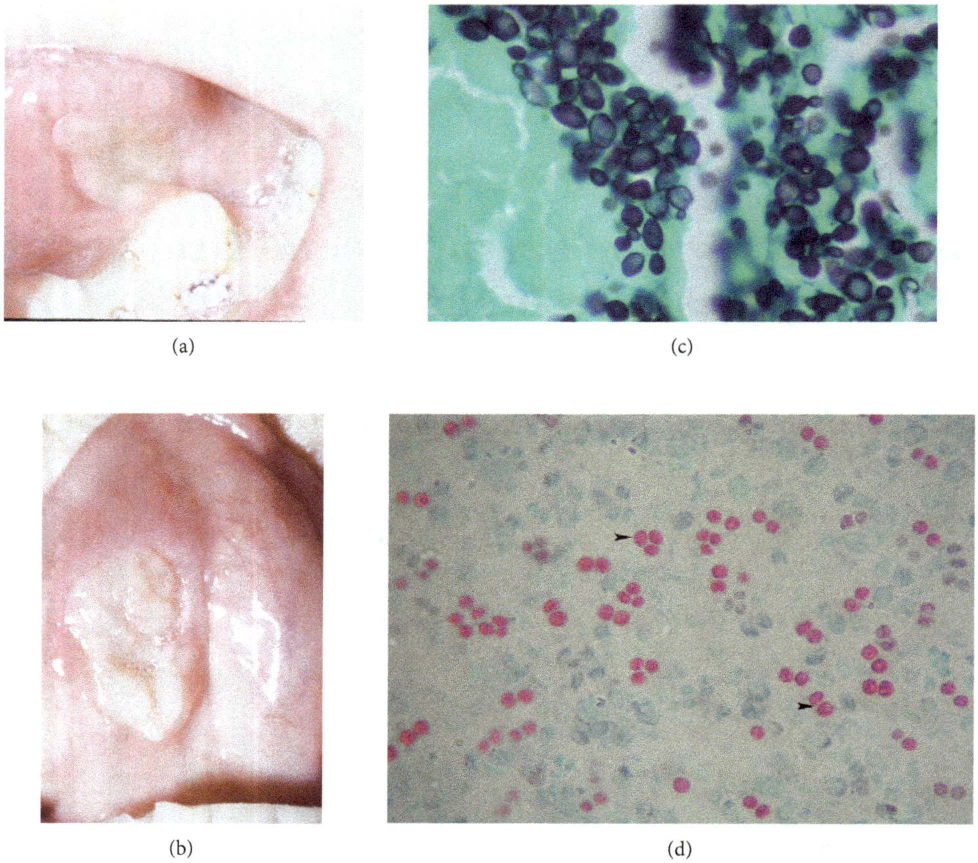

Figure 1: (a, b) Lesions on the tongue (4×2 cm and 3×2 cm) with slightly rolled and raised edges. (c) High-power view of a Gomori methenamine silver stain (GMS). Biopsy from ulcerated vocal cord lesion demonstrates spherical to oval yeast cells, some of which are budding. (d) High-power view of a Kinyoun stain. Round ascospores (arrowhead) inside the asci that are characteristic of *S. cerevisiae*.

Right vocal cord biopsy showed ulcerated squamous mucosa with polymorphonuclear leukocytes, and monocytes and macrophages indicating acute and chronic inflammation. No stromal fibrosis to indicate effects of radiation therapy was noted. Abundant extracellular oval budding yeast forms were seen on hematoxylin and eosin and Grocott's methenamine silver stains (Figure 1(c)). Tissue culture on Sabouraud dextrose agar at 30°C grew a creamy moist colony that was evident after 72 hours. This was then placed on Cornmeal agar, and a Vitek card identified it as *Saccharomyces cerevisiae*. Microscopic examination revealed multilateral ellipsoidal budding yeasts without a capsule with a largest diameter of 7–9 μm and occasional pseudohyphae. Kinyoun stain revealed oval asci with 1–4 ascospores inside, a characteristic finding of *Saccharomyces* genus (Figure 1(d)). Using the broth microdilution method of the Clinical and Laboratory Standards Institute [4], the isolate was found to have fluconazole MIC ≤ 8 μg/mL.

Given lack of response to oral fluconazole 400 mg/day after 2 weeks despite low fluconazole MIC, the dose was increased to 800 mg/day. Significant improvement in the tongue lesions was seen within 1 week with 50% reduction in the size of the lesions. After 4 weeks, one of the tongue lesions had resolved completely, and the other showed 90% clearance. Repeat laryngoscopy also showed significant improvement, and fluconazole was continued for 6 weeks until the oral lesions had resolved completely.

3. Discussion

To our knowledge, this is the first case report of a patient with laryngitis due to *S. cerevisiae* who also had oral lesions presumably due to the same infectious agent given their similar appearance. *Saccharomyces* genus was identified based on microscopy, and *S. cerevisiae* was confirmed by Vitek. Acute and chronic inflammation seen on the vocal cord biopsy indicated that it was a true infection and not just colonization. Inflammation combined with lack of fibrosis makes it unlikely that the pathological changes were due to radiation therapy.

Head and neck XRT is associated with increased risk of oral fungal infections. Oropharyngitis has been reported in a 65-year-old male, but this was after receiving both chemotherapy and XRT for head and neck carcinoma [5]. Interestingly, the prevalence of oral candidiasis during head and neck XRT (37.4%) is similar to that during chemotherapy (38%) [6]. But there are no reports on *Saccharomyces* infection or colonization following head and neck XRT. Possible mechanisms for increased risk of oral fungal infections, including *Saccharomyces*, may be hyposalivation and local tissue damage although these were not found in our patient.

Upon reviewing 22 documented cases of *S. cerevisiae* infections in patients with cancer, we found four where on probiotics while on chemotherapy that have been the source of infection [5, 7]. Other possible sources include locally brewed beer [8] and, as in our patient, grapes [9]. A detailed history of probiotic supplement intake, food, and drink may reveal possible sources in patients with *S. cerevisiae* infections.

Saccharomyces boulardii, a component of several probiotic supplements, was initially classified as a novel species of the genus *Saccharomyces*. Although there are some physiological differences, comparative gene analysis has characterized it as a strain of *S. cerevisiae* [10]. Probiotics labeled as containing *S. boulardii* have resulted in fungemia due to yeast identified as *S. cerevisiae* var. *boulardii* [11]. For clinical purposes, the two can be considered to be the same.

Diagnosis of *S. cerevisiae* is facilitated by matrix-assisted laser desorption/ionization time-of-flight mass spectrometry (MALDI-TOF MS) for rapid and accurate identification of *S. cerevisiae* [12]. Cultures should be obtained in high-risk patients with fever of unknown origin, leukocytosis despite antibiotic therapy, and a history of probiotic use or beer consumption. Our case is from 2003 when MALDI-TOF MS was unavailable and diagnosis was based on culture and special stains showing the characteristic ascospores (Figure 1(d)) and Vitek.

S. cerevisiae is consistently susceptible to amphotericin B (0.5–1 mg/mL), but mean MIC^{90} and ranges of susceptibility to fluconazole (2/0.1–128) and itraconazole (0.5/0.015–64) are much more variable [3, 13]. However, no therapeutic failures have been clearly attributable to high fluconazole MIC. In our patient, despite low fluconazole MIC, a higher dose of 800 mg/day was required. In cases with severe infection, combination therapy with amphotericin B and fluconazole is associated with better outcomes compared to monotherapy with amphotericin B alone [3]. Poor outcomes were mostly associated with older age, delayed detection and treatment, disseminated infection, and associated critical conditions such as pancreatic cancer, aplastic anemia, myelodysplastic syndrome, relapsing acute lymphocytic leukemia, cardiac surgery, and neurosurgery. Management should include discontinuation of probiotics containing *Saccharomyces*, central venous catheter (CVC) removal, and consideration of combination antifungal therapy.

In conclusion, *S. cerevisiae* should be considered as a potential pathogen when recovered from patients with cancer, immunosuppression, presence of CVC, and other critical illnesses. In addition, since contaminated vascular catheters may be the point of entry in some cases, probiotic treatments containing *Saccharomyces* should be carefully handled to avoid aerosolization and cross contamination [14]. In case of fever of unknown origin in high-risk patients, fungal cultures must be considered and performed early to avoid a delay in treatment. Finally, in cases of documented fungemia, management should include antifungals, removal of CVC, and discontinuation of probiotics. With rise in probiotic use [15], more *S. cerevisiae* infections can be expected and should be considered in the differential diagnosis.

References

[1] A. G. Billoo, M. A. Memon, S. A. Khaskheli et al., "Role of a probiotic (*Saccharomyces boulardii*) in management and prevention of diarrhoea," *World Journal of Gastroenterology*, vol. 12, no. 28, pp. 4557–4560, 2006.

[2] B. Posteraro, M. Sanguinetti, G. D'Amore, L. Masucci, G. Morace, and G. Fadda, "Molecular and epidemiological characterization of vaginal *Saccharomyces cerevisiae* isolates," *Journal of Clinical Microbiology*, vol. 37, no. 7, pp. 2230–2235, 1999.

[3] P. Munoz, E. Bouza, M. Cuenca-Estrella et al., "*Saccharomyces cerevisiae* fungemia: an emerging infectious disease," *Clinical Infectious Diseases*, vol. 40, no. 11, pp. 1625–1634, 2005.

[4] M. Cuenca-Estrella, W. Lee-Yang, M. A. Ciblak et al., "Comparative evaluation of NCCLS M27-A and EUCAST broth microdilution procedures for antifungal susceptibility testing of *Candida* species," *Antimicrobial Agents and Chemotherapy*, vol. 46, no. 11, pp. 3644–3647, 2002.

[5] S. Henry, L. D'Hondt, M. Andre, X. Holemans, and J. L. Canon, "*Saccharomyces cerevisiae* fungemia in a head and neck cancer patient: a case report and review of the literature," *Acta Clinica Belgica*, vol. 59, no. 4, pp. 220–222, 2004.

[6] R. V. Lalla, M. C. Latortue, C. H. Hong et al., "A systematic review of oral fungal infections in patients receiving cancer therapy," *Supportive Care in Cancer*, vol. 18, no. 8, pp. 985–992, 2010.

[7] S. Cesaro, P. Chinello, L. Rossi, and L. Zanesco, "*Saccharomyces cerevisiae* fungemia in a neutropenic patient treated with *Saccharomyces boulardii*," *Supportive Care in Cancer*, vol. 8, no. 6, pp. 504–505, 2000.

[8] W. J. Olver, S. A. James, A. Lennard et al., "Nosocomial transmission of *Saccharomyces cerevisiae* in bone marrow transplant patients," *Journal of Hospital Infection*, vol. 52, no. 4, pp. 268–272, 2002.

[9] C. M de Ponzzes-Gomes, D. L. de Melo, C. A. Santana et al., "*Saccharomyces cerevisiae* and non-*Saccharomyces* yeasts in grape varieties of the Sao Francisco Valley," *Brazilian Journal of Microbiology*, vol. 45, no. 2, pp. 411–416, 2014.

[10] I. Khatri, R. Tomar, K. Ganesan, G. S. Prasad, and S. Subramanian, "Complete genome sequence and comparative genomics of the probiotic yeast *Saccharomyces boulardii*," *Scientific Reports*, vol. 7, no. 1, p. 371, 2017.

[11] M. C. Appel-da-Silva, G. A. Narvaez, L. R. R. Perez, L. Drehmer, and J. Lewgoy, "*Saccharomyces cerevisiae* var. *boulardii* fungemia following probiotic treatment," *Medical Mycology Case Reports*, vol. 18, pp. 15–17, 2017.

[12] C. Cassagne, A. C. Normand, L. Bonzon et al., "Routine identification and mixed species detection in 6,192 clinical yeast isolates," *Medical Mycology*, vol. 54, no. 3, pp. 256–265, 2016.

[13] A. Enache-Angoulvant and C. Hennequin, "Invasive *Saccharomyces* infection: a comprehensive review," *Clinical Infectious Diseases*, vol. 41, no. 11, pp. 1559–1568, 2005.

[14] M. Cassone, P. Serra, F. Mondello et al., "Outbreak of *Saccharomyces cerevisiae* subtype *boulardii* fungemia in patients neighboring those treated with a probiotic preparation of the organism," *Journal of Clinical Microbiology*, vol. 41, no. 11, pp. 5340–5343, 2003.

[15] S. H. Yi, J. A. Jernigan, and L. C. McDonald, "Prevalence of probiotic use among inpatients: a descriptive study of 145 U.S. hospitals," *American Journal of Infection Control*, vol. 44, no. 5, pp. 548–553, 2016.

4

Infection of a Ventricular Septal Defect Patch with *Acremonium* Species

Nosheen Nasir,[1] Kauser Jabeen,[2] Joveria Farooqi,[2] Binish Arif Sultan,[2] Afia Zafar,[2] Aamir Hameed Khan,[1] Muneer Amanullah,[3] and Farheen Ali[1]

[1]*Department of Medicine, Aga Khan University, Karachi, Pakistan*
[2]*Department of Pathology and Microbiology, Aga Khan University, Karachi, Pakistan*
[3]*Department of Surgery, Aga Khan University, Karachi, Pakistan*

Correspondence should be addressed to Nosheen Nasir; nosheenasir@yahoo.com

Academic Editor: Sinésio Talhari

A ventricular septal defect (VSD) patch infection with *Acremonium* species isolated from vegetation and blood culture is described. Antifungal treatment was discontinued after 3 months and patient developed relapse. Surgery with prolonged oral voriconazole was instituted with recovery. We emphasize importance of surgery and prolonged therapy to treat such infections.

1. Background

Acremonium species are present in the environment and mostly cause superficial and locally invasive infections after traumatic inoculation. Invasive infections are rare and are mainly reported in immunocompromised patients. It has been reported to cause osteomyelitis, sinusitis, arthritis, peritonitis, and less frequently central nervous system infections [1]. Nosocomial and postsurgical invasive infections have also been described, in particular *Acremonium* fungemia associated with central line infection and pacemaker infection [2, 3]. As invasive infections with *Acremonium* species are rare, reliable diagnosis and optimal management of these infections is challenging. Additionally, the species of *Acremonium* are morphologically very similar to each other, and thus their exact identification is not always possible despite use of modern DNA based methods. Hence, in most case reports, the agent is reported only as an *Acremonium* sp. [4]. Therapy too is challenging as high MICs against all systemic antifungals used to treat invasive mycoses have been reported [5]. Due to inherent resistance and variable clinical response to antifungals, poor outcome generally is reported in invasive *Acremonium* infections. Anecdotal evidence suggests a combination of surgical intervention, when possible, and amphotericin B for a favorable outcome [5]. Reports describing cardiac infections are even rarer. We are reporting a case of a 21-year-old male with an infected ventricular septal defect (VSD) patch, after Tetralogy of Fallot repair, with *Acremonium* species associated with fungemia and septic emboli to the lung, kidneys, liver, and spleen.

2. Case Report

A 21-year-old male with a history of Tetralogy of Fallot (TOF) repair (with Dacron Patch over a large ventricular septal defect (VSD)) was admitted with complaints of fever and weight loss for 2 months and left sided abdominal pain since 1 week. He was recently admitted with similar complaints to another hospital where he was found to have a right sided pneumonia and was being treated with intravenous ceftriaxone. Later, suspecting infective endocarditis, gentamicin was added but as the patient was still having persistent fevers of 40°C, he was referred to our hospital. On examination, the patient was of lean built with grade IV clubbing without cyanosis, and there were no peripheral stigmata of infective endocarditis. He had a loud pansystolic murmur on the left sternal edge and had tenderness on palpation of the left upper abdomen. His initial investigations showed a high white blood cell count and C-reactive protein (CRP) (Table 1). A chest X-ray showed

Table 1: Serial white blood cell count (WBC) and inflammatory markers erythrocyte sedimentation rate (ESR) and C-reactive protein (CRP).

Labs	On presentation	After 3 months of treatment	At relapse	After 1 year of treatment
WBC (×10^9 per liter (L))	17.7	7.6	8.8	8.9
ESR (mm/hr)	65	14	87	18
CRP (mg/L)	22.1	<0.3	10.8	<0.1

left mid and right lower lung zone infiltrates, and an ultrasound of the upper abdomen showed an ill-defined splenic lesion without internal vascularity suggesting either an abscess or infarct. Three sets of blood cultures were subsequently negative. Echocardiogram showed vegetation on the VSD patch along with dehiscence, a large VSD, and moderate right ventricular outflow obstruction. A CT abdomen with contrast was done which showed multiple liver, splenic, and lung abscesses with infarcted left kidney and thrombus at the bifurcation of the aorta secondary to the septic embolic phenomenon. Cardiothoracic surgery consultation was sought, and the patient underwent a redo-sternotomy and removal of vegetations from right ventricular outflow tract site, removal of Dacron Patch, and complete repair of TOF. Postoperative echocardiogram did not show any residual VSD or vegetation, only mild left ventricular dysfunction and moderately reduced right ventricle function was seen. The vegetation removed from right outflow tract and Dacron Patch was sent for bacterial, mycobacterial, and mycology cultures. Chocolate, Sheep Blood (SBA), and MacConkey Agar plates were incubated at 37°C for aerobic culture and a SBA plate incubated anaerobically. For fungal culture, tissue was stabbed onto the surface of Sabouraud's dextrose (SDA), potato dextrose (PDA), and Mycosel agar plates incubated at 25°C and an additional SDA and SBA incubated at 37°C. The initial Gram stain and 10% potassium hydroxide (KOH) preparation revealed clusters of oval conidia and hyphae mistaken for yeast cells and pseudohyphae as well as septate hyphae. Patient was empirically started on intravenous amphotericin deoxycholate at 1 mg/kg (40 mg/dose), his fever gradually subsided, and the patient was discharged on amphotericin and oral voriconazole. Bacterial cultures remained negative, and a filamentous mould grew from the vegetation at 48 h that was finally identified phenotypically as *Acremonium* species (Figure 1). It grew on all plates except MacConkey agar. Mycobacterial cultures remained negative. Susceptibilities were performed by E-test® (bioMerieux, France) on RPMI agar, and the isolate showed an MIC of >32 mcg/ml against amphotericin and 2 mcg/ml against voriconazole. After final identification amphotericin, deoxycholate was discontinued and oral voriconazole 200 mg twice daily was continued. However, treatment was discontinued at 3 months based on clinical improvement and due to inability of the patient to bear the cost of the treatment. After 2 months of stopping therapy, patient had recurrence of symptoms along with new vegetation on the pulmonary valve. Blood cultures were submitted in BD BACTEC™ aerobic and anaerobic bottles and incubated in the BD BACTEC 9240 system, as BD BACTEC MYCO/F Lytic system was not available. The bottles flagged positive after 3 days of incubation and two sets of blood cultures grew *Acremonium* species with similar antifungal susceptibilities (Figure 2). The mould was identified on the colony and microscopic morphology. It was a hyaline mould appearing in 3 days on solid media, with cream coloured wrinkled surface and an off-white to tan reverse. By day 6, the colonies became slightly floccose. On microscopic examination, the hyphae were thin, hyaline, and septate, with short non-septate conidiophores giving rise to elliptical conidia clinging to the philaides in wet masses of 10–20. Molecular confirmation could not be made; however, the isolate was phenotypically differentiated from *Fusarium* and *Phialemonium* species due to colony appearance, absence of macroconidia, and septations at the base of conidiophores.

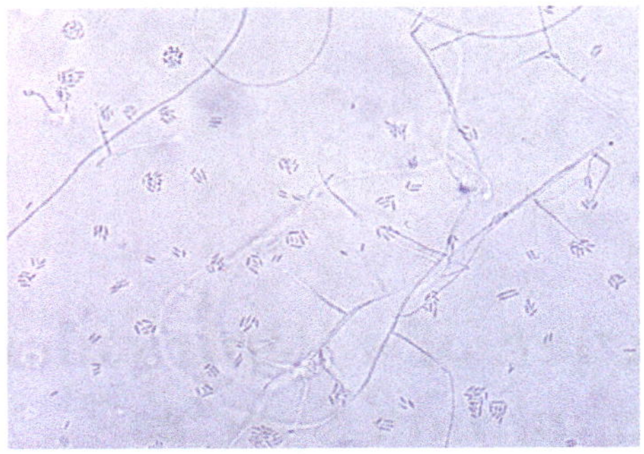

Figure 1: Microscopic image of the slide culture of the isolate from the prosthetic valve.

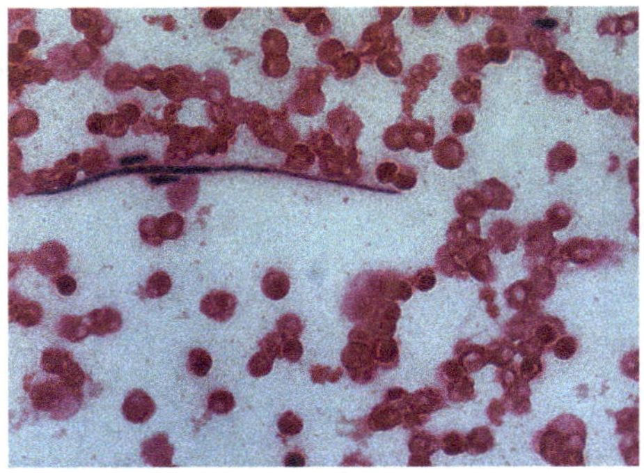

Figure 2: Gram stain from the blood culture bottle when the patient relapsed showing septate hyphae and ellipsoidal blastoconidium of *Acremonium*, mimicking pseudohyphae of candida.

Voriconazole was restarted and surgical excision of the pulmonary valve was performed two months later with growth of the similar fungus. The patient was continued on oral voriconazole for a period of one year with clinical improvement, improvement in inflammatory biomarkers, no residual vegetation on repeat echocardiogram, and serially negative blood cultures.

3. Discussion

A rare case of fungal infection of a VSD repair patch with *Acremonium* species is described. Diagnosis of this case was

TABLE 2: Summary of case reports of *Acremonium* endocarditis.

Case reports	This case	Panzaru et al. [12]	Guarro et al. [9]	Heitmann et al. [3]	Lacaz Cda et al. [10]	Degeorges et al. [11]
Age/gender	21 years/male	51 years/male	73 years/male	80 years/male	47 years/male	31 years/male
Risk factors	TOF repair with Dacron Patch over VSD	Immunocompetent, admitted with pneumonia and CHF	Severe COPD on steroids, prosthetic mitral valve	Had been on steroids for inflammatory eye disease, pacemaker	Prosthetic valve	Aortic stenosis
Species isolated	*Acremonium* spp.	*Acremonium* spp.	*Acremonium strictum*	*Acremonium* spp.	*Acremonium kiliense*	*Acremonium* spp.
Valve involved	No valves, VSD patch only	Pulmonary and tricuspid valves	Prosthetic mitral valve	Pacemaker related tricuspid valve	Prosthetic mitral valve	Aortic valve
Treatment given	Amphotericin deoxycholate and voriconazole for 3 months then voriconazole for 12 months, removal of Dacron Patch	Fluconazole 400 mg twice daily for 30 days	Caspofungin followed by voriconazole	Voriconazole for 6 weeks	Amphotericin B, 5 flucytosine, surgery	Amphotericin B
Outcome	Recovered	Recovered	Died	Recovered	Died	Died

established by visualization of fungal elements on microscopy of vegetation tissue and later from culture. Relapse was confirmed by growth of a similar fungus in pulmonary valve tissue and two sets of blood cultures. Identification of all isolated fungi was determined by the conventional method. Although ITS region sequencing was performed on the blood culture isolates, it was not able to give reliable identification.

Although there have been reports of *Acremonium* species, particularly *Acremonium kiliense* causing peritonitis [6], involvement of lung and disseminated infection in immunocompromised patients [7], there are only few case reports of cardiac infection with *Acremonium* species (Table 2). In almost all cases, the infection was of a prosthetic valve or pacemaker [3, 8–10]. However, there have also been reports of native valve infective endocarditis with this organism [11, 12]. There have been several reports of fungemia usually associated with central line associated blood stream infection and mostly occurring in immunocompromised patients, but none complicated by associated endocarditis [2, 4, 13]. *Acremonium* endocarditis has resulted in mortality despite surgical treatment and intravenous amphotericin (Table 2). In a case of *Acremonium strictum* colonization of a prosthetic mitral valve, the patient died of multiorgan failure despite treatment with intravenous caspofungin and later voriconazole [9]. However, there have been reports of patients recovering successfully with azole treatment as well [3, 12]. The treatment duration has varied for both the cases that were treated successfully. Intravenous fluconazole at high doses was given for one month with success, and in another case, patient was treated with intravenous voriconazole initially and later with an oral formulation for six weeks duration and had an uneventful recovery [3]. Our patient was treated with surgical intervention as well as with voriconazole for three months initially but unfortunately relapsed and was subsequently treated for a whole year.

The case report that we have described is the first one from our region and unlike most other cases with adverse outcome, our patient recovered despite having advanced disease. Based on our review of other case reports as well as our own experience, we would recommend surgical intervention along with voriconazole therapy for a prolonged duration for better outcome in patients having *Acremonium* endocarditis.

Acknowledgments

This project is supported through grants from the Higher Education Commission and United States Agency for International Development (HEC/USAID).

References

[1] R. M. Fincher, J. F. Fisher, R. D. Lovell, C. L. Newman, A. Espinel-Ingroff, and H. J. Shadomy, "Infection due to the fungus *Acremonium* (cephalosporium)," *Medicine*, vol. 70, no. 6, pp. 398–409, 1991.

[2] F. A. Diaz-Couselo and M. Zylberman, "Catheter-related *Acremonium kiliense* fungemia in a patient with ulcerative colitis under treatment with infliximab," *Case Reports in Infectious Diseases*, vol. 2011, Article ID 710740, 2 pages, 2011.

[3] L. Heitmann, A. Cometta, M. Hurni, N. Aebischer, I. Tschan-Schild, and J. Bille, "Right-sided pacemaker-related endocarditis due to *Acremonium* species," *Clinical Infectious Diseases*, vol. 25, no. 1, pp. 158–60, 1997.

[4] Z. C. Rodriguez and M. G. Ramos, "*Acremonium* species associated fungemia: a novel pathogen in the immunosuppressed patient," *Boletín de la Asociación Médica de Puerto Rico*, vol. 106, no. 3, pp. 29–31, 2014.

[5] J. Guarro, W. Gams, I. Pujol, and J. Gene, "*Acremonium* species: new emerging fungal opportunists–in vitro antifungal susceptibilities and review," *Clinical Infectious Diseases*, vol. 25, no. 5, pp. 1222–1229, 1997.

[6] Z. Khan, K. Al-Obaid, S. Ahmad, A. A. Ghani, L. Joseph, and R. Chandy, "*Acremonium* kiliense: reappraisal of its clinical

significance," *Journal of Clinical Microbiology*, vol. 49, no. 6, pp. 2342–2347, 2011.

[7] H. Perdomo, D. A. Sutton, D. Garcia et al., "Spectrum of clinically relevant *Acremonium* species in the United States," *Journal of Clinical Microbiology*, vol. 49, no. 1, pp. 243–256, 2011.

[8] N. Kouvousis, G. Lazaros, E. Christoforatou et al., "Pacemaker pocket infection due to *Acremonium* species," *Pacing and Clinical Electrophysiology*, vol. 25, no. 3, pp. 378-379, 2002.

[9] J. Guarro, A. Del Palacio, J. Gene, J. Cano, and C. G. Gonzalez, "A case of colonization of a prosthetic mitral valve by *Acremonium strictum*," *Revista Iberoamericana de Micología*, vol. 26, no. 2, pp. 146–148, 2009.

[10] S. Lacaz Cda, E. Porto, J. J. Carneiro, I. O. Pazianni, and W. P. Pimenta, "Endocarditis in dura mater prosthesis caused by *Acremonium kiliense*," *Revista do Instituto de Medicina Tropical de São Paulo*, vol. 23, no. 6, pp. 274–279, 1981.

[11] M. Degeorges, C. Heintz, J. Valty, E. Drouhet, J. F. Acar, and G. Leduc, "Infectious endocarditis due to Listeria monocytogenes and Cephalosporium," *Presse Médicale*, vol. 79, no. 30, pp. 1377–1380, 1971.

[12] C. Panzaru, M. Dan, M. O. Balasanian, G. Coada, G. Tinica, and E. R. Dabija, "Subacute fungal endocarditis due to *Acremonium* spp: a case study and review of the literature," *Revista Medico-Chirurgicală a Societăţii de Medici şi Naturalişti din Iaşi*, vol. 118, no. 1, pp. 182–185, 2014.

[13] E. Roilides, E. Bibashi, E. Acritidou et al., "*Acremonium* fungemia in two immunocompromised children," *Pediatric Infectious Disease Journal*, vol. 14, no. 6, pp. 548–550, 1995.

5

Cutaneous Fusariosis in a Patient with Job's (Hyper-IgE) Syndrome

Ahmed M. Altibi,[1,2] Radhika Sheth,[1] Ayman Battisha,[3] and Vivek Kak[1]

[1]*Henry Ford Allegiance Health (HFAH), Jackson, MI, USA*
[2]*Harvard T. H. Chan School of Public Health, Harvard University, Boston, MA, USA*
[3]*University of Massachusetts Medical School-Baystate, Springfield, MA, USA*

Correspondence should be addressed to Vivek Kak; vkak1@hfhs.org

Academic Editor: Gloria Taliani

Fusarium is a filamentous fungus that is ubiquitous in nature and can cause severe opportunistic infections in immunocompromised hosts. The association between *Fusarium* and hyper-IgE syndrome is exceedingly rare and has only been documented in a single report previously. A 44-year-old male, working as marijuana grower, with prior diagnosis of hyper-IgE syndrome and recurrent infections presented with enlarging right knee ulcer that did not respond to antimicrobial treatment. The patient was diagnosed with cutaneous fusariosis, confirmed with punch biopsy and positive wound cultures. The patient was managed with extended antifungal therapy (i.e., posaconazole) and surgical debridement resulting in remarkable improvement with wound healing leaving a pale scar. *Fusarium* should be considered in differential for cutaneous and invasive fungal infections in presence of cutaneous manifestations. Exposure to *Cannabis* plants is a noticeable risk factor. Multimodal approach involving systemic antifungals and wound debridement is essential for favorable outcome. Posaconazole was demonstrated to be a highly efficacious antifungal choice.

1. Introduction

Fusarium is a genus of filamentous fungi that can cause superficial, locally invasive, or disseminated infections in humans [1, 2]. Superficial infections typically occur in immunocompetent individuals, with the two classic infections being fungal keratitis and onychomycosis [3, 4]. On the contrary, invasive and disseminated infections occur almost exclusively in immunocompromised, particularly in profoundly neutropenic and T-cell deficient individuals. Patients with hematological malignancies and hematopoietic stem cell transplant recipients represent the majority of severe reported fusarial cases [5]. In immunocompromised individuals, the most common presentation for fusarial infections is prolonged fever refractory to antimicrobials in the setting of profound neutropenia; hence, it should be considered in differential for neutropenic fever. Other forms of infections include cutaneous fusariosis, sinusitis, pneumonia, endophthalmitis, and fusarial fungemia [6–8].

Cutaneous fusarial infections can be localized or disseminated. While the vast majority of immunocompromised individuals (88%) present with disseminated cutaneous lesions, only a minority of immunocompetent individuals (7%) develop disseminated cutaneous lesions [9]. Cutaneous involvement in the setting of an invasive fungal infection (e.g., fungemia) should raise suspicion for *Fusarium* as a potential culprit pathogen since skin involvement exists in 70% of patients with fusariosis [9]. The most commonly reported skin manifestations in cutaneous fusariosis include multiple painful erythematous papules/nodules, with or without central necrosis. Necrotic lesions tend to be associated with lesions resembling ecthyma gangrenosum, some with evolution into target lesions [9]. Other less common cutaneous manifestations include onychomycosis and periungual cellulitis.

In this clinical report, we describe a rare case of cutaneous fusarial infection in a patient with hyper-IgE syndrome (i.e., Job's syndrome). The association of fusarial infection with this rare immune disorder had only been previously reported in a single report in the literature [10]. We also shed light on successfully treating this case with oral posaconazole as monotherapy for fusariosis.

2. Case Report

This is a 44-year-old Caucasian male patient with past history significant for hyper-IgE syndrome (confirmed with positive STAT3 mutation) and recurrent infections since childhood, including soft tissue infections (i.e., abscesses and osteomyelitis), recurrent pulmonary infections (i.e., empyemas), and recurrent staphylococcal infections. The patient presented to the infectious disease clinic with a progressively enlarging skin lesion on the lateral aspect of the right knee for two months. The lesion initially started as a quarter-sized ulcerative lesion associated with intermittent purulent discharge and pain upon palpation. Initial evaluation showed a temperature of 36.6°C (97.7°F), blood pressure of 108/60 mmHg, pulse of 80 beats/minute, and respiratory rate of 16/minute. On examination, the patient was well-developed and well-nourished. Cardiopulmonary and abdominal examinations were unremarkable. Upon skin inspection, the patient had several scars on his neck and back (Figure 1(a)), reflecting prior staphylococcal furunculosis previously treated with linezolid. Remarkably, the patient also had onychomycosis (Figure 1(b)), affecting several fingernails and toenails.

The primary skin lesion on the lateral aspect of the right knee (Figure 2) was measuring 7.5 cm × 6.0 cm × 0.1 cm. The wound bed was mostly filled with eschar with very little granulation tissue. The surrounding skin was edematous, erythematous, and with mildly tender edges but did not show signs of cellulitis. Debridement was attempted during the initial encounter, but it was limited by the thick eschar tissue. Subsequently, wound culture and a punch biopsy of the lesion was obtained. The patient was scheduled for a follow-up visit with the wound clinic. Beyond the primary skin lesion, the patient denied having fever, chills, recent trauma, and animal/tick bites. He also denied a history of malignancy, chemotherapy, or hematopoietic stem cell transplant.

He has previously been treated for an HPV infection and had a negative hepatitis C and HIV screening tests recently. The patient had a recent travel to Hawaii one month prior to his initial encounter. During the trip, he indulged in aquatic sports, including swimming in pools and the ocean. Of notice, the patient has recently started a marijuana dispensary business, which also involved growing *Cannabis* plants. He reported that his marijuana plants were "damaged by mold" after which he had to bring new plants to grow.

2.1. Investigations

2.1.1. Laboratory Findings. Initial workup showed a hemoglobin of 14.2 g/dl, white blood cell count of 3.9 k/ul (neutrophils: 56%, lymphocytes: 19%, monocytes: 15%, and eosinophils: 8%), and platelets of 214 k/ul. ESR and CRP were both within normal range at 13 mm/hour and <0.1 mg/L, respectively. Liver studies showed an ALT of 29 IU/L, AST of 35 IU/L, alkaline phosphatase of 57 IU/L, total bilirubin of 0.5 mg/dl, albumin of 5.0 g/dl, globulins of 3.4 g/dl, and total protein of 7.4 g/dl. Upon reviewing immunoglobulins levels, the patient was noticed to have a markedly elevated IgG (1,838 mg/dl, normally <200) and IgE levels (4,242 mg/dl, normally <300).

2.1.2. Histopathology. A punch biopsy of the right knee lesion was performed during the initial encounter and showed an ulcer and abscess in the upper and mid-dermis. The deep dermis also exhibited suppurative inflammation within the subcutaneous tissue. Most remarkably, digestive PAS stain revealed the presence of numerous fungal hyphae consistent with deep fungal infection (Figure 3). Gram stain appeared negative for bacterial organisms.

2.1.3. Microbiology. Wound cultures from the right knee lesion obtained on initial encounter isolated *Fusarium* species on the aerobic culture. However, no bacterial growth was observed on Gram stain or anaerobic cultures. Wound swab culture was repeated four days later which again identified *Fusarium* species as well as coagulase-negative staphylococci, likely representing cross contamination.

Sabouraud dextrose agar (SDA), the standard media for most fungi, was used to cultivate the organism. The VITEK-2 automated system was utilized for fungal identification, and *Fusarium* species were identified. In addition, lactophenol cotton blue (LPCB) wet-mount preparation was used for direct visualization of fungal structures, and structures consistent with *Fusarium* species were recognized (e.g., *Fusarium* species hyphae) under slide preparation. Further identification of the fusarial subspecies was attempted; however, the cost of processing was prohibitive.

2.2. Treatment and Outcomes. Since *Fusarium* species were isolated from wound culture, the patient was initiated on antifungal therapy with *posaconazole* (300 mg once daily) for a planned treatment duration of 4–6 months. Since azole antifungals are notorious for hepatotoxicity, patient's liver functions were monitored monthly and were persistently normal. In addition, serum levels of posaconazole were monitored during the treatment duration to ensure achieving the target therapeutic range (>0.7 mcg/ml). Wound debridement was attempted; however, it was initially limited by the thick eschar tissue (Figure 4).

One week after initiating treatment, granulation tissues started to appear, and serosanguinous discharge continued to show on the ulcer base (Figure 4). On subsequent visits, surgical debridement was performed until almost all eschar tissue was removed. A month later, the ulcer showed hypergranulation with sloughing around the periphery, without eschar tissue or serosanguinous discharge (Figure 4). The patient continued to be free of symptoms during

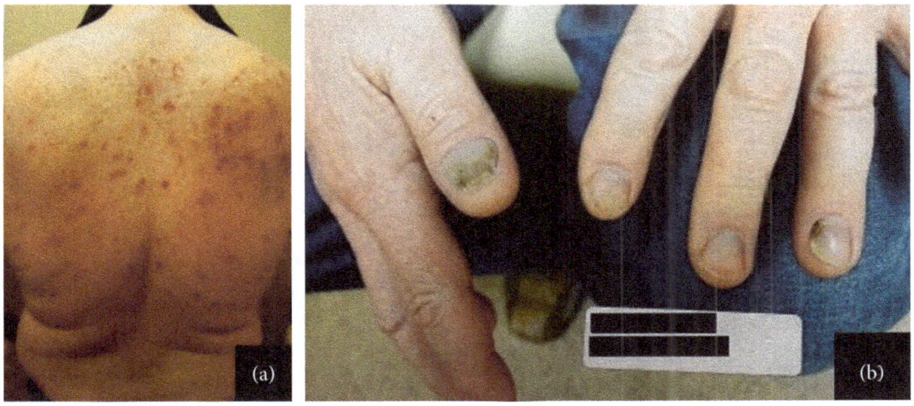

FIGURE 1: (a) Several scars on the patient's back resembling healing of old staphylococcal furunculosis; (b) distal subungual onychomycosis affecting multiple fingernails.

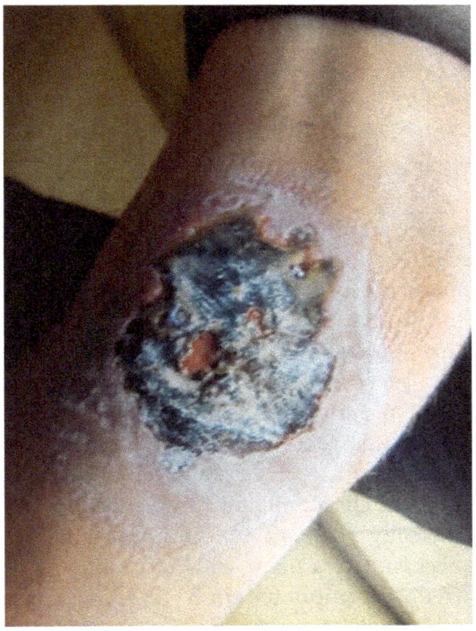

FIGURE 2: Ulcerative and necrotic lesion on the lateral aspect of the right knee measuring $7.5 \times 6.0 \times 0.1$ cm. The wound base was mostly filled with eschar tissue with minimal granulation tissue.

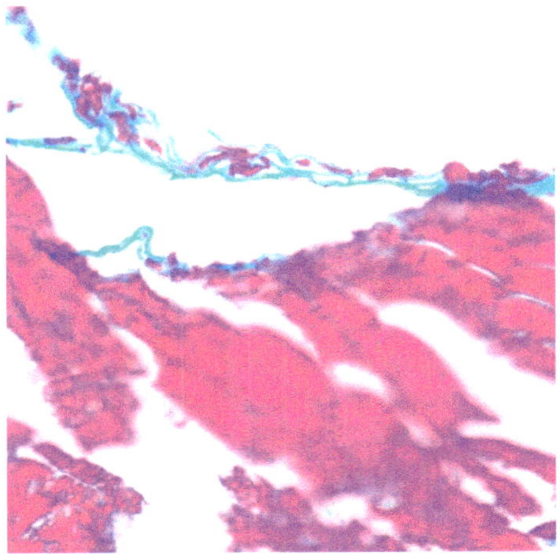

FIGURE 3: Punch excision skin biopsy obtained from a right lower extremity ulcer. Digestive PAS stain demonstrating the presence of numerous fungal hyphae consistent with fungal infection. Gram stain appeared negative for bacterial organisms.

that time and was able to tolerate posaconazole without adverse events. After six weeks of treatment, the ulcer had reduced to 6.0×4.0 cm with visible pink granulation tissue at the base; no further surgical debridement was needed. By the third month, the wound healed completely leaving pale and raised scar tissue at the site of the lesion (Figure 4). The patient continued on *posaconazole* for a total of four months before it was discontinued.

3. Discussion

Fusarium is an opportunistic fungal pathogen that can cause localized, invasive, or disseminated infections in severely immunocompromised (IC) individuals [6]. The two most commonly reported risk factors for invasive fusariosis include neutropenia and hematological malignancies. In this article, we describe a case of cutaneous fusariosis in a patient with AD-HIES (a.k.a. Job's syndrome). While patients with Job's syndrome are prone to invasive opportunistic infections, an infection with fusariosis is an exceedingly rare event that had only been documented in a single report in the literature [10].

Individuals with hyper-IgE syndrome have a genetic mutation of the signal transducer and activator of transcription 3 (*STAT3*), a component of the *JAK-STAT* pathway that is required for the activation of a number of different immune cells [11]. A defect in *STAT3* impairs the cytokine signaling for differentiation of Th17 cells and chemotaxis of neutrophils [12]. Hence, patients with defective *STAT3* are susceptible to staphylococcal and fungal infections. Our patient had been suffering from recurrent staphylococcal abscesses, empyemas, and recurrent osteomyelitis since childhood—all attributed to his AD-HIES.

Interestingly, our patient has been growing marijuana in his home yard and reported that all his plants "died out because of the mold". Hence, it is possible that exposure

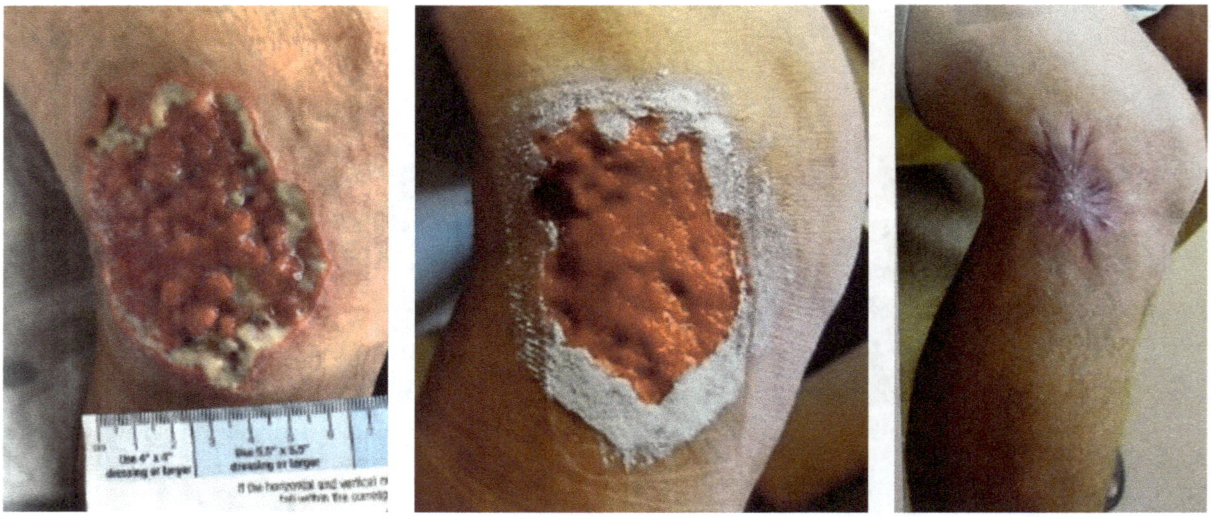

(a) (b) (c)

FIGURE 4: (a) Granulation tissue started to appear and serosanguineous discharge continued to show on the ulcer base (8.1 × 6.4 cm). (b) Progressive healing evidenced by hypergranulation with sloughing around the periphery (no serosanguinous discharge and no eschar tissue). (c) The size of the lesion had significantly reduced to 1.8 × 1.4 cm, and the wound healed completely leaving a pale and raised scar tissue at the site of the lesion.

occurred upon contact with the infested *Cannabis* plants in his yard with subsequent inoculation of the *Fusarium* spores. The unique route of exposure to this rare fungus in the setting of an equally rare immunodeficiency disorder (i.e., Job's syndrome) is what makes this case intriguing.

While interrupting culture results, one should be thoughtful about the clinical context of these results [2]. For instance, *Fusarium* species growing in skin scraping of an immunocompetent patient likely represents contamination or colonization, whereas *Fusarium spp.* in respiratory secretion from an immunocompromised individual should be considered diagnostic for fusariosis [7]. *Fusarium* is also a well-known etiologic agent for onychomycosis responsible for 10–40% of cases caused by fungi other than dermatophytes [13, 14]. Fusarial infection in our case was associated with onychomycosis; however, a microbiologic confirmation for the causative organism was not sought.

Fusarium can invade blood vessels causing hematogenous spread—the hallmark of "disseminated" fusariosis [15]. A definitive diagnosis of "disseminated" disease requires two positive culture from either internal organs, blood cultures, or both [16]. On the contrary, a fusarial infection is classified as "local" when there is a histological evidence of invasion confirmed by a positive culture from the same site without systemic involvement [1]. In our case, the patient had histological and microbiological diagnosis for *Fusarium*, but with negative blood cultures or distant organ involvement; hence, the infection was classified to be "local".

In histopathology sections, *Fusarium* species often appears similar to *Aspergillus* and *Pseudallescheria* species, with septate hyphae branching at an acute angle. It is important to distinguish between them as the latter two tends to be more resistant to the commonly used antifungals.

So far, there are no well-established treatment guidelines for fusarial infections, given the rarity of the disease and the species-dependent susceptibility to antifungals. Most data in the literature are derived from case reports and limited observational studies in immunocompromised patients [7]. In general, a successful treatment strategy entails a composite of systemic antifungals, surgical debridement, and source control (e.g., removal of potential source catheters). Fusarial species tend to be resistant to most antifungals in vitro; hence, the choice of antifungal can be challenging. While universally resistant to echinocandins (i.e., caspofungin), successful treatment with favorable outcomes had been reported with amphotericin B [12, 13, 17], voriconazole [18, 19], and posaconazole [20–22]. Optimum treatment duration remains obscure, but generally antifungals are recommended to be continued at least until all clinical signs of infection resolve. Patients with nonlocalized fusariosis typically require prolonged course of treatment (i.e., months). For instance, the case by Belcher et al. required eight months of aggressive systemic therapy, while in our case, treatment with oral posaconazole extended for a total of four months. Nonetheless, this can largely vary based on the extent of dissemination of infection and the immune status of the patient. Further studies are required to explore the ideal antifungal treatment and also the therapeutic efficacy of posaconazole in fusarial infections.

4. Conclusion

We highlighted a case of cutaneous fusariosis in the setting of a rare entity "Job's syndrome." *Fusarium* species should especially be considered in the differential for local and invasive fungal infections in presence of cutaneous manifestations. In addition to immune deficiency, exposure to

Cannabis plants might be a noticeable risk factor. A multimodal approach involving systemic antifungals and wound debridement is essential for a more favorable outcome. Fusarial infections tend to require prolonged treatment duration (i.e., months). Posaconazole was demonstrated in our case to be a highly efficacious antifungal choice. Yet, further large-scale studies are required to characterize the optimum antifungal regimen and duration of therapy.

Authors' Contributions

Ahmed M. Altibi and Radhika Sheth contributed equally to this manuscript.

References

[1] R. Nir-Paz, J. Strahilevitz, M. Shapiro et al., "Clinical and epidemiological aspects of infections caused by *Fusarium* species: a collaborative study from Israel," *Journal of Clinical Microbiology*, vol. 42, no. 8, pp. 3456–3461, 2004.

[2] M. Nucci and E. Anaissie, "*Fusarium* infections in immunocompromised patients," *Clinical Microbiology Reviews*, vol. 20, no. 4, pp. 695–704, 2007.

[3] G. Walther, S. Stasch, K. Kaerger et al., "*Fusarium* keratitis in Germany," *Journal of Clinical Microbiology*, vol. 55, no. 10, pp. 2983–2995, 2017.

[4] R. Baran, A. Tosti, and B. M. Piraccini, "Uncommon clinical patterns of *Fusarium* nail infection: report of three cases," *British Journal of Dermatology*, vol. 136, no. 3, pp. 424–427, 1997.

[5] M. Z. Hayashida, C. A. Seque, M. M Enokihara, and A. M. Porro, "Disseminated fusariosis with cutaneous involvement in hematologic malignancies: report of six cases with high mortality rate," *Anais Brasileiros de Dermatologia*, vol. 93, no. 5, pp. 726–729, 2018.

[6] F. Nucci, S. A. Nouér, D. Capone et al., "*Fusarium*," *Seminars in Respiratory and Critical Care Medicine*, vol. 36, no. 5, pp. 706–714, 2015.

[7] M. Muhammed, T. Anagnostou, A. Desalermos et al., "*Fusarium* infection," *Medicine*, vol. 92, no. 6, p. 1, 2013.

[8] A. Tupaki-Sreepurna and A. J. Kindo, "*Fusarium*: the versatile pathogen," *Indian Journal of Medical Microbiology*, vol. 36, no. 1, p. 8, 2018.

[9] M. Nucci and E. Anaissie, "Cutaneous infection by *Fusarium* species in healthy and immunocompromised hosts: implications for diagnosis and management," *Clinical Infectious Diseases*, vol. 35, no. 8, pp. 909–920, 2002.

[10] M. D. Belcher, L. Ishii, J. E. Turrentine, and J. E. Turrentine, "Multimodal therapy for recalcitrant cutaneous *Fusarium* solani infection in a patient with hyper-IgE syndrome," *Dernatology Archives*, vol. 1, 2017.

[11] C. Woellner, E. M. Gertz, A. A. Schäffer et al., "Mutations in STAT3 and diagnostic guidelines for hyper-IgE syndrome," *Journal of Allergy and Clinical Immunology*, vol. 125, no. 2, pp. 424–432, 2010.

[12] H. D. Ochs, M. Oukka, and T. R. Torgerson, "TH17 cells and regulatory T cells in primary immunodeficiency diseases," *Journal of Allergy and Clinical Immunology*, vol. 123, no. 5, pp. 977–983, 2009.

[13] K. Diongue, M. Ndiaye, M. C. Seck et al., "Onychomycosis caused by *Fusarium* spp. in dakar, Senegal: epidemiological, clinical, and mycological study," *Dermatology Research and Practice*, vol. 2017, Article ID 1268130, 4 pages, 2017.

[14] M. Guevara-Suarez, J. F. Cano-Lira, M. C. Cepero de García et al., "Genotyping of *Fusarium* isolates from onychomycoses in Colombia: detection of two new species within the *Fusarium* solani species complex and in vitro antifungal susceptibility testing," *Mycopathologia*, vol. 181, no. 3-4, pp. 165–174, 2016.

[15] B. E. Shields, M. Rosenbach, Z. Brown-Joel et al., "Angioinvasive fungal infections impacting the skin: background, epidemiology, and clinical presentation," *Journal of the American Academy of Dermatology*, vol. 80, no. 4, pp. 869–880, 2019.

[16] E. I. Boutati and E. J. Anaissie, "*Fusarium*, a significant emerging pathogen in patients with hematologic malignancy: ten years' experience at a cancer center and implications for management," *Blood*, vol. 90, no. 3, pp. 999–1008, 1997.

[17] J. R. Perfect, "Treatment of non-Aspergillus moulds in immunocompromised patients, with Amphotericin *B* lipid complex," *Clinical Infectious Diseases*, vol. 40, no. 6, pp. S401–S408, 2005.

[18] A. Meyer and M. Jones, "Treatment of a locally invasive cutaneous *Fusarium* species infection with voriconazole and liposomal Amphotericin *B* in a patient with relapsed acute myeloid leukemia," *Journal of the Advanced Practitioner in Oncology*, vol. 8, no. 5, 2017.

[19] J. R. Perfect, K. A. Marr, T. J. Walsh et al., "Voriconazole treatment for less-common, emerging, or refractory fungal infections," *Clinical Infectious Diseases*, vol. 36, no. 9, pp. 1122–1131, 2003.

[20] I. I. Raad, R. Y. Hachem, R. Herbrecht et al., "Posaconazole as salvage treatment for invasive fusariosis in patients with underlying hematologic malignancy and other conditions," *Clinical Infectious Diseases*, vol. 42, no. 10, pp. 1398–1403, 2006.

[21] N. P. Wiederhold, L. K. Najvar, R. Bocanegra et al., "Efficacy of posaconazole as treatment and prophylaxis against *Fusarium* solani," *Antimicrobial Agents and Chemotherapy*, vol. 54, no. 3, pp. 1055–1059, 2010.

[22] A. Tanase, A. Colita, G. Ianosi et al., "Rare case of disseminated fusariosis in a young patient with graft vs. host disease following an allogeneic transplant," *Experimental and Therapeutic Medicine*, vol. 12, no. 4, pp. 2078–2082, 2016.

6

Fusarium Infection in a Kidney Transplant Recipient Successfully Treated with Voriconazole

Ahmed M. Alkhunaizi,[1] Ali M. Bazzi,[2] Ali A. Rabaan,[2] and Elwaleed A. Ahmed[3]

[1] *Nephrology Section, Specialty Medicine Department, Johns Hopkins Aramco Healthcare, Dhahran, Saudi Arabia*
[2] *Department of Pathology, Johns Hopkins Aramco Healthcare, Dhahran, Saudi Arabia*
[3] *Infectious Diseases Section, Specialty Medicine Department, Johns Hopkins Aramco Healthcare, Dhahran, Saudi Arabia*

Correspondence should be addressed to Ahmed M. Alkhunaizi; aalkhunaizi@gmail.com

Academic Editor: Raul Colodner

Fusarium infections in solid-organ transplant recipients are rare and carry high mortality. We report a case of a kidney transplant recipient who developed infection with *Fusarium* species. The patient received treatment with oral voriconazole for five months with good response.

1. Introduction

Opportunistic infections are common complications in patients with hematologic malignancies, bone marrow transplant patients, and recipients of solid-organ transplants [1]. Invasive fungal infections are particularly serious complications and carry a high mortality rate in immunocompromised hosts [2, 3]. *Fusarium* species are ubiquitous molds that thrive in soil and decomposing vegetation. Infection with *Fusarium* species among solid-organ transplant recipients is an uncommon event. In this report, we describe the case of a kidney transplant recipient who developed infection with *Fusarium* species and was successfully managed with voriconazole.

2. Case Report

A 55-year-old male patient presented with a history of hypertension and type 2 diabetes mellitus. He developed end-stage renal disease (ESRD) and was started on hemodialysis in July 2016. In August 2016, he underwent a living unrelated kidney transplantation in another country. He received induction therapy with antithymocyte globulin and was subsequently maintained on a triple immunosuppressive regimen consisting of tacrolimus, mycophenolate mofetil, and prednisone. His postoperative course was complicated by the development of a perinephric hematoma, acute tubular necrosis, and urinary tract infection with extended-spectrum beta-lactamase producing *Escherichia coli*. Evacuation of the hematoma was performed using percutaneous drainage. In January 2017, he developed fever and abdominal pain localized to the kidney graft. Ultrasonography showed complex fluid collection surrounding the kidney measuring $20 \times 9 \times 8$ cm. A percutaneous drain was inserted and revealed purulent fluid. Gram stain of the fluid showed many white cells and rare Gram-positive bacilli. Calcofluor white stain and KOH method showed fungal elements. The fluid culture was positive for *Fusarium* species (Figure 1).

There were no skin lesions, and the blood culture was negative. The immunosuppression regimen was modified with discontinuation of mycophenolate mofetil and reduction of the dose of tacrolimus. In addition, the patient was started on voriconazole at a maintenance dose of 4 mg/kg every 12 hours. After completing a treatment period of five months, the infection was considered cured and voriconazole was discontinued. Repeat ultrasound showed remnant cavity with septations. No adverse events were noted during the treatment period. The patient remained

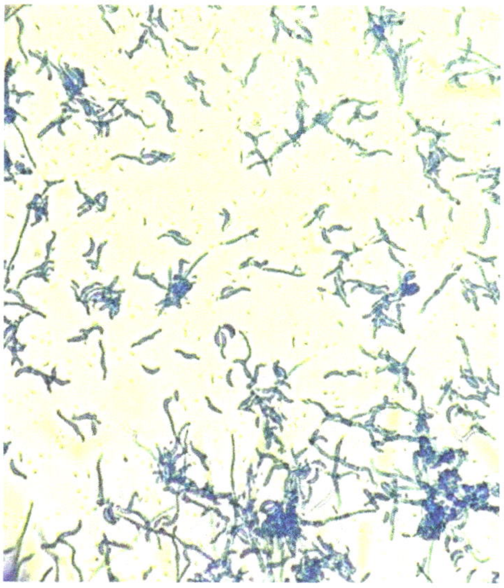

FIGURE 1: Sickle-shaped, multicell macroconidia (40x) of *Fusarium* species stained with lactophenol cotton blue counterstain from a perinephric fluid collection.

free of recurrent infection, and the kidney graft function remained stable with a serum creatinine of 0.9 mg/dl (normal range 0.7–1.2) 18 months after transplantation.

3. Discussion

Our patient developed infection with *Fusarium* species. The infection was localized to a perinephric cavity as a result of perinephric hematoma. The presence of a percutaneous drain in the setting of heavy immunosuppression in the early post-renal transplantation period was a predisposing factor. There was no other tissue or organ involvement, and therefore, we could not establish tissue invasion histologically.

Reduction of the dose of immunosuppressive medications together with a prolonged administration of voriconazole led to a cure and preservation of the renal allograft function. Susceptibility testing was not performed; however, the response to treatment indicates that the organism was sensitive to voriconazole.

Fungal infections, localized or invasive, are serious complications following organ transplantation. The consequences include prolonged hospitalization, allograft dysfunction, and high mortality, in addition to the high cost of treatment [4, 5]. Most of the fungal infections are caused by *Candida* species followed by aspergillosis and cryptococcosis [5]. The overall incidence during the first year after transplantation has been estimated at 3%; however, this varies depending on the type of organ transplantation [5]. Risk factors are related to the net state of immunosuppression, environmental exposure/colonization, and use of prophylactic antifungal agents. We have previously reported series of fungal infections related to transplant tourism similar to this case [4]. Transplant tourism is unfortunately still practiced in some parts of the world despite the commitment of many countries to the Declaration of Istanbul that aimed to combat this type of practice [6].

Fusarium species are ubiquitous, widely distributed in air, water, soil, and subterranean and aerial plant parts, and may occasionally infect animals and humans [7, 8]. In humans, they can cause a broad spectrum of infections including skin, eye, locally invasive infections, and in immunocompromised hosts, disseminated infections which carry a high mortality rate [2, 9]. Portals of entry include the respiratory and the gastrointestinal tracts, catheter tips, indwelling central venous catheters, and cutaneous sites [8, 10]. The most frequent species causing infections in humans are *Fusarium solani*, *Fusarium oxysporum*, and *Fusarium moniliforme* [8]. Most of the affected individuals are either bone marrow transplant recipients or have bone marrow suppression as a result of hematologic malignancy [11–14]. In contrast, infection with *Fusarium* species has been rarely reported in kidney transplant recipients, and most of the cases were related to skin infection (Table 1) [15–19]. Skin lesions can result either from direct skin invasion or through hematogenous spread in case of disseminated disease. The diagnosis of *Fusarium* infection may be made on histopathology, Gram stain, tissue culture, blood culture, or serology. Obtaining a susceptibility profile is not always possible, due to the nature of fusarial species and the inoculate size and prolonged incubation period during the susceptibility testing [20, 21]. However, all attempts should be made to perform susceptibility testing either locally or by sending the specimen to a center with experience in fungal diseases.

Treatment of fusariosis depends on the site and extent of infection. While surgical intervention may play an important role in cases of localized diseases, invasive fusariosis is more difficult to treat and poses a challenge to clinicians. Amphotericin B is effective in vitro against *Fusarium* species and historically was used to eradicate disseminated fusarial infection [22]. However, its use is limited by side effects such as nephrotoxicity especially in renal transplant recipients. More recently, voriconazole, the first available second-generation triazole, has added a new and improved therapeutic option as a primary therapy of invasive fungal infections such as aspergillosis, yeast infections, and other molds [23]. It has been used alone or in combination with other antifungal agents such as amphotericin B and terbinafine with success in treating fusarial infection [3, 24–30]. The good bioavailability of voriconazole and favorable safety profile make it easy to administer orally for a prolonged period of time. As an azole antifungal agent, voriconazole is known to inhibit cytochrome P450 3A enzymes. Drug-drug interaction with calcineurin inhibitors (CNIs) such as tacrolimus or cyclosporine is a very important consideration in treating organ transplant recipients. For example, voriconazole has been shown to inhibit the metabolism of tacrolimus by 50% [31]. Therefore, close monitoring of the blood concentration and adjustment of the dose of CNI are warranted when transplant patients receiving CNI are treated with voriconazole.

Table 1: *Fusarium* infection in kidney transplant recipients.

Reference	Age (years)	Gender	Site of infection	Time at diagnosis	Treatment	Outcome
Young and Meyers [15]	30	F	Localized, skin	5 years after transplantation	Surgical excision	Cure
Heinz et al. [16]	45	M	Localized, skin	21 weeks after transplantation	Surgical amputation	Cure
Girardi et al. [17]	50	M	Localized, skin	2 years after transplantation	Surgical debridement	Poor response
Cocuroccia et al. [18]	53	M	Localized, skin	4 years after transplantation	Itraconazole	Cure
Garbino et al. [19]	56	F	Peritoneal cavity	Pretransplantation	Voriconazole for 2 months	Cure
Present report	55	M	Perinephric	One month	Voriconazole for 5 months	Cure

Disclosure

Opinions expressed in this article are those of the authors and not necessarily of Johns Hopkins Aramco Healthcare.

Acknowledgments

The authors acknowledge the use of Johns Hopkins Aramco Healthcare (JHAH) facilities for research data used in this article.

References

[1] J. A. Fishman, "Infection in solid-organ transplant recipients," *New England Journal of Medicine*, vol. 357, no. 25, pp. 2601–2614, 2007.

[2] M. Nucci, E. J. Anaissie, F. Queiroz-Telles et al., "Outcome predictors of 84 patients with hematologic malignancies and *Fusarium* infection," *Cancer*, vol. 98, no. 2, pp. 315–319, 2003.

[3] M. Muhammed, T. Anagnostou, A. Desalermos et al., "*Fusarium* infection: report of 26 cases and review of 97 cases from the literature," *Medicine*, vol. 92, no. 6, pp. 305–316, 2013.

[4] A. M. Alkhunaizi, A. A. Amir, and J. A. Al-Tawfiq, "Invasive fungal infections in living unrelated renal transplantation," *Transplantation Proceedings*, vol. 37, no. 7, pp. 3034–3037, 2005.

[5] P. G. Pappas, B. D. Alexander, D. R. Andes et al., "Invasive fungal infections among organ transplant recipients: results of the Transplant-Associated Infection Surveillance Network (TRANSNET)," *Clinical Infectious Diseases*, vol. 50, no. 8, pp. 1101–1111, 2010.

[6] International Summit on Transplant Tourism and Organ Trafficking Convened, "The Declaration of Istanbul on organ trafficking and transplant tourism," *Clinical Journal of the American Society of Nephrology*, vol. 3, no. 5, pp. 1227–1231, 2008.

[7] M. Nucci and E. Anaissie, "*Fusarium* infections in immunocompromised patients," *Clinical Microbiology Reviews* vol. 20, no. 4, pp. 695–704, 2007.

[8] P. E. Nelson, M. C. Dignani, and E. J. Anaissie, "Taxonomy, biology, and clinical aspects of *Fusarium* species," *Clinical Microbiology Reviews*, vol. 7, no. 4, pp. 479–504, 1994.

[9] M. Nucci and E. Anaissie, "Cutaneous infection by *Fusarium* species in healthy and immunocompromised hosts: implications for diagnosis and management," *Clinical Infectious Diseases*, vol. 35, no. 8, pp. 909–920, 2002.

[10] A. K. Gupta, R. Baran, and R. C. Summerbell, "*Fusarium* infections of the skin," *Current Opinion in Infectious Diseases*, vol. 13, no. 2, pp. 121–128, 2000.

[11] E. I. Boutati and E. J. Anaissie, "*Fusarium*, a significant emerging pathogen in patients with hematologic malignancy: ten years' experience at a cancer center and implications for management," *Blood*, vol. 90, no. 3, pp. 999–1008, 1997.

[12] C. Hennequin, V. Lavarde, J. L. Poirot et al., "Invasive *Fusarium* infections: a retrospective survey of 31 cases," *Medical Mycology*, vol. 35, no. 2, pp. 107–114, 1997.

[13] A. S. Gamis, T. Gudnason, G. S. Giebink, and N. K. Ramsay, "Disseminated infection with *Fusarium* in recipients of bone marrow transplants," *Reviews of Infectious Diseases*, vol. 13, no. 6, pp. 1077–1088, 1991.

[14] M. Campo, R. E. Lewis, and D. P. Kontoyiannis, "Invasive fusariosis in patients with hematologic malignancies at a cancer center: 1998–2009," *Journal of Infection*, vol. 60, no. 5, pp. 331–337, 2010.

[15] C. N. Young and A. M. Meyers, "Opportunistic fungal infection by *Fusarium oxysporum* in a renal transplant patient," *Medical Mycology*, vol. 17, no. 3, pp. 219–223, 1979.

[16] T. Heinz, J. Perfect, W. Schell, E. Ritter, G. Ruff, and D. Serafin, "Soft-tissue fungal infections: surgical management of 12 immunocompromised patients," *Plastic and Reconstructive Surgery*, vol. 97, no. 7, pp. 1391–1399, 1996.

[17] M. Girardi, E. J. Glusac, and S. Imaeda, "Subcutaneous *Fusarium* foot abscess in a renal transplant patient," *Cutis*, vol. 63, no. 5, pp. 267–270, 1999.

[18] B. Cocuroccia, J. Gaido, E. Gubinelli, G. Annessi, and G. Girolomoni, "Localized cutaneous hyalohyphomycosis caused by a *Fusarium* species infection in a renal transplant patient," *Journal of Clinical Microbiology*, vol. 41, no. 2, pp. 905–907, 2003.

[19] J. Garbino, I. Uckay, P. Rohner, D. Lew, and C. Van Delden, "*Fusarium* peritonitis concomitant to kidney transplantation successfully managed with voriconazole: case report and review of the literature," *Transplant International*, vol. 18, no. 5, pp. 613–618, 2005.

[20] M. Azor, J. Gene, J. Cano, and J. Guarro, "Universal in vitro antifungal resistance of genetic clades of the *Fusarium solani* species complex," *Antimicrobial Agents and Chemotherapy*, vol. 51, no. 4, pp. 1500–1503, 2007.

[21] N. I. Paphitou, L. Ostrosky-Zeichner, V. L. Paetznick, J. R. Rodriguez, E. Chen, and J. H. Rex, "In Vitro activities of investigational triazoles against *Fusarium* species: effects of inoculum size and incubation time on broth microdilution susceptibility test results," *Antimicrobial Agents and Chemotherapy*, vol. 46, no. 10, pp. 3298–3300, 2002.

[22] M. A. Wolff and R. Ramphal, "Use of amphotericin B lipid complex for treatment of disseminated cutaneous *Fusarium* infection in a neutropenic patient," *Clinical Infectious Diseases*, vol. 20, no. 6, pp. 1568-1569, 1995.

[23] H. W. Boucher, A. H. Groll, C. C. Chiou, and T. J. Walsh, "Newer systemic antifungal agents : pharmacokinetics, safety and efficacy," *Drugs*, vol. 64, no. 18, pp. 1997–2020, 2004.

[24] S. Consigny, N. Dhedin, A. Datry, S. Choquet, V. Leblond, and O. Chosidow, "Successful voriconazole treatment of disseminated *Fusarium* infection in an immunocompromised patient," *Clinical Infectious Diseases*, vol. 37, no. 2, pp. 311–313, 2003.

[25] D. Y. Ho, J. D. Lee, F. Rosso, and J. G. Montoya, "Treating disseminated fusariosis: amphotericin B, voriconazole or both?," *Mycoses*, vol. 50, no. 3, pp. 227–231, 2007.

[26] M. Stanzani, N. Vianelli, G. Bandini et al., "Successful treatment of disseminated fusariosis after allogeneic hematopoietic stem cell transplantation with the combination of voriconazole and liposomal amphotericin B," *Journal of Infection*, vol. 53, no. 6, pp. e243–e246, 2006.

[27] J. Y. Liu, W. T. Chen, B. S. Ko et al., "Combination antifungal therapy for disseminated fusariosis in immunocompromised patients: a case report and literature review," *Medical Mycology*, vol. 49, no. 8, pp. 872–878, 2011.

[28] S. Inano, M. Kimura, J. Iida, and N. Arima, "Combination therapy of voriconazole and terbinafine for disseminated fusariosis: case report and literature review," *Journal of Infection and Chemotherapy*, vol. 19, no. 6, pp. 1173–1180, 2013.

[29] J. M. Stempel, S. P. Hammond, D. A. Sutton, L. M. Weiser, and F. M. Marty, "Invasive fusariosis in the voriconazole era: single-center 13-year experience," *Open Forum Infectious Diseases*, vol. 2, no. 3, article ofv099, 2015.

[30] H. A. Carneiro, J. J. Coleman, A. Restrepo, and E. Mylonakis, "*Fusarium* infection in lung transplant patients: report of 6 cases and review of the literature," *Medicine*, vol. 90, no. 1, pp. 69–80, 2011.

[31] S. Zhang, V. C. Pillai, S. R. Mada, S. Strom, and R. Venkataramanan, "Effect of voriconazole and other azole antifungal agents on CYP3A activity and metabolism of tacrolimus in human liver microsomes," *Xenobiotica*, vol. 42, no. 5, pp. 409–416, 2012.

7

Rare Case of Four Osseous Lesions of the Skull in a Patient with Secondary Syphilis

Jace Kusler[1] and **Supha Arthurs**[2]

[1]*University of North Dakota School of Medicine and Health Sciences, 1301 N. Columbia Rd., Grand Forks, ND 58203, USA*
[2]*CHI St. Alexius Health, 900 E. Broadway Ave., Bismarck, ND 58503, USA*

Correspondence should be addressed to Jace Kusler; jace.e.kusler19@gmail.com

Academic Editor: Antonella Marangoni

Syphilis is a sexually transmitted infection that is caused by the bacterium *Treponema pallidum*. Syphilis can present as primary, secondary, tertiary, or congenital. It can have an effect on many different organ systems and tissues leading to a wide variety of symptoms and complications; one rare manifestation is bone involvement. The patient in this case was diagnosed with secondary and early neurosyphilis and was also found to have skull lesions that were due to *Treponema pallidum*. There are guidelines for the treatment of primary, secondary, tertiary, and congenital syphilis; however, there are currently no guidelines for the treatment of syphilis with bone involvement.

1. Introduction

Bone involvement is an unusual manifestation of syphilis, which is caused by the bacterium *Treponema pallidum*. Although there are not currently guidelines for treatment, the literature has shown treatment with high-dose penicillin therapy to have favorable outcomes. This report details a case of secondary and early neurosyphilis with four osseous lesions of the skull. Of particular significance, this case demonstrates the rare finding of osseous lesions with secondary syphilis and successful treatment with 14 days of 24 million units per day of IV penicillin G.

2. Case Report

A 50-year-old Native American female presented to the ER with a bladder infection, and a urine culture grew *E. coli*. She was treated with trimethoprim/sulfamethoxazole and developed a diffuse rash including the palms and soles. There was no lymphadenopathy present upon physical exam. One month later, she presented to the clinic with a month of severe pounding headaches, blurry vision in the right eye, and pain over the temporal area on the right side. Her ESR was elevated with a normal CRP. The suspected diagnosis was giant cell arteritis, and she was started on 60 mg of oral prednisone daily that helped the headaches. A temporal artery biopsy was done and showed no evidence of vasculitis. The patient was tapered from the steroid and started having progressive blurry vision and floaters. Three months later, the patient presented to the emergency department and was admitted to the hospital due to the blurry vision and floaters at which time she had a positive fluorescent treponemal antibody absorption test. She was HIV negative. The patient had a Venereal Disease Research Laboratory test of the cerebral spinal fluid done which came back negative. Her cerebral spinal fluid cell count was 178 nucleated cells with 164 lymphocytes, and protein was 53 mg/dl. She had a serum rapid plasma reagin titer of 1 : 1024. She was diagnosed with secondary and early neurosyphilis for which she was started on 24 million units per day of IV penicillin G, and severe uveitits for which she was started on 60 mg of oral prednisone and 1% prednisolone acetate eye drops. The uveitis was likely secondary to the syphilis infection. A CT scan of the head showed four osseous lesions (Figures 1–4). An immunohistochemical stain of a skull biopsy was done which came back positive for *Treponema pallidum*, thus

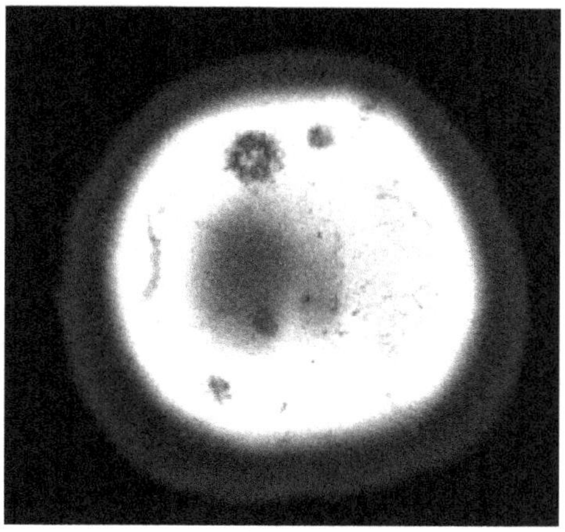

FIGURE 1: Lesion of right parietal bone.

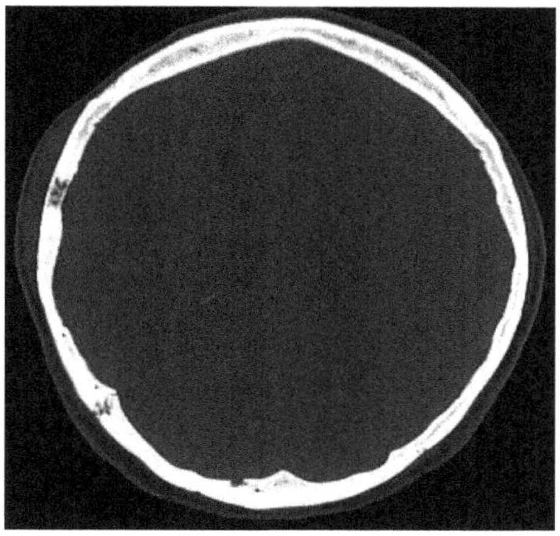

FIGURE 2: Lesion of right temporal bone.

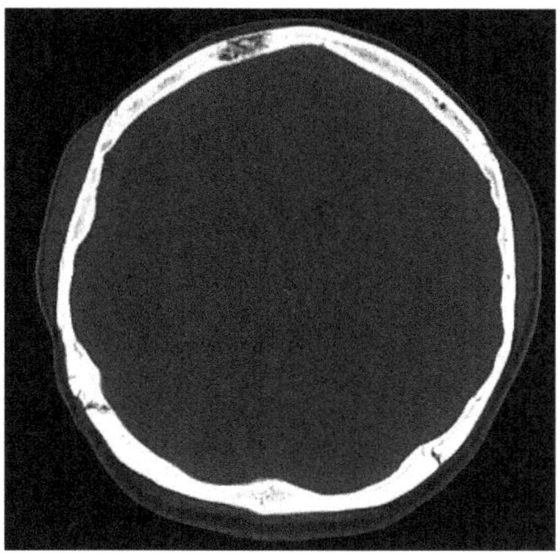

FIGURE 3: Lesion of right frontal bone.

confirming syphilis as the cause of the bone lesions. An echocardiogram was performed which did not show any significant cardiac defect. The patient completed 14 days of 24 million units per day of IV penicillin G, and there was no evidence of a Jarish–Hexheimer reaction. Upon follow-up,

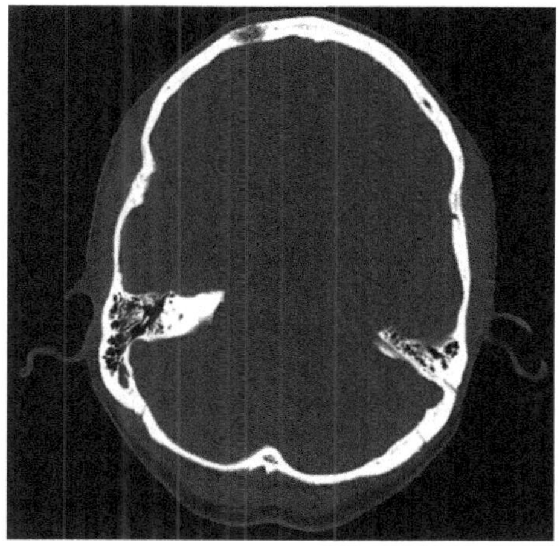

FIGURE 4: Lesion of right frontal bone.

the patient still complained of blurry motion, but denied a headache or skin rash. The eye exam showed improvement and showed no signs of ocular syphilis. Four months after discharge from the hospital, her blood rapid plasma reagin titer was 1 : 256 that is more than a fourfold decrease from her baseline, and a CT scan of the head showed the osseous lesions were unchanged from the previous CT scan. Three months after her previous follow-up, her serum rapid plasma reagin titer was 1 : 128. A repeat lumbar puncture showed 18 nucleated cells with 16 lymphocytes, and protein was 42 mg/dl. A repeat Venereal disease research laboratory test of the cerebral spinal fluid was done and came back positive with a 1 : 8 titer that was negative on the previous exam, which is hypothesized to be a false negative result. The patient was lost to further follow-up.

3. Discussion

Bones can be affected at all stages of syphilis, but it is more common in tertiary and congenital infection [1]. Cases of syphilis with bone involvement have been reported in patients who are HIV positive as well as patients who are HIV negative [2]. Bone lesions can occur without any clinical signs or symptoms; however, the most common presentation is bone pain [2–4]. In some cases when skull lesions are present, patients report headaches [1].

The long bones and skull are most commonly affected by syphilis; however, there have been cases affecting the ribs, clavicle, spine, and sternum [2]. Bone lesions can be detected with plain radiography, CT scan, MRI, or bone scintigraphy [5]. Identification of spirochetes in bone lesions with dark-field microscopy, silver stain, immunoperoxidase stain, or polymerase chain reaction is uncommon and occurs even less in late-stage disease [2, 5].

The current guidelines for treatment of syphilis is parenteral penicillin G. Patients with primary, secondary, or early latent syphilis are to be treated with a single intramuscular dose of 2.4 million units of benzathine penicillin G. Patients with tertiary and late latent syphilis are to be treated with 7.2 million total units of benzathine penicillin G, and patients with neurosyphilis are to be treated with 18–24 million units per day for 10–14 days of aqueous crystalline penicillin G [6]. There are currently no treatment guidelines for syphilis with bone lesions; however, 2.4 million units of intramuscular benzathine penicillin G for two to four weeks has been shown to be an effective treatment [1–3]. Symptomatic relief occurs rapidly after the start of therapy. After completion of appropriate therapy, there can be complete radiographic resolution of the lesions; however, the osseous lesions can persist for 7–11 months [5, 7].

Although bone involvement is a rare complication of syphilis, it is important to include syphilis in the differential diagnosis as a cause of bone pain or radiographic osseous lesions. There are currently no treatment guidelines for syphilis with bone lesions; however, there have been cases that have shown successful treatment with 2.4 million units of intramuscular benzathine penicillin G for two to four weeks. In this case, 14 days of 24 million units per day of IV penicillin G was given due to early neurosyphilis, and this treatment was effective in resolving the patient's bone pain and reducing her rapid plasma reagin titer by fourfold; however, the patient was lost to follow-up and thus follow-up imaging was not obtained.

References

[1] I. Herrera-Herrera, C. Escalona-Huerta, J. D. Valle Zapico, J. Montoya Bordon, C. Ordonez Gonzalez, and B. Sobrino Guijarro, "Secondary syphilis with bone involvement of the skull: a case report," *OMICS Journal of Radiology*, vol. 6, p. 4, 2017.

[2] K.-H. Park, M. S. Lee, I. K. Hong et al., "Bone involvement in secondary syphilis: a case report and systematic review of the literature," *Sexually Transmitted Diseases*, vol. 41, no. 9, pp. 532–537, 2014.

[3] S. H. Kang, S. W. Park, K. Y. Kwon, and W. J. Hong, "A solitary skull lesion of syphilitic osteomyelitis," *Journal of Korean Neurosurgical Society*, vol. 48, no. 1, pp. 85–87, 2010.

[4] Z. Liu, Y. Zhang, and K. Qui, "Osteomyelitis as the only manifestation of late latent syphilis; case report and literature review," *International Journal of STD and AIDS*, vol. 22, no. 6, pp. 353–355, 2011.

[5] I. Huang and J. L. Leach, "Osteomyelitis of the skull in early-acquired syphilis: evaluation by MR imaging and CT," *American Journal of Neuroradiology*, vol. 28, no. 2, pp. 307-308, 2007.

[6] Centers for Disease Control and Prevention, *2015 Sexually Transmitted Diseases Treatment Guidelines*, Centers for Disease Control and Prevention, Atlanta, GA, USA, 2016.

[7] I. A. Gurland, L. Korn, L. Edelman, and F. Wallach, "An unusual manifestation of acquired syphilis," *Clinical Infectious Diseases*, vol. 32, no. 4, pp. 667–669, 2001.

8

Cystoisospora belli Gallbladder Infection in a Liver Transplant Donor

Clifford Akateh,[1] **Christina A. Arnold**,[2] **Dathe Benissan-Messan**,[1] **Anthony Michaels**,[3] **and Sylvester M. Black**[4]

[1]*General and Gastrointestinal Surgery, Department of Surgery, The Ohio State University Wexner Medical Center, Columbus, OH 43210, USA*
[2]*Department of Pathology, The Ohio State University Wexner Medical Center, Columbus, OH 43210, USA*
[3]*Division of Gastroenterology, Hepatology and Nutrition, Department of Internal Medicine, The Ohio State University Wexner Medical Center, Columbus, OH 43210, USA*
[4]*Division of Transplant Surgery, Department of Surgery, The Ohio State University Wexner Medical Center, Columbus, OH 43210, USA*

Correspondence should be addressed to Clifford Akateh; clifford.akateh@osumc.edu

Academic Editor: Raul Colodner

Introduction. Cystoisospora belli (previously *Isospora belli*) is a parasitic protozoan of the human gastrointestinal system. It rarely causes symptoms in immunocompetent hosts but can cause severe diarrhea in immunocompromised patients, with a rate of recurrence and risk of dissemination. Gallbladder infections are however rare. The treatment of choice for symptomatic patients is a 7–10-day course of trimethoprim-sulfamethoxazole. *Case.* In this case, we report on an incidental finding of *Cystoisospora belli* organisms in the donor gallbladder following a transplant cholecystectomy. There was no report of symptoms in the donor. The recipient was treated with a course of trimethoprim-sulfamethoxazole, without evidence of cystoisosporiasis. Given the risk of recurrence in immunocompromised hosts, the patient will continue to be monitored for reactivation in the future. *Conclusion.* Despite advances in transplant protocols and screening, disease transmission from the donor to recipient still occurs in about 0.2% of all organ transplants. With the increased use of organs from drug overdose victims and other high-risk donors, practitioners (including pathologists, hepatologists, and surgeons) must maintain a high index of suspicion for such potentially harmful organisms.

1. Introduction

Cystoisospora belli, previously called *Isospora belli* (*C. belli*), is an intracellular protozoan of the intestinal epithelium. Although present worldwide, it is a less common cause of protozoal diarrhea, compared to *Toxoplasma* and *Cryptosporidium*. It is most prevalent in the tropical regions [1–3]. In the West, *Cystoisospora belli* is associated with HIV/AIDS infection and occasionally diarrhea in travelers [4–8]. It is transmitted by the ingestion of contaminated produce or water [3]. The oocysts can be seen on light microscopy with hematoxylin and eosin stain of tissue samples. Modified acid-fast stains can also be used in challenging ova in stool samples [9]. In addition, PCR assays to detect the organism in stool samples exist [10, 11].

In immunocompetent individuals, the protozoan occasionally causes mild episodes of watery diarrhea, fever, nausea, vomiting, and malabsorption, but overall is typically asymptomatic [12]. On the other hand, immunocompromised patients experience more severe and prolonged symptoms [13]. In 1994, Benator et al., reported on the first case of *C. belli*-induced acalculous cholecystitis [14]. Extraintestinal manifestations have also been reported in these patients as well, including gallbladder and biliary tract infections [13–17]. In recent years, there have been case reports of *C. belli* infections in immunocompetent individuals. Most of these cases involve a recent immigrant from the subtropics [5, 7, 8]. Surprisingly, there are growing reports of biliary infection in immunocompetent individuals as well, including cases of acute and chronic cholecystitis [18–20].

C. belli infections have equally been seen in patients following solid organ transplant [21–24]. More recently, there was a case of *C. belli* infection reported in a patient who underwent a small bowel transplant [25]. In these cases, the patients were successfully treated, without further sequelae and had no reports of extraintestinal manifestations. However, given the need for chronic immunosuppression use in these patients, reactivation remains a concern [26]. Also, it is not clear whether *C. belli* infections in these solid organ transplant recipients were derived from the donor or contracted independently by the recipient. There has been one previous report incidentally found *C. belli* in donor gallbladders, during a retrospective pathologic review of gallbladders [27]. Unfortunately, no further information was available on the recipients or donors in these cases.

2. Case Report

2.1. Recipient. The patient is a 59-year-old male who had struggled with oxalate nephrolithiasis since the age of 13, without formal workup. He previously underwent multiple lithotripsies, as well as a partial nephrectomy and remained relatively controlled with a baseline creatinine of 1.2-1.3 mg/dL (reference range: 0.70–1.30 mg/dL). Unfortunately, in September 2016, the patient progressed to chronic kidney disease, after an episode of dehydration. He was seen in our institution in November 2016 after presenting with an episode of acute on chronic renal failure. He had no renal reserve and was initiated on hemodialysis. Further history revealed a daughter with oxalate stones disease as well, raising concern for hereditary oxalosis; other serological studies were negative, and biopsy confirmed acute tubular necrosis (ATN) with oxalate nephropathy. Genetic testing was pursued, and the results showed an AGXT mutation consistent with a type 1 primary hyperoxaluria. All preoperative liver testing results were within the normal limits. Given this diagnosis, the patient was evaluated by the transplant committee, and a combined liver-kidney transplant was recommended [28, 29]. The patient underwent a combined orthotopic liver (OLT)-kidney transplant in July 2017. A donor cholecystectomy was done as per the standard protocol. Pathologic examination revealed *Cystoisospora belli* organisms. The patient was treated with trimethoprim/sulfamethoxazole (TMP/SMX) DS 800–160 mg every 6 hours for ten days followed twice daily for three weeks. There is currently no evidence of *C. belli* reactivation.

2.2. Donor. The donor was a 20-year-old Caucasian male who suffered an anoxic brain injury. He had no history of biliary disease/symptoms and had no evidence of acute or chronic cholecystitis, biliary disease, or other biliary disease

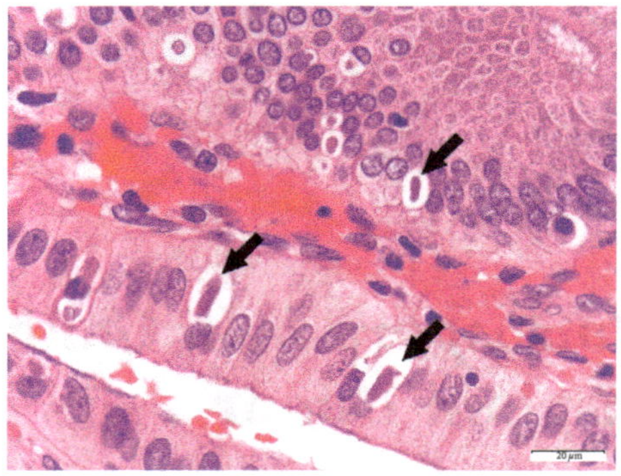

Figure 1: Donor gallbladder, H&E, 1000x. The characteristic morphology of *Cystoisospori belli* includes its banana-shape and perinuclear parasitophorous vacuoles (arrows) within the gallbladder epithelium, as seen here.

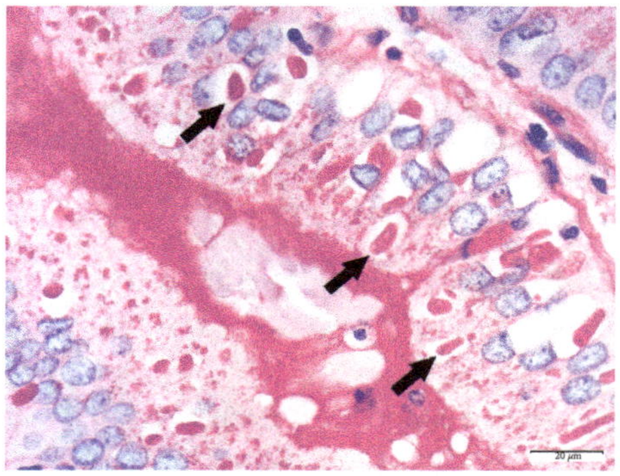

Figure 2: Donor gallbladder, periodic acid–Schiff stain with diastase (PAS/d), 1000x. Although not required for diagnosis, the parasites can be highlighted by a PAS/d special stain (arrows).

at the time of donation. There was no reported history of acute or chronic diarrhea, and he was otherwise immunocompetent. He had no medical comorbidities, no prior surgeries, no history IV drug use, or other risky behaviors. He had no history of recent travel outside of the United States. Notable pretransplantation labs included bilirubin of 0.5, AST 62, ALT 76, and alkaline phosphatase of 49.

2.3. Pathologic Review. The donor gallbladder specimen measured 5.6 × 2.1 × 0.6 cm. It had a tan-gray and smooth serosa, with a limited amount of attached adipose tissue. There were no pericystic lymph nodes, and the cystic duct was not obstructed. The lumen had no calculi and no erosion, and mucosa was tan-brown, with an average wall thickness of 0.3 cm. This was consistent with a grossly normal gallbladder. On H&E staining, oval-shaped intracellular structures, measuring approximately 20 μm, were identified within the cytoplasm of the biliary epithelium, consistent with *C. belli.* (Figure 1) The background gallbladder was otherwise unremarkable [27, 30, 31]. The organisms were highlighted by the PAS/D special stain. (Figure 2). The liver histologic evaluation was otherwise unremarkable, with no significant fat, fibrosis, or inflammation. (Figure 3).

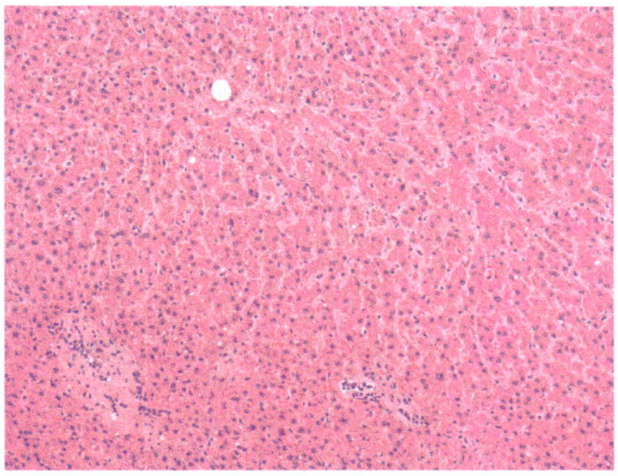

FIGURE 3: Native liver explant, H&E, 20x. Sections show an unremarkable liver with no significant fat, fibrosis, or inflammation.

3. Discussion

C. belli infection is a rare cause of diarrhea, even in immunocompromised individuals. This is likely due to the rarity of the organism especially in the West, as well as improvement in prophylaxis in transplant patients and severely immunocompromised HIV patients. However, there is increasing awareness of the disease among practitioners [27]. There are multiple causes of infectious diarrhea in transplant patients including CMV, noroviruses, bacterial infections, and protozoans like cryptosporidium, Giardia, and toxoplasmosis [32–34]. In this case, the histologic diagnosis of *C. belli* was challenging because the background gallbladder was essentially unremarkable, requiring careful high-power examination to identify the parasite.

Luckily, liver transplant patients undergo a cholecystectomy at the time of transplant. However, in addition to the high rate of recurrent infection in immunocompromised (and some immunocompetent) patients [26, 35], *C. belli* infections are associated with extraintestinal dissemination and have been linked to arthritis [17], thrombotic thrombocytopenic purpura (TTP) and hemolytic uremic syndrome (HUS) [36]. In this case, the histologic diagnosis of *C. belli* was challenging because the background gallbladder was mostly unremarkable, requiring careful high-power examination to identify the parasite. The typical features described in the literature include epithelial disarray and vacuolated epithelium [14, 27], features not seen in all cases. However, if identified, the patient can be easily treated and given prophylaxis [37] against future reactivation. Additionally, if reactivation does occur, the clinician will have a higher index of suspicion than otherwise.

This case study equally highlights the ever-present concern of donor to recipient infection transmission in solid organ transplantation [38, 39]. The absence of specific protocols and guidelines to check for protozoal and intracellular infections, such as these, means that surgeons rely on the physician's index of suspicion to adequately screen for such organisms. Given the increasing use of high-risk donors [40–42] in organ transplantation, one must be aware of these below-the-radar type infections in order to decrease posttransplant complications. This case is important to raise awareness of *C. belli*, which is a challenging diagnosis to make and has only been rarely reported in the literature. To date, there have been two reports [21, 43] of *C. belli* infection after liver transplant. One occurred after eight months and the other after four years (with recurrence in two months). Although these were likely contracted through ingestion of contaminated water or food, reactivation from infected donor tissue is a possibility as this has not been previously recognized.

4. Conclusion

C. belli is an infectious protozoan, which rarely produces symptoms in immunocompetent individuals, but can cause severe, life-threatening diarrhea and dehydration, as well as extraintestinal symptoms in immunocompromised hosts. Posttransplant immunosuppression put liver transplant patients at risk of contracting the disease, not only through the usual routes but also through the process of organ transfer. Thus, a high index of suspicion is required when assessing donors and donor specimens to prevent the risks of transmission of this protozoan, as well as, other infectious agents during transplantation.

Abbreviations

HIV/AIDS: Human immunodeficiency virus/acquired immunodeficiency syndrome
PCR: Polymerase chain reaction
ATN: Acute tubular necrosis
AGXT: Alanine-glyoxylate aminotransferase
OLT: Orthotopic liver transplantation
TMP/SMX DS: Trimethoprim/sulfamethoxazole double strength
AST: Aspartate aminotransferase
ALT: Alanine aminotransferase
H&E: Hematoxylin and eosin
PAS/D: Periodic acid–schiff–diastase
CMV: Cytomegalovirus
TTP: Thrombotic thrombocytopenic purpura
HUS: Hemolytic uremic syndrome.

References

[1] P. Legua and C. Seas, "*Cystoisospora* and *Cyclospora*," *Current Opinion in Infectious Diseases*, vol. 26, no. 5, pp. 479–483, 2013.

[2] R. W. Goodgame, "Understanding intestinal spore-forming protozoa: *Cryptosporidia*, *Microsporidia*, *Isospora*, and *Cyclospora*," *Annals of Internal Medicine*, vol. 124, no. 4, pp. 429–441, 1996.

[3] CDC, *Cystoisosporiasis 1600 Clifton Road Atlanta, GA 30329-4027 USA: Global Health*, 2017, https://www.cdc.gov/dpdx/cystoisosporiasis/index.html.

[4] F. J. Sorvillo, L. E. Lieb, J. Seidel, P. Kerndt, J. Turner, and L. R. Ash, "Epidemiology of *Isosporiasis* among persons with acquired immunodeficiency syndrome in Los Angeles County," *American Journal of Tropical Medicine and Hygiene*, vol. 53, no. 6, pp. 656–659, 1995.

[5] S. A. Woon, R. Yang, U. Ryan, P. Boan, and D. Prentice, "Chronic *Cystoisospora belli* infection in an immunocompetent Myanmar refugee—microscopy is not sensitive enough," *BMC Infectious Diseases*, vol. 16, no. 1, p. 221, 2016.

[6] D. C. Assis, D. V. Resende, M. Cabrine-Santos, D. Correia, and M. B. Oliveira-Silva, "Prevalence and genetic characterization of *Cryptosporidium* spp. and *Cystoisospora belli* in HIV-infected patients," *Revista do Instituto de Medicina Tropical de São Paulo*, vol. 55, no. 3, pp. 149–154, 2013.

[7] P. Agnamey, D. Djeddi, Z. Oukachbi, A. Totet, and C. P. Raccurt, "*Cryptosporidium hominis* and *Isospora belli* diarrhea in travelers returning from West Africa," *Journal of Travel Medicine*, vol. 17, no. 2, pp. 141-142, 2010.

[8] A. Pérez-Ayala, B. Monge-Maíllo, M. Díaz-Menéndez, F. Norman, J. A. Pérez-Molina, and R. López-Vélez, "Self-limited travelers' diarrhea by *Isospora belli* in a patient with dengue infection," *Journal of Travel Medicine*, vol. 18, no. 3, pp. 212-213, 2011.

[9] R. Bialek, N. Binder, K. Dietz, J. Knobloch, and U. E. Zelck, "Comparison of autofluorescence and iodine staining for detection of *Isospora belli* in feces," *American Journal of Tropical Medicine and Hygiene*, vol. 67, no. 3, pp. 304-305, 2002.

[10] R. J. ten Hove, L. van Lieshout, E. A. T. Brienen, M. A. Perez, and J. J. Verweij, "Real-time polymerase chain reaction for detection of *Isospora belli* in stool samples," *Diagnostic Microbiology and Infectious Disease*, vol. 61, no. 3, pp. 280–283, 2008.

[11] M. Taniuchi, J. J. Verweij, and O. Sethabutr, "Multiplex polymerase chain reaction method to detect *Cyclospora*, *Cystoisospora*, and *Microsporidia* in stool samples," *Diagnostic Microbiology and Infectious Disease*, vol. 71, no. 4, pp. 386–390, 2011.

[12] CDC, *Cystoisosporiasis*, 2017, https://www.cdc.gov/parasites/cystoisospora/index.html.

[13] J. A. DeHovitz, J. W. Pape, M. Boncy, and W. D. Johnson Jr., "Clinical manifestations and therapy of *Isospora belli* infection in patients with the acquired immunodeficiency syndrome," *New England Journal of Medicine*, vol. 315, no. 2, pp. 87–90, 1986.

[14] D. A. Benator, A. L. French, L. M. Beaudet, C. S. Levy, and J. M. Orenstein, "*Isospora belli* infection Associated with Acalculous Cholecystitis in a patient with AIDS," *Annals of Internal Medicine*, vol. 121, no. 9, pp. 663-664, 1994.

[15] B. G. Gellin and R. Soave, "Coccidian infections in AIDS: *Toxoplasmosis*, *Cryptosporidiosis*, and *Isosporiasis*," *Medical Clinics of North America*, vol. 76, no. 1, pp. 205–234, 1992.

[16] E. Bernard, P. Delgiudice, M. Carles et al., "Disseminated *Isosporiasis* in an AIDS patient," *European Journal of Clinical Microbiology and Infectious Diseases*, vol. 16, no. 9, pp. 699–701, 1997.

[17] J. González-Dominguez, R. Roldán, J. L. Villanueva, J. M. Kindelán, R. Jurado, and J. Torre-Cisneros, "*Isospora belli* reactive arthritis in a patient with AIDS," *Annals of the Rheumatic Diseases*, vol. 53, no. 9, pp. 618-619, 1994.

[18] Z. Walther and M. D. Topazian, "*Isospora* cholangiopathy: case study with histologic characterization and molecular confirmation," *Human Pathology*, vol. 40, no. 9, pp. 1342–1346, 2009.

[19] M. G. Martelli and J. Y. Lee, "Parasitic Infection of the Gallbladder: *Cystoisospora belli* infection as a cause of chronic abdominal pain and acalculous cholecystitis," *Journal of the Mississippi State Medical Association*, vol. 57, no. 6, pp. 174–176, 2016.

[20] H. Takahashi, G. A. Falk, M. Cruise, and G. Morris-Stiff, "Chronic cholecystitis with *Cystoisospora belli* in an immunocompetent patient," *BMJ Case Reports*, vol. 2015, Article ID bcr2015209966, 2015.

[21] M. Atambay, M. R. Bayraktar, U. Kayabas, S. Yilmaz, and Y. Bayindir, "A rare diarrheic parasite in a liver transplant patient: *Isospora belli*," *Transplantation Proceedings*, vol. 39, no. 5, pp. 1693–1695, 2007.

[22] O. Koru, R. E. Araz, Y. A. Yilmaz et al., "Case report: *Isospora belli* infection in a renal transplant recipient," *Turkiye Parazitol Derg*, vol. 31, no. 2, pp. 98–100, 2007.

[23] A. Marathe and K. Parikh, "Severe diarrhoea due to *Cystoisospora belli* in renal transplant patient on immunosuppressive drugs," *Indian Journal of Medical Microbiology*, vol. 31, no. 2, pp. 185–187, 2013.

[24] B. F. Sanches, J. Morgado, N. Carvalho, and R. Anjos, "Multiple parasitic infections in a cardiac transplant recipient," *BMJ Case Reports*, vol. 2015, Article ID bcr2014207033, 2015.

[25] F. Gruz, C. Fuxman, A. Errea et al., "*Isospora belli* infection after isolated intestinal transplant," *Transplant Infectious Disease*, vol. 12, no. 1, pp. 69–72, 2010.

[26] S. Jongwutiwes, P. Sampatanukul, and C. Putaporntip, "Recurrent isosporiasis over a decade in an immunocompetent host successfully treated with pyrimethamine," *Scandinavian Journal of Infectious Diseases*, vol. 34, no. 11, pp. 859–862, 2002.

[27] K. K. Lai, H. E. Goyne, D. Hernandez-Gonzalo et al., "*Cystoisospora belli* infection of the gallbladder in immunocompetent patients," *American Journal of Surgical Pathology*, vol. 40, no. 8, pp. 1070–1074, 2016.

[28] P. Cochat, S. A. Hulton, C. Acquaviva et al., "Primary hyperoxaluria type 1: indications for screening and guidance for diagnosis and treatment," *Nephrology Dialysis Transplantation*, vol. 27, no. 5, pp. 1729–1736, 2012.

[29] P. Cochat and G. Rumsby, "Primary hyperoxaluria," *New England Journal of Medicine*, vol. 369, no. 7, pp. 649–658, 2013.

[30] J. N. Velásquez, S. Carnevale, M. Mariano et al., "Isosporosis and unizoite tissue cysts in patients with acquired immunodeficiency syndrome," *Human Pathology*, vol. 32, no. 5, pp. 500–505, 2001.

[31] A. C. K. Rao, V. Geetha, R. Kudva, S. Vidhyalakshmi, and S. Rupashree, "Histology as a diagnostic tool for intestinal isosporiasis in immunocompromised patients," *Asian Pacific Journal of Tropical Disease*, vol. 2, no. 3, pp. 251-252, 2012.

[32] P. M. Ginsburg and P. J. Thuluvath, "Diarrhea in liver transplant recipients: etiology and management," *Liver Transplantation*, vol. 11, no. 8, pp. 881-890, 2005.

[33] J. H. Helderman and S. Goral, "Gastrointestinal complications of transplant immunosuppression," *Journal of the American Society of Nephrology*, vol. 13, no. 1, pp. 277–287, 2002.

[34] H. Arslan, E. K. Inci, O. K. Azap, H. Karakayali, A. Torgay, and M. Haberal, "Etiologic agents of diarrhea in solid organ recipients," *Transplant Infectious Disease*, vol. 9, no. 4, pp. 270–275, 2007.

[35] T. H. Boyles, J. Black, G. Meintjes, and M. Mendelson, "Failure to eradicate *Isospora belli* diarrhoea despite immune reconstitution in adults with HIV-a case series," *PLoS One*, vol. 7, no. 8, Article ID e42844, 2012.

[36] P. Auwaeter, *Cystoisospora belli*, *Johns Hopkins Guides*, 2016, https://www.hopkinsguides.com/hopkins/view/Johns_Hopkins_ABX_Guide/540152/all/Cystoisospora_belli.

[37] J. W. Pape, R. I. Verdier, and W. D. Johnson, "Treatment and prophylaxis of *Isospora belli* infection in patients with the

acquired immunodeficiency syndrome," *New England Journal of Medicine*, vol. 320, no. 16, pp. 1044–1047, 1989.
[38] A. G. Melissa, J. K. Matthew, and A. F. Jay, "Infectious disease transmission during organ and tissue transplantation," *Emerging Infectious Disease journal*, vol. 18, no. 8, p. e1, 2012.
[39] I. A. Echenique and M. G. Ison, "Update on donor-derived infections in liver transplantation," *Liver Transplantation*, vol. 19, no. 6, pp. 575–585, 2013.
[40] E. Izadi, *So Many People are Dying of Drug Overdoses that They're Easing the Donated Organ Shortage*, 2016, https://www.washingtonpost.com/news/to-your-health/wp/2016/05/09/one-out-of-every-11-organ-donors-last-year-died-of-a-drug-overdose/.
[41] M. Bebinger, *Organ Donations Spike in the Wake of the Opioid Epidemic: @NPR*, 2016, https://www.npr.org/sections/health-shots/2016/10/14/497799446/organ-donations-spike-in-the-wake-of-the-opioid-epidemic.
[42] S. Sternberg, *Drug Overdose Deaths Leading to More Organ Donors: @USNews*, 2016, https://www.usnews.com/news/articles/2016-04-28/drug-overdose-deaths-leading-to-more-organ-donors.
[43] S. Usluca, T. Inceboz, T. Unek, and U. Aksoy, "*Isospora belli* in a patient with liver transplantation," *Turkish Journal of Parasitology*, vol. 36, no. 4, pp. 247–250, 2012.

9

Unusual Radiographic Presentation of *Pneumocystis* Pneumonia in a Patient with AIDS

Brian L. Block,[1] Tejas Mehta,[2] Gabriel M. Ortiz,[3] Sean P. Ferris,[4] Thienkhai H. Vu,[5] Laurence Huang,[1,6] and Adithya Cattamanchi[1]

[1]*Division of Pulmonary and Critical Care Medicine, University of California, San Francisco, CA, USA*
[2]*SBKS Medical Institute and Research Centre, Gujarat, India*
[3]*Division of Hospital Medicine, Priscilla Chan and Mark Zuckerberg San Francisco General Hospital and Trauma Center, San Francisco, CA, USA*
[4]*Division of Pathology and Laboratory Medicine, University of California, San Francisco, CA, USA*
[5]*Department of Radiology and Biomedical Imaging, Priscilla Chan and Mark Zuckerberg San Francisco General Hospital and Trauma Center and University of California, San Francisco, CA, USA*
[6]*HIV, Infectious Diseases, and Global Medicine Division, University of California, San Francisco, CA, USA*

Correspondence should be addressed to Brian L. Block; brian.block@ucsf.edu

Academic Editor: Sinésio Talhari

Pneumocystis jirovecii pneumonia (PCP) typically presents as an interstitial and alveolar process with ground glass opacities on chest computed tomography (CT). The absence of ground glass opacities on chest CT is thought to have a high negative predictive value for PCP in individuals with AIDS. Here, we report a case of PCP in a man with AIDS who presented to our hospital with subacute shortness of breath and a nonproductive cough. While his chest CT revealed diffuse nodular rather than ground glass opacities, bronchoscopy with bronchoalveolar lavage and transbronchial biopsies confirmed the diagnosis of PCP and did not identify additional pathogens. PCP was not the expected diagnosis based on chest CT, but it otherwise fit well with the patient's clinical and laboratory presentation. In the era of combination antiretroviral therapy, routine prophylaxis for PCP, and increased use of computed tomography, it may be that PCP will increasingly present with nonclassical chest radiographic patterns. Clinicians should be aware of this presentation when selecting diagnostic and management strategies.

1. Introduction

Pneumocystis jirovecii pneumonia (PCP) is a potentially life-threatening infection that most often occurs in immunocompromised hosts. PCP was the most frequent complication of HIV/AIDS in the early phases of the epidemic, and while its incidence has declined substantially in the current era of combination antiretroviral therapy, it remains one of the most common HIV-associated opportunistic infections.

Generally, the diagnosis of PCP is suggested by a subacute illness featuring fever, nonproductive cough, malaise, and progressive shortness of breath [1]. Dyspnea and hypoxemia can be profound. Lung auscultation and chest roentgenogram can both be normal, but computed tomography (CT) of the chest typically demonstrates "ground glass opacities" [2, 3]. This is likely due to the accumulation of cellular debris, fibrin, and organisms within the alveolar spaces [2], as well as interstitial inflammation. Other radiographic patterns of PCP include a predilection for upper lobes (particularly in patients who use aerosolized pentamidine for prophylaxis), a preference for central rather than peripheral zones, and a tendency to form cysts [1, 4, 5]. Several serum tests can be used to help determine the likelihood of PCP, but microscopic visualization of induced sputum or bronchoalveolar lavage fluid specimens remains the gold standard for diagnosis [6].

A previous publication from our institution suggested that the presence of ground glass on high-resolution chest CT (HRCT) is 100% sensitive for PCP in patients with AIDS [7]. In other words, the absence of ground glass

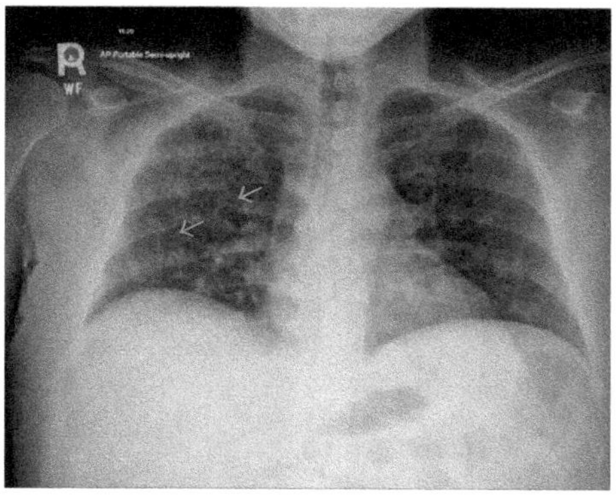

Figure 1: Chest roentgenogram at referring hospital. AP chest radiograph at outside hospital performed 4 days prior. Diffuse micronodules greater in the right lung are seen. Hint of small cavities is noted (blue arrows).

opacities on HRCT ruled out the diagnosis of PCP in such patients. Based on these data, our standard clinical practice has been to recommend against additional diagnostic testing and empiric PCP therapy for HIV-infected patients when their chest HRCT does not contain ground glass opacities, even in the setting of a clinical syndrome suggestive of PCP [8].

Here, we report a case of PCP with an unusual radiographic appearance consisting of nodular opacities without ground glass on chest CT. While the clinical syndrome was convincing for PCP, the radiographic presentation made PCP seem unlikely and led to an interruption of PCP therapy.

2. Case Presentation

A 57-year-old man was admitted to our hospital with a four-week history of nonproductive cough and dyspnea. His past medical history was notable for type II diabetes mellitus, chronic kidney disease with a baseline creatinine of 1.3 mg/dL, and untreated HIV/AIDS, which had been diagnosed 20 years previously. Prior opportunistic infections included oral candidiasis and cryptococcal meningitis. He was allergic to sulfonamides and had been prescribed dapsone for PCP prophylaxis, but he was not taking it reliably. His most recent known CD4 count and HIV viral load, 11 months prior to admission, were 15 cells/uL and 148,582 copies/mL, respectively.

Four days prior to presenting to our emergency department, the patient was admitted to another hospital with the same symptoms of nonproductive cough and shortness of breath. Chest radiograph at that time showed diffuse micronodules, greater in the right lung (Figure 1). There, he was empirically treated for both community-acquired pneumonia and PCP with ceftriaxone, azithromycin, clindamycin, primaquine, and steroids. He was also given fluconazole for thrush. Unfortunately, he left that facility against medical advice after 48 hours. He took no further treatment before coming to our hospital two days later.

When he subsequently came to our emergency department complaining of ongoing shortness of breath and cough, temperature was 35.9 degree Celsius, heart rate 119

Table 1: Initial laboratory studies.

Lab name	Value at outside hospital (4 days prior to admission)	Value on admission to our hospital (day 0)	Reference range
WBC (k/uL)	7.0	6.2	3.9–11.7
Neutrophils (%)	—	63	44–68
Lymphocytes (%)	—	19	25–44
Monocytes (%)	—	13	0–7
Eosinophils (%)	—	3	0–4
Bands (%)	12	0	0
Hemoglobin (g/dL)	10.3	10.1	13.3–17.7
Glucose (mg/dL)	293	71	70–199
Creatinine (mg/dL)	2.4	1.7	0.70–1.30
Troponin (ng/mL)	—	<0.04	<0.04
Lactate (mmol/L)	4.7	1.7	0.5–2.2
Lactate dehydrogenase (u/L)	—	385	100–190
Beta-D-glucan (pg/mL)	—	398	<60 negative 61–79 indeterminate >80 positive
Cryptococcal antigen	—	Negative	Negative
Coccidioides antibody (complement fixation)	—	<1 : 2, Negative	Negative
Coccidioides antibody (immunodiffusion)	—	Negative	Negative
CD4+ T-cells (cells/uL)	—	15	420–1250
HIV viral load (copies/mL)	—	173,887	0

beats per minute, blood pressure 107/71 mmHg, respiratory rate 18 breaths per minute, and oxygen saturation 96% while breathing ambient air. He was ill-appearing with conjunctival pallor and oral thrush. The remainder of his physical examination was normal, including chest auscultation, which revealed good air movement without wheezing, rales, or rhonchi. Laboratory analysis was notable for white blood cell count of 6,200 cells/uL with 63% neutrophils, 19% lymphocytes, 13% monocytes, and 3% eosinophils, elevated lactate dehydrogenase of 385 u/L, and positive beta-D-glucan of 389 pg/mL (Table 1). Chest roentgenogram revealed diffuse micronodules with confluent areas of nodular opacities (Figure 2). On the basis of these findings, the patient was admitted to our medical service and treated empirically for community-acquired pneumonia with ceftriaxone and doxycycline, for thrush with fluconazole, and for PCP with clindamycin and primaquine.

On hospital day 2, the patient developed worsening shortness of breath with hypoxemia requiring supplemental oxygen. A noncontrast, volumetric chest CT scan (Figure 3) revealed diffuse micronodules with central cavitation and bronchial wall thickening, most suspicious

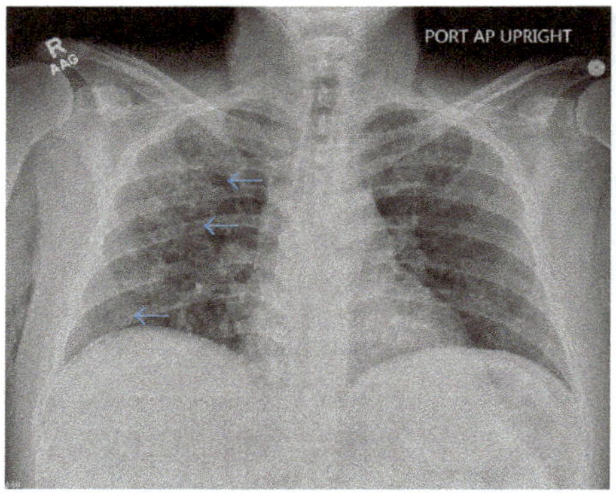

FIGURE 2: Chest roentgenogram on admission to our hospital. AP chest radiograph at presentation. Again seen are diffuse micronodules with confluent areas in the right upper and lower lungs. Hint of small cavities is again noted (blue arrows).

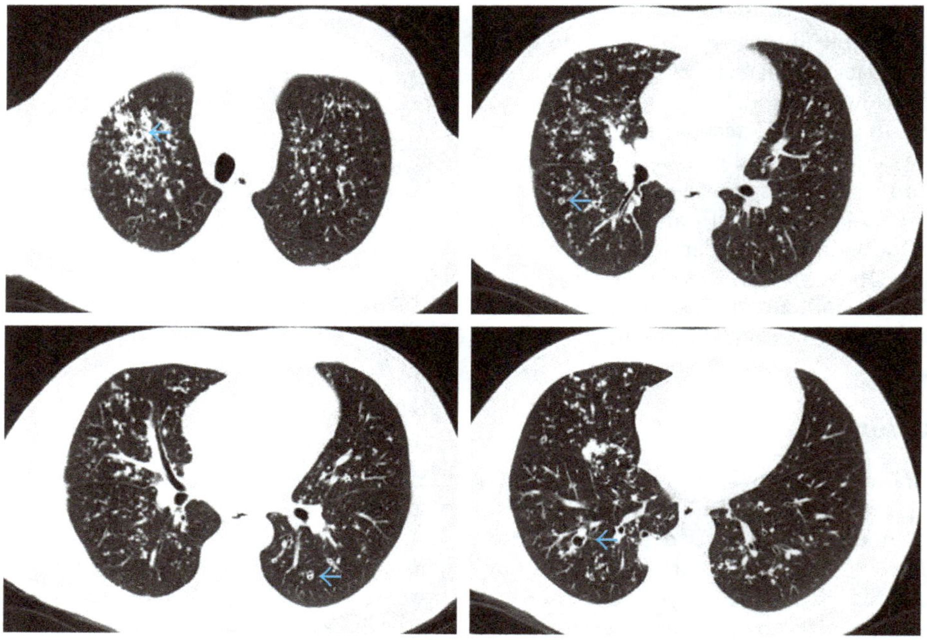

FIGURE 3: Selected images of computed tomography (CT) scan of the chest on admission to our hospital. Axial images in lung window confirm diffuse micronodules with central cavitation of varying sizes (blue arrows).

for mycobacterial or fungal infection. Notably, there were no ground glass opacities. Based on this CT and the lack of ground glass opacities, the treating team discontinued PCP therapy, initiated tuberculosis treatment, and consulted the pulmonary service for assistance and consideration of bronchoscopy. The patient underwent bronchoscopy with bronchoalveolar lavage (BAL) and transbronchial biopsy the following day. Pathologic analysis of the transbronchial biopsy specimen demonstrated foamy exudates on hematoxylin and eosin- (H&E-) stained sections, and silver stain revealed *Pneumocystis jirovecii*-type fungal organisms confirming the diagnosis to be PCP [9] (Figure 4). No concurrent infections were found on cultures or pathologic samples (Table 2). The patient was treated with three weeks of clindamycin, primaquine, and prednisone. He was discharged home on hospital day 10 without requiring supplemental oxygen and did well thereafter, with a resolution of radiographic abnormalities on imaging obtained four months later (Figure 5).

3. Discussion

Although the incidence of PCP has decreased since the advent of combination antiretroviral therapy in the 1990s, it remains among the most common pulmonary opportunistic infections in patients with AIDS. PCP should be suspected in the clinical setting of subacute dyspnea, nonproductive cough, and fever. While microscopic visualization of bronchoalveolar lavage fluid is the gold standard for diagnosing PCP, chest CT is increasingly being used to make clinical decisions about empiric treatment, and whether to pursue bronchoscopy.

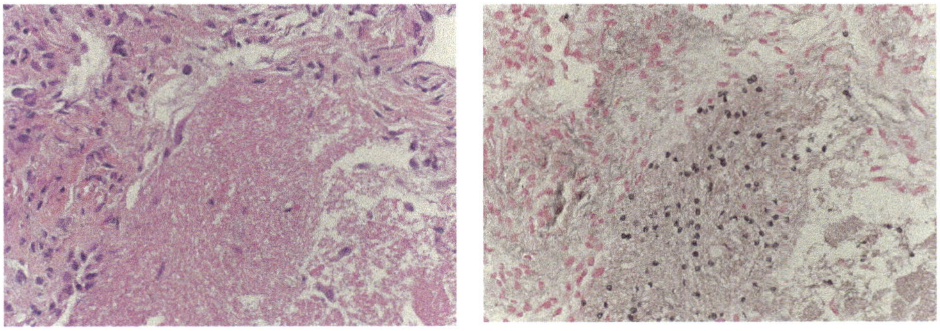

(a) (b)

FIGURE 4: Transbronchial biopsy pathologic results. Pathologic evidence for PCP infection from the patient's transbronchial biopsy specimen. (a) Hematoxylin and eosin- (H&E-) stained section demonstrates classic intra-alveolar eosinophilic foamy exudates. (b) Gomori methenamine silver (GMS) special stain demonstrates nonbudding cysts with thin walls and intracystic capsular dots, consistent with *Pneumocystis jirovecii*-type fungal organisms.

TABLE 2: Microbiology studies.

Test name	Hospital day collected	Result
Blood culture x2	0	Negative
Nasopharynx influenza RNA	0	Negative
Blood for acid-fast bacilli	1	Negative at 42 days
Induced sputum for acid-fast bacilli	2	Negative at 56 days
Induced sputum for acid-fast bacilli	3	Negative at 56 days
Induced sputum for MTb PCR	3	Negative
Induced sputum for bacterial culture	2	Few oronasal flora
Induced sputum for fungal culture	2	*Candida albicans***
BAL fluid for PCP examination	4	Many clumps of trophozoites and cysts. No viral inclusions seen. No fungi seen.
BAL fluid for fungal culture	4	*Candida albicans***
BAL fluid for acid-fast bacilli	4	Negative at 56 days
BAL fluid for bacterial culture	4	No organisms seen
Serum cryptococcal antigen	1	Negative
Coccidioides antibody (complement fixation)	1	<1 : 2, Negative
Coccidioides antibody (immunodiffusion)	1	Negative
Transbronchial biopsy for acid-fast bacilli culture	4	Negative at 28 days
Transbronchial biopsy for bacterial culture	4	Negative at 56 days

**Patient had thrush, and this was felt to be an upper airway contaminant.

The radiographic appearance of PCP can vary from person to person. The "classic" presentation on plain film is of bilateral, symmetric opacities in an interstitial or alveolar pattern [3, 10]. Chest CT in patients with AIDS who develop PCP most often shows ground glass opacities [2, 4, 11, 12]. However, PCP has also been described to present infrequently with additional findings including cystic lung disease, pneumothoraces, and nodules, among other patterns [2, 3, 13].

It is not entirely surprising that PCP can have a variety of radiographic presentations. As a pathogen that primarily causes disease in the immunosuppressed, PCP often occurs in lungs that have been damaged by prior infections, distorting their architecture. Moreover, it is not uncommon for PCP to co-occur with another infection in an immunocompromised host. In such a circumstance, the radiographic signature of PCP may be subsumed by the coinfecting pathogen.

At our institution where we have extensive experience caring for patients with HIV/AIDS, a chest CT without ground glass is generally thought to "rule out" PCP in patients with AIDS. This is based on a 1997 study of 51 patients with AIDS and a clinical syndrome consistent with PCP but normal chest roentgenogram who underwent HRCT of the chest [7]. In this cohort, the absence of ground glass opacities on chest CT had a perfect negative predictive value for *Pneumocystis* pneumonia (i.e., the presence of ground glass was 100% sensitive for PCP). Knowing these data and subsequent clinical experience, the team treating the described patient was surprised to learn that the patient had PCP, and PCP alone—as the absence of ground glass

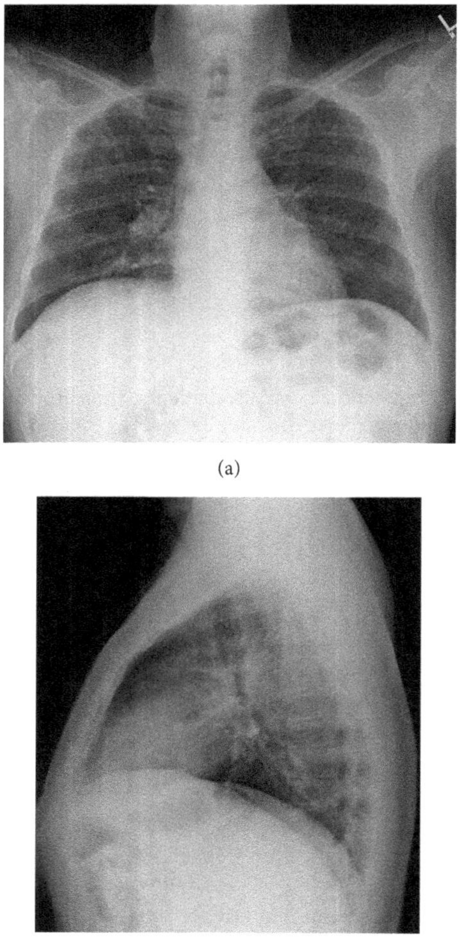

(a)

(b)

FIGURE 5: Chest roentgenogram four months after hospitalization. (a) PA and (b) lateral chest radiographs post treatment four months later demonstrated marked improvements.

opacities on chest CT was highly unusual. Indeed, the treating clinicians decided to discontinue PCP-directed therapy on the basis of the CT findings.

While highly atypical, the radiographic appearance of the described patient's PCP is not entirely without precedent. Some of the previously mentioned publications do describe rare instances of PCP presenting as nodules [2–4, 10]. Still, such described presentations were the exception rather than the rule, and over the past 20 years, all cases of PCP that we have seen at our institution have consistently manifested as ground glass opacities on chest CT (when obtained).

It is likely that we, and others, will encounter more cases of PCP with "atypical" radiographic presentations. The increased access to CT scanners means more patients are undergoing chest CT for indications that previously may not have led to such imaging. Our patient, for example, with subacute cough, dyspnea, fevers, and malaise had a clinical history consistent with PCP, and his chest roentgenogram with regions of confluent nodular opacities could have been interpreted as typical of PCP. Based on the inclusion criteria for the aforementioned 1997 study [7] from our institution, our patient would have proceeded directly to sputum induction or bronchoscopy on the basis of his clinical history and chest roentgenogram, without first having undergone chest CT. If that course had been taken, he would have been discovered to have PCP in the setting of a compatible clinical history and imaging (plain film) and his presentation would have been considered entirely typical. We would not have appreciated the exclusively nodular aspect of his disease.

Beyond the increased availability of cross-sectional imaging with chest CT, increased access to combination antiretroviral therapy and PCP prophylaxis may also alter the radiographic appearance of PCP [3]. Even in patients with inconsistent treatment adherence, the degree of immunosuppression, extent of opportunistic infection, and radiographic presentation of PCP may not be directly comparable to those with HIV who are treatment-naive.

In the case of the patient we describe, his two days of therapy with clindamycin and primaquine at the referring hospital could theoretically have altered his chest CT finding and explained the lack of ground glass opacities. However, this seems highly unlikely because (1) his plain films on admission to each institution were similar and (2) he worsened clinically after receiving the initial PCP-directed therapy. This worsening, which is often seen with PCP, suggests a robust alveolar and interstitial inflammatory response, which we would expect to cause more, not fewer, ground glass opacities on chest CT.

In summary, we describe a case of PCP in a patient with AIDS, with classic presenting symptoms but an unusual radiographic pattern on chest CT featuring nodular opacities and no ground glass. The lack of ground glass opacities resulted in brief PCP treatment interruption. CT scan findings alone should not be used to discontinue PCP-specific treatment, particularly in patients with a clinical syndrome that is otherwise consistent with PCP.

Authors' Contributions

Brian L. Block and Tejas Mehta contributed equally to this work.

References

[1] C. F. Thomas Jr. and A. H. Limper, "*Pneumocystis* pneumonia," *New England Journal of Medicine*, vol. 350, no. 24, pp. 2487–2498, 2004.

[2] J. P. Kanne, D. R. Yandow, and C. A. Meyer, "*Pneumocystis jirovecii* pneumonia: high-resolution CT findings in patients with and without HIV infection," *American Journal of Roentgenology*, vol. 198, no. 6, pp. W555–W561, 2012.

[3] J. E. Kuhlman, "*Pneumocystis* infections: the radiologist's perspective," *Radiology*, vol. 198, no. 3, pp. 623–635, 1996.

[4] P. M. Boiselle, C. A. Crans Jr., and M. A. Kaplan, "The changing face of *Pneumocystis carinii* pneumonia in AIDS patients," *American Journal of Roentgenology*, vol. 172, no. 5, pp. 1301–1309, 1999.

[5] J. E. Kuhlman, M. Kavuru, E. K. Fishman, and S. S. Siegelman, "*Pneumocystis carinii* pneumonia: spectrum of parenchymal CT findings," *Radiology*, vol. 175, no. 3, pp. 711–714, 1990.

[6] J. Kovacs, K. Crothers, H. Furrer et al., "Guidelines for the prevention and treatment of opportunistic infections in HIV-infected adults and adolescents," 2017, https://aidsinfo.nih.gov/contentfiles/lvguidelines/glchunk/glchunk_321.pdf.

[7] J. F. Gruden, L. Huang, J. Turner et al., "High-resolution CT in the evaluation of clinically suspected *Pneumocystis carinii* pneumonia in AIDS patients with normal, equivocal, or nonspecific radiographic findings," *American Journal of Roentgenology*, vol. 169, no. 4, pp. 967–975, 1997.

[8] L. Huang, A. Cattamanchi, J. L. Davis et al., "HIV-associated *Pneumocystis* pneumonia," *Proceedings of the American Thoracic Society*, vol. 8, no. 3, pp. 294–300, 2011.

[9] P. H. Hartel, K. Shilo, M. Klassen-Fischer et al., "Granulomatous reaction to *Pneumocystis jirovecii*: clinicopathologic review of 20 cases," *American Journal of Surgical Pathology*, vol. 34, no. 5, pp. 730–734, 2010.

[10] L. J. DeLorenzo, C. T. Huang, G. P. Maguire, and D. J. Stone, "Roentgenographic patterns of *Pneumocystis carinii* pneumonia in 104 patients with AIDS," *Chest*, vol. 91, no. 3, pp. 323–327, 1987.

[11] C. J. Bergin, R. L. Wirth, G. J. Berry, and R. A. Castellino, "*Pneumocystis carinii* pneumonia: CT and HRCT observations," *Journal of Computer Assisted Tomography*, vol. 14, no. 5, pp. 756–759, 1990.

[12] T. E. Hartman, S. L. Primack, N. L. Muller, and C. A. Staples, "Diagnosis of thoracic complications in AIDS: accuracy of CT," *American Journal of Roentgenology*, vol. 162, no. 3, pp. 547–553, 1994.

[13] G. P. Cornalba, P. Mariani, E. Colombo, R. Bianco, and S. Vona, "Atypical radiological images in *Pneumocystis carinii* infection in HIV-positive patients," *La Radiologia Medica*, vol. 87, no. 6, pp. 763–767, 1994.

Primary *Klebsiella pneumoniae* Osteomyelitis with Bacteremia and Sepsis in a Patient with Cirrhosis

Akshay Khatri[1], **Naga Sasidhar Kanaparthy**[1], **Bright Jebaraj Selvaraj**[1], **Eunna Cho**[1] **and Marc Y. El Khoury**[1,2]

[1]*Department of Medicine, New York Medical College at Westchester Medical Center, Valhalla, NY 10595, USA*
[2]*Division of Infectious Diseases, New York Medical College at Westchester Medical Center, Valhalla, NY 10595, USA*

Correspondence should be addressed to Akshay Khatri; akshay.khatri@wmchealth.org

Academic Editor: Larry M. Bush

Osteomyelitis is commonly caused by *Staphylococci*, *Streptococci*, *Escherichia coli*, and anaerobes. There have been cases of rare organisms like *Klebsiella pneumoniae* (*Kp*) being initially overlooked as causes of osteomyelitis. We report a case of an elderly cirrhotic adult male transferred for further management of liver failure, who was subsequently diagnosed with *Kp* osteomyelitis and sepsis. He had a history of blunt leg trauma, and MRI of the leg revealed osteomyelitis, with a negative workup for other sources of infection. *Kp* osteomyelitis is reported in less than 100 cases, mainly in pediatric and sickle-cell patients. There are no pathognomonic imaging findings. Lesions may be metastatic, with rapid widespread destruction and exuberant periosteal reaction. *Kp* is a rare, under recognized cause of osteomyelitis in immune-suppressed adults. Given its pathogenicity, early identification is critical.

1. Introduction

Osteomyelitis is a progressive infectious process involving various bone components— the periosteum, cortical bone, and medullary cavity. It is characterized by progressive inflammatory destruction of bone, necrosis, and new bone apposition [1].

There are three main types of osteomyelitis, that is, due to local spread from a contiguous source of infection; secondary to vascular insufficiency; and hematogenous osteomyelitis, with seeding of injured bone from bacteria present in the blood [2]. The most common microorganism is *Staphylococcus aureus*. Other microrgansims include coagulase-negative staphylococci, beta-hemolytic streptococci, *Streptococcus viridans*, enterococci, aerobic Gram-negative bacilli (*Pseudomonas* and *Enterobacter* sp. and *Escherichia coli*), anaerobes, and *Mycobacterium tuberculosis* [2, 3]. Hematogenous osteomyelitis is usually monomicrobial, whereas osteomyelitis related to contiguous spread or inoculation may be monomicrobial or polymicrobial [4].

Klebsiella pneumoniae (*Kp*) is a rare cause of osteomyelitis, especially in adults. We report a case of *Kp* osteomyelitis and sepsis in a patient with cirrhosis.

2. Case Presentation

A 64-year-old African American man, resident of a correctional facility, was transferred from an outside hospital for further management of liver failure. He was initially admitted at an outside hospital when routine blood tests showed leukocyte count 24,000/μL, platelet count 123,000/μL, serum sodium level 127 meq/L, aspartate aminotransferase (AST) 169 U/L, alanine aminotransferase (ALT) 116 U/L, alkaline phosphatase (ALP) 230 U/L, total bilirubin 17.7 mg/dL, and direct bilirubin 13 mg/dL. His past medical and surgical history was significant for decompensated alcohol-induced cirrhosis with untreated chronic hepatitis C; recurrent ascites; hypertension; schizophrenia; cholecystectomy; and appendectomy. He is a current smoker (40 pack-year) but quit drinking alcohol and using intravenous drugs 6 years ago. The patient complained of mild diffuse abdominal pain with several episodes of watery, nonbloody, nonfoul-smelling diarrhea. He denied fevers, chills, vomiting, melena, or hematochezia. He also reported an unintentional weight loss of 18 pounds over the last 6 months. The rest of the review of the system was negative.

On examination, he was alert and oriented, with temperature 37.3 degrees Celsius, pulse 113/min, blood pressure 103/71 mmHg, respiratory rate 18/min, and saturation 96% on room air. He had icteric sclera. Heart and lung exam was normal. Abdomen was mildly distended, nontender, and tympanic with no shifting dullness. Extremities were warm, with left foot and leg-pitting edema and severe tenderness without erythema. On direct questioning, the patient recalled hurting his left leg 8 days prior to admission while removing his boots, followed 3 days later by swelling, pain in the left foot and ankle that progressed to the leg. No skin lesions or wounds were noted.

His admission labs were significant for a leukocyte count of 14,700/μL, hemoglobin 12.1 g/dL, platelet count 137,000/μL, sedimentation rate 20 mm/hr, C-reactive protein 16mg/dL (normal range 0–0.5 mg/dl), AST 161 U/L, ALT 99 U/L, ALP 177 U/L, total bilirubin 15 mg/dL, direct bilirubin 10.7 mg/dL, albumin 1.5 g/dL, and INR 1.54. HIV antibodies were negative. Hepatitis C virus (HCV) RNA was 184,000 copies/mL.

Six hours after admission, the patient developed worsening tachycardia (125/min) with hypotension. He was given 2 liters of intravenous normal saline boluses and started on vancomycin and cefepime empirically. Blood cultures grew a mucoid strain of *K. pneumoniae*, in both aerobic and anaerobic cultures within 8 hours of collection, resistant only to ampicillin. Vancomycin was discontinued, and further serotype testing was not performed at that time.

A diagnostic paracentesis revealed ascites leukocyte count 358/mL with 66% neutrophils, and peritoneal fluid cultures were negative. A transthoracic echocardiogram was normal. A CT scan of the chest was done showing mild lower lung atelectasis. A triple-phase CT scan of the liver showed an enlarged left hepatic lobe with a shrunken right lobe with cirrhotic morphology, a small right hepatic lobe cyst, and moderate ascites. Magnetic resonance imaging of the left foot and leg without contrast revealed intraosseous abscess in the second metatarsal and marrow edema within the cuneiforms and second through fourth metatarsal bases suggestive of osteomyelitis (Figures 1–3). There was extensive edema within the subcutaneous soft tissues of the leg and dorsum of the foot, with infiltration of subcutaneous fat compatible with cellulitis (Figures 3 and 4).

The patient's hospital course was complicated by encephalopathy requiring transient intubation for airway protection and acute kidney injury secondary to sepsis and hepatorenal syndrome requiring hemodialysis. The patient sepsis and bacteremia resolved; his mental status improved but remained in renal failure. He was discharged to a correctional facility to complete 8 weeks of intravenous ceftazidime.

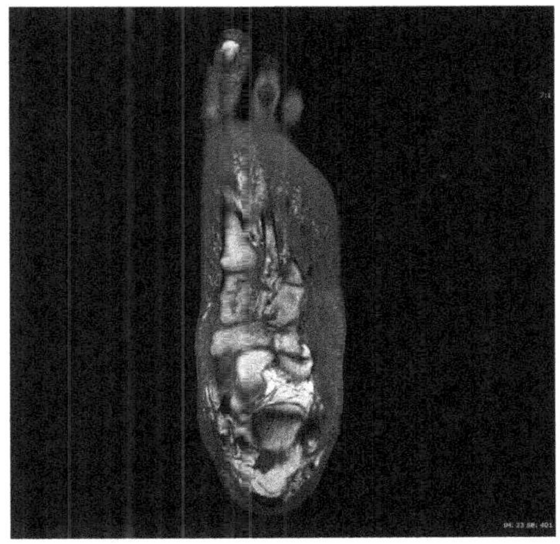

FIGURE 1: T1-weighted axial image of MRI of left foot without contrast, showing decreased signals (hypointensities) of cuneiforms and metatarsals, reflecting medullary edema and osteomyelitis.

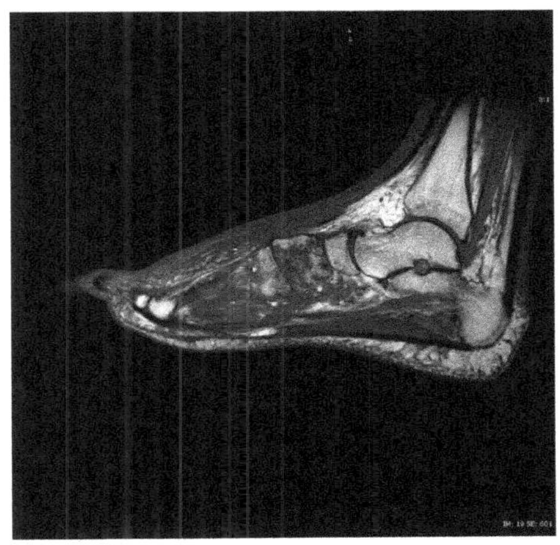

FIGURE 2: T1-weighted sagittal image of MRI of left foot without contrast, showing medullary edema and osteomyelitis of cuneiforms and metatarsals.

3. Discussion

Klebsiella pneumoniae (*Kp*)— also known as Friedlander's bacillus—was first identified in 1882 as an etiological agent in lobar pneumonia [5]. It is one of the few Gram-negative bacilli that can cause primary lobar pneumonia leading in many instances to cavitation [6]. It is the second most common cause of Gram-negative bacteremia [7]. *Kp* is classified into approximately 80 serotypes based on its capsular lipopolysaccharide [8], which is considered a critical virulence factor [9]. *Kp* primarily colonizes the gastrointestinal tract and sometimes the oropharynx [10]. Its presence on the skin is usually considered a transient phenomenon [11] and is sometimes overlooked as a cause of cellulitis or osteomyelitis [12].

Predisposing factors leading to *Kp*-related community-acquired infections include diabetes mellitus, alcoholism, malignancy, or hepatobiliary disease [8, 13]. Diabetes

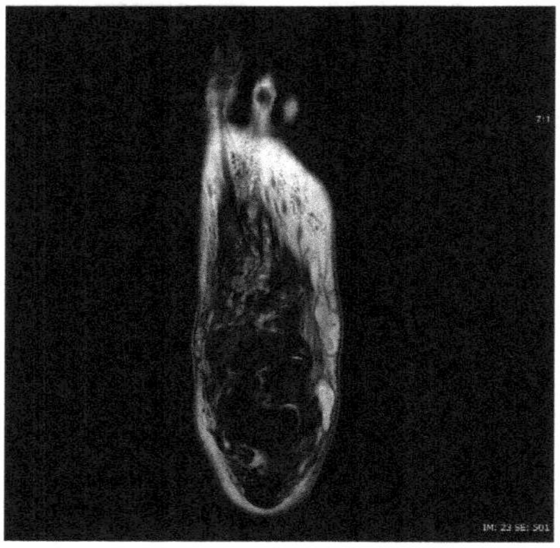

FIGURE 3: T2-weighted axial image of MRI of left foot without contrast, showing increased signals in soft tissues (compatible with cellulitis), as well as deep-seated multilocular collection at Lisfranc's joints and second metatarsophalangeal joints.

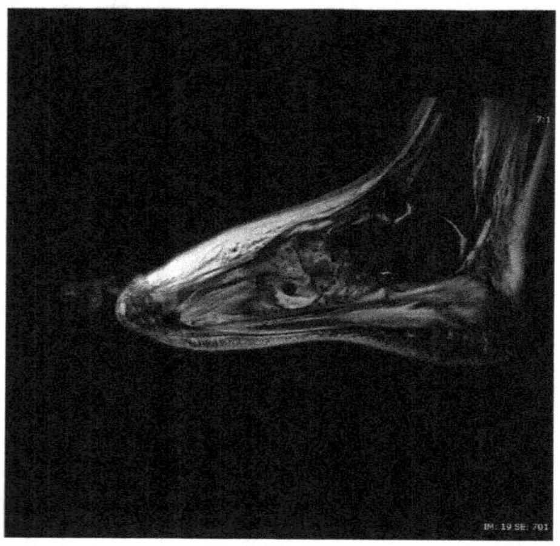

FIGURE 4: T2-weighted sagittal image of MRI of left foot without contrast, showing cellulitis of soft tissues, as well as deep-seated multilocular collection at Lisfranc's joints and second metatarsophalangeal joints.

mellitus is the most common predisposing factor as hyperglycemia facilitates the growth of the capsular polysaccharide and promotes resistance to phagocytosis [13].

Nosocomially acquired *Kp* infections are more common in patients with malignancies or following urinary catheterization, chemotherapy, mechanical ventilation, central venous catheter insertion and recent surgery. Antimicrobial resistance is more common, with higher expected morbidity and mortality [13].

In patients with cirrhosis, *Kp* infections are commonly related to spontaneous bacterial peritonitis, urinary tract infections, and community-acquired pneumonia [14]. The incidence of *Kp* infections in cirrhotics is uncommon and variable—one study reported it in 1.9% of patients [15], while another reported it as 8.51% of all organisms isolated [16].

Cellulitis has been diagnosed in 10.5–12.5% of patients with cirrhosis [17, 18]. The exact prevalence of *Kp* osteomyelitis in adults is not known, with axial skeleton involvement (mandible, vertebrae, spine, and pelvic bones) being most commonly reported [19, 20]. *Kp* osteomyelitis was first reported in 1938 in which seven patients with osteomyelitis of the femur, tibia, humerus, or mastoid were described. Five of the seven had a preceding or simultaneous infection with *Kp* at another site [21]. In our case, the patient had no apparent remote source of infection to account for hematogenous seeding; thus, we believe that infection started locally following minor trauma to the skin.

Unlike in adults, *Kp* osteomyelitis and septic arthritis have commonly been reported in children, infants, and neonates [22]. In both adults and children, some cases had a clear source of primary infection [23, 24]; others had no apparent risk factors except minor trauma which was often missed or under reported [25, 26].

Kp osteomyelitis is characterized by a tendency to rapid evolution, being multifocal with long bone involvement, widespread destruction, and exuberant periosteal reaction [27]. In addition, in the setting of emerging nosocomially acquired multidrug-resistant *Kp* infection, a microbiologic diagnosis becomes of upmost importance with either bone aspiration or biopsy [6] when blood cultures are negative and when no apparent source is identified [12].

In recent years, new hypervirulent *Kp* strains (in particular, *Kp* serotypes K1 and K2) have been associated with life-threatening infections (bacteremia, liver abscess, and meningitis) with distant metastasis in younger immune-competent hosts [12, 28, 29]. The increased virulence is related to the presence of the capsular (K) antigen, producing a hyperviscous capsule leading to the growth of mucoid colonies on culture plates that resists phagocytosis [12, 30].

Our patient had an infection with a mucoid *Kp* strain sensitive to all antibiotics except ampicillin suggesting a hypervirulent strain. The *Kp* capsular serotype remains unknown as such testing is not routinely performed at our hospital, and it was not requested since the patient had a favorable clinical response to early antimicrobial therapy.

4. Conclusion

Kp is a rare cause of osteomyelitis in adults, affecting mainly those with underlying immunosuppression. Given its pathogenic nature, early identification and therapy remains a key step in management.

Acknowledgments

The authors gratefully acknowledge the assistance of Jeffrey Gnerre, MD (Department of Radiology, Westchester Medical Center), in the interpretation of the MRI images.

References

[1] D. P. Lew and F. A. Waldvogel, "Acute and chronic osteomyelitis," in *Clinical Infectious Disease*, D. Schlossberg, Ed., pp. 479-484, Cambridge Unversity Press, NewYork, NY, USA, 1st edition, 2008

[2] D. P. Lew and F. A. Waldvogel, "Osteomyelitis," *The Lancet*, vol. 364, no. 9431, pp. 369–379, 2004.

[3] S. K. Schmitt, "Osteomyelitis," *Infectious Disease Clinics of North America*, vol. 31, no. 2, pp. 325–338, 2017.

[4] J. T. Mader, M. Ortiz, and J. H. Calhoun, "Update on the diagnosis and management of osteomyelitis," *Clinics in Podiatric Medicine and Surgery*, vol. 13, no. 4, pp. 701–724, 1996.

[5] R. G. Weber and B. F. Ansell, "A report of a case of *Klebsiella pneumoniae* arthritis and a review of extrapulmonary *Klebsiella* infections," *Annals of Internal Medicine*, vol. 57, no. 2, pp. 281–289, 1962.

[6] J. A. Sanders, "*Kiebsiella pneumoniae* osteomyelitis: demonstration by three-phase radionucide bone imaging," *Journal of Nuclear Medicine*, vol. 30, pp. 1412–1414, 1989.

[7] C. S. Bryan, K. L. Reynolds, and E. R. Brenner, "Analysis of 1,186 episodes of gram-negative bacteremia in non-university hospitals: the effects of antimicrobial therapy," *Clinical Infectious Diseases*, vol. 5, no. 4, pp. 629–638, 1983.

[8] A. S. Shon, R. P. Bajwa, and T. A. Russo, "Hypervirulent (hypermucoviscous) *Klebsiella pneumoniae*: a new and dangerous breed," *Virulence*, vol. 4, no. 2, pp. 107–118, 2013.

[9] H. Baer and L. Ehrenworth, "The pathogenicity of *Klebsiella pneumoniae* for mice: the relationship to the quantity and rate of production of type-specific capsular polysaccharide," *Journal of Bacteriology*, vol. 72, no. 5, pp. 713–717, 1956.

[10] H. D. Rose and J. Schreier, "The effect of hospitalization and antibiotic therapy on the gram-negative fecal flora," *American Journal of the Medical Sciences*, vol. 255, no. 4, pp. 228–236, 1968.

[11] W. E. Kloos and M. S. Musselwhite, "Distribution and persistence of *Staphylococcus* and *Micrococcus* species and other aerobic bacteria on human skin," *Applied Microbiology*, vol. 30, no. 3, pp. 381–385, 1975.

[12] B. C. Prokesch, M. TeKippe, J. Kim et al., "Primary osteomyelitis caused by hypervirulent *Klebsiella pneumoniae*," *Lancet Infectious Diseases*, vol. 16, no. 9, pp. e190–e195, 2016.

[13] R. W. Tsay, L. K. Siu, C. P. Fung, and F. Y. Chang, "Characteristics of bacteremia between community-acquired and nosocomial *Klebsiella pneumoniae* infection: risk factor for mortality and the impact of capsular serotypes as a herald for community-acquired infection," *Archives of Internal Medicine*, vol. 162, no. 9, pp. 1021–1027, 2002.

[14] R. Podschun and U. Ullmann, "*Klebsiella* spp. as nosocomial pathogens: epidemiology, taxonomy, typing methods, and pathogenicity factors," *Clinical Microbiology Reviews*, vol. 11, pp. 589–603, 1998.

[15] J. Fernández, M. Navasa, J. Gómez et al., "Bacterial infections in cirrhosis: epidemiological changes with invasive procedures and norfloxacin prophylaxis," *Hepatology*, vol. 35, no. 1, pp. 140–148, 2002.

[16] W. R. Caly and E. Strauss, "A prospective study of bacterial infections in patients with cirrhosis," *Journal of Hepatology*, vol. 18, no. 3, pp. 353–358, 1993.

[17] P. Mohan, B. Ramu, E. Bhasker, and J. Venkataraman, "Prevalence and risk factors for bacterial skin infection and mortality in cirrhosis," *Annals of Hepatology*, vol. 10, pp. 15–20, 2011.

[18] J. H. Kim, J. S. Lee, S. H. Lee et al., "Renal dysfunction induced by bacterial infection other than spontaneous bacterial peritonitis in patients with cirrhosis: incidence and risk factor," *Gut and Liver*, vol. 3, no. 4, pp. 292–297, 2009.

[19] E. R. Halsband, P. L. Maloney, and H. C. Doku, "Gram-negative osteomyelitis. Report of a case," *Oral Surgery, Oral Medicine, Oral Pathology*, vol. 29, no. 6, pp. 806–811, 1970.

[20] R. S. Fishbach, J. E. Rosenblatt, and J. G. Dahigren, "Pyogenic vertebral osteomyelitis in heroin addicts," *California Medical*, vol. 119, pp. 1–4, 1973.

[21] A. Talbot and M. Parlange, "Lea osteomyelitis a pneumo bacille de Friedlander," *Revue de Chirurgie Paris*, vol. 76, pp. 271–289, 1938.

[22] A. A. Adeyemo, J. A. Akindele, and S. I. Omokhodion, "Klebsiella septicemia, osteomyelitis and septic arthritis in neonates in Ibadan, Nigeria," *Annals of Tropical Paediatrics*, vol. 13, no. 3, pp. 285–289, 1993.

[23] L. C. Chew, "Septic monoarthritis and osteomyelitis in an elderly man following *Klebsiella pneumoniae* genitourinary infection: case report," *Annals of the Academy of Medicine, Singapore*, vol. 35, pp. 100–103, 2006.

[24] J. M. Goldman and J. K. Kowalec, "Hepatic abscess and osteomyelitis from *Klebsiella pneumoniae*," *JAMA: The Journal of the American Medical Association*, vol. 240, no. 24, p. 2660, 1978.

[25] L. Dubey, K. Krasinski, and M. Hernanz-Schulman, "Osteomyelitis secondary to trauma or infected contiguous soft tissue," *Pediatric Infectious Disease Journal*, vol. 7, no. 1, pp. 26–34, 1988.

[26] M. S. Ritter, H. Mroch, and M. J. Burns, "Soaring suppurative sea shells from the sea shore: *Pseudomonas aeruginosa* and *Klebsiella pneumoniae* septic arthritis after marine sea shell injury," *Pediatric Emergency Care*, vol. 9, no. 5, pp. 289–291, 1993.

[27] R. O. Murray and H. G. Jacobson, *The Radiology of Skeletal Disorders*, Livingstone, Vol. 2, Livingstone, London, UK, 2nd edition, 1977.

[28] C. T. Fang, Y. P. Chuang, C. T. Shun, S. C. Chang, and J. T. Wang, "A novel virulence gene in *Klebsiella pneumoniae* strains causing primary liver abscess and septic metastatic complications," *Journal of Experimental Medicine*, vol. 199, no. 5, pp. 697–705, 2004.

[29] S. Kishibe, Y. Okubo, S. Morino et al., "Pediatric hypervirulent *Klebsiella pneumoniae* septic arthritis," *Pediatrics International*, vol. 58, no. 5, pp. 382–385, 2016.

[30] B. Li, Y. Zhao, C. Liu et al., "Molecular pathogenesis of *Klebsiella pneumoniae*," *Future Microbiology*, vol. 9, no. 9, pp. 1071–1081, 2014.

11

A Rare and Potentially Catastrophic Infection: Primary Intestinal Aspergillosis—Case Report in an HIV Patient

Cátia Dias, Filipa Duarte-Ribeiro, Sara Pipa, and Margarida Mota

Department of Internal Medicine, Centro Hospitalar Vila Nova de Gaia/Espinho, Espinho, Portugal

Correspondence should be addressed to Cátia Dias; kati.diass@gmail.com

Academic Editor: Raul Colodner

Aspergillus species are ubiquitous in nature; however, infection is uncommon, except in immunocompromised or immunosuppressed hosts. We present the case of a 71-year-old woman with a history of human immunodeficiency virus infection who presented with fever, weight loss, and diarrhea, posteriorly diagnosed with intestinal aspergillosis after examination of a segmental enterectomy piece. The diagnosis was made postmortem once the patient died after fast and progressive deterioration in the postoperative period.

1. Introduction

Aspergillosis is the disease caused by species of *Aspergillus* spp. These are ubiquitous in nature and their inhalation is common in the general population. However, tissue invasion and consequent infection are uncommon and usually involves some degree of immunosuppression, which alters the immune response to inhaled species. We present the case of a 71-year-old woman with a history of human immunodeficiency virus infection who was diagnosed postmortem with intestinal aspergillosis after histological examination of a segmental enterectomy piece.

2. Case Description

A 71-year-old woman with a past medical history of uterine cancer 25 years before, herpes-zoster infection two years before, recent diagnosis of human immunodeficiency virus (HIV) infection, and cervical adenopathies under investigation presented at the first medical appointment at the Infectious Diseases Unit referring a 3-week history of fever, weight loss of 20 kg, and hemoptoic cough, as well as diarrhea with one year of evolution. On physical examination, she was cachectic and weak, had axillary temperature of 38°C, blood pressure of 112/80 mmHg, respiration rate of 40 per minute, heart rate of 142 beats per minute, and oxygen saturation of 95% in room air. She also presented with pain and tenderness at the palpation of the hypogastric region, and during the consultation, she presented cardiorespiratory arrest. Advanced life support with favorable response was performed, and she was subsequently transferred to the emergency room where it was necessary to initiate aminergic support and proceed to orotracheal intubation and mechanical invasive ventilation. The complementary diagnostic exams revealed white blood cell count 14,740/μL with absolute neutrophil count 13,180/μL (89.4%) and absolute lymphocyte count 970/μL (6.6%) with 113 CD4+/μL cells, hemoglobin level 11.3 g/d, and platelet count 2,33,000/μL. She presented with blood creatinine 1.34 mg/dL, pancreatic amylase 222 U/L (4 times above the upper limit of normal), pancreatic lipase 174 U/L (3 times above the upper limit of normal), and seric lactates 6.5 mmol/L. Viral load of HIV by polymerase chain reaction was 2,330,220 copies/mL. Thoracic, abdominal, and pelvic computed tomography (CT) revealed pneumoperitoneum, peritonitis, diffuse parietal thickening, and dilatation of the intestinal loops of the jejunum with splenic infarction (Figure 1).

An emerging surgery exploratory laparotomy was performed having been found enteric peritonites of the large cavity, occlusion with transition point at the level of the distal jejunum and poor perfusion, and thickening of the distal loops and perforation at the level of the distal

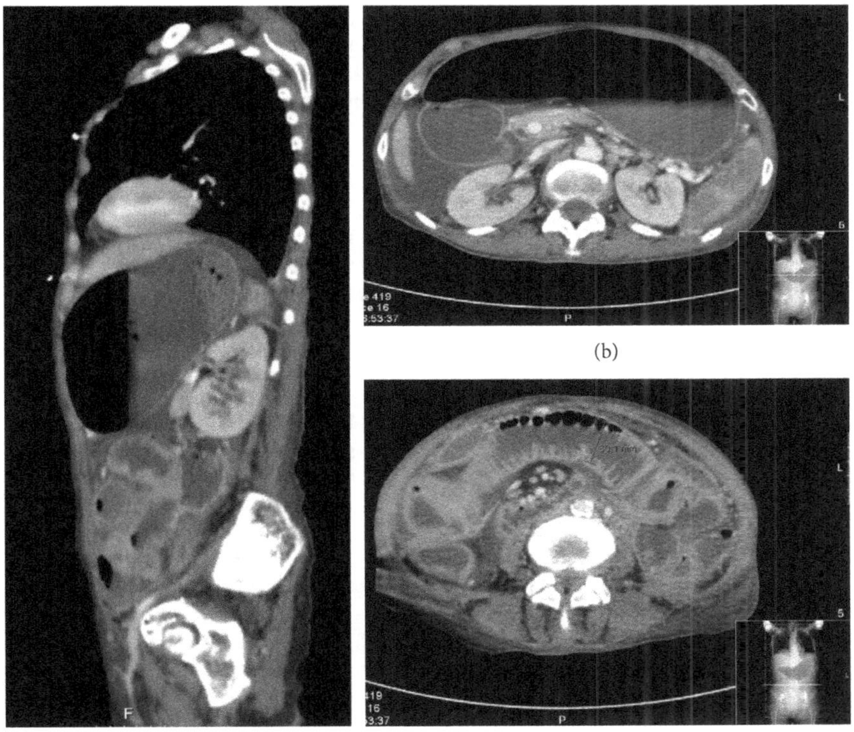

(a) (b) (c)

FIGURE 1: Thoracic, abdominal, and pelvic CT from the day of admission in (a) sagittal and (b, c) transverse planes.

ileum. Segmental enterectomy of approximately 35 cm of jejunum/ileum has been performed, including ischemic loop and ileal perforation. In the postoperative period, she was admitted to the intensive care unit, and broad-spectrum antibiotic therapy has been initiated. Nevertheless, she evolved with progressive clinical deterioration with increasing need of amines and without favorable hemodynamic response. The patient passed away the same day. The histological examination of the segmental enterectomy piece and available postmortem revealed acute transmural inflammation of the enteric wall, with suppuration and necrosis and extensive lesions of acute fibrinoexudative serositis with fungal hyphae of the *Aspergillus* spp. type. There were no images of angioinvasion, epithelioid granulomas, or signs of malignancy. The culture of peritoneal fluid obtained during surgery revealed polybacterial and fungal overinfection with *Enterococcus faecium*, *Escherichia coli*, and *Candida albicans*.

3. Discussion

Aspergillosis may refer to several types of diseases such as allergic disease, invasion of the upper or lower airways, skin infection, or extrapulmonary disease, which may be due to tissue invasion and hematogenous dissemination, which can lead to disseminated infection. Invasive aspergillosis (IA) occurs almost exclusively in situations where cellular immunity is severely compromised. In fact, when immunity is intact, *Aspergillus* conidia and hyphae are inhaled but destroyed by alveolar macrophages and polymorphonuclear leukocytes. When there is a qualitative or quantitative defect of these cells, there may be angioinvasive growth with hemorrhage, thrombosis, hypoxia, necrosis, and dissemination [1]. The majority of cases of IA are described in patients submitted to allogeneic hematopoietic cell transplant or solid organ transplant, those with severe and prolonged neutropenia, and those in need of high doses of glucocorticoids or immunosuppressive regimens [2]. HIV infection, although infrequent, is one of the risk factors for IA, being present in approximately 4% of the cases of IA described [2], even though IA occurs in less than 1% of HIV-infected patients [3, 4].

In this group of patients, IA has a high morbidity and mortality, with fatality rates around 86% [2, 5]. The risk of occurrence of IA increases with highest degree of immunosuppression or in those with other risk factors for invasive disease, such as neutropenia or use of corticoids [6]. The incidence is higher in patients with CD4+ cells below 100/μL and with one or more opportunistic diseases (acquired immunodeficiency syndrome (AIDS)-defining) [6]. However, in the highly active antiretroviral therapy (HAART) era, this paradigm has changed, with more cases being identified in patients with CD4+ cells higher then 100/μL [7]. It should be noted that in the present case, none of the other risk factors presented above were present, with the exception of low CD4+ cells.

Most cases of invasive aspergillosis occur in the lungs and respiratory tract, and patients with HIV infection are no exception (approximately 61.2% of the cases). Cases of intestinal IA described in the literature are extremely rare, constituting only isolated clinical cases. Although other routes of entry to IA other than pulmonary are only speculative, it is thought that in the intestine, the invasion may be through local inoculation and there are, as in the case of the patient presented, some cases described in patients with proven intestinal IA but without pulmonary disease [8–10]. Intestinal aspergillosis may manifest as enterocolitis, appendicitis, colonic ulcers, abdominal pain, and gastrointestinal bleeding.

The diagnosis of IA is considered "proven" when the hyphae of *Aspergillus* spp. are observed together with evidence of tissue injury (as presented in this case), or when a positive culture for *Aspergillus* spp. is obtained from a specimen obtained by sterile procedure and from a normally sterile site [11]. Whenever possible, microbiological cultures and histology should be obtained; however, isolated positive cultures may only be related to contamination of the samples.

4. Conclusion

Although very rare, patients with HIV infection/AIDS are susceptible to *Aspergillus* infection, which can lead to disseminated disease with high rates of morbidity and mortality, with most cases of extrapulmonary infections being documented postmortem. This case emphasizes the importance of early consideration of this differential diagnosis when approaching HIV-infected patients with symptoms similar to those of the patient under discussion.

References

[1] R. Ben-Ami, R. E. Lewis, and D. P. Kontoyiannis, "Enemy of the (immunosuppressed) state: an update on the pathogenesis of *Aspergillus fumigatus* infection," *British Journal of Haematology*, vol. 150, no. 4, pp. 406–417, 2010.

[2] S. J. Lin, J. Schranz, and S. M. Teutsch, "Aspergillosis case-fatality rate: systematic review of the literature," *Clinical Infectious Diseases*, vol. 32, no. 3, pp. 358–366, 2001.

[3] K. B. Tong, C. J. Lau, K. Murtagh, A. J. Layton, and R. Seifeldin, "The economic impact of aspergillosis: analysis of hospital expenditures across patient subgroups," *International Journal of Infectious Diseases*, vol. 13, no. 1, pp. 24–36, 2009.

[4] M. Cornet, L. Fleury, C. Maslo, J.-F. Bernard, and G. Brücker, "Epidemiology of invasive aspergillosis in France: a six-year multicentric survey in the Greater Paris area," *Journal of Hospital Infection*, vol. 51, pp. 288–296, 2002.

[5] E. Mylonakis, T. F. Barlam, T. Flanigan, and J. D. Rich, "Pulmonary Aspergillosis and invasive disease in AIDS: review of 342 cases," *Chest*, vol. 114, no. 1, pp. 251–262, 1998.

[6] K. J. Holding, M. S. Dworkin, P. C. Wan et al., "Aspergillosis among people infected with human immunodeficiency virus: incidence and survival. Adult and Adolescent Spectrum of HIV Disease Project," *Clinical Infectious Diseases*, vol. 31, no. 5, pp. 1253–1257, 2000.

[7] B. Denis, M. Guiguet, N. de Castro et al., "Relevance of EORTC criteria for the diagnosis of invasive aspergillosis in hiv-infected patients, and survival trends over a 20-year period in France," *Clinical Infectious Diseases*, vol. 61, no. 8, pp. 1273–1280, 2015.

[8] P. Eggimann, J. C. Chevrolet, M. Starobinski et al., "Primary invasive aspergillosis of the digestive tract: report of two cases and review of the literature," *Infection*, vol. 34, no. 6, pp. 333–338, 2006.

[9] M. González-Vicent, M. A. Díaz, I. Colmenero, J. Sevilla, and L. Madero, "Primary gastrointestinal aspergillosis after autologous peripheral blood progenitor cell transplantation: an unusual presentation of invasive aspergillosis," *Transplant Infectious Disease*, vol. 10, no. 3, pp. 193–196, 2008.

[10] D. P. Kontoyiannis, M. Mathur, Y. B. Chen et al., "Case records of the Massachusetts General Hospital. Case 13-2014. A 41-year-old man with fever and abdominal pain after stem-cell transplantation," *New England Journal of Medicine*, vol. 370, no. 17, pp. 1637–1646, 2014.

[11] B. De Pauw, T. J. Walsh, J. P. Donnelly et al., "Revised definitions of invasive fungal disease from the European Organization for Research and Treatment of Cancer/Invasive Fungal Infections Cooperative Group and the National Institute of Allergy and Infectious Diseases Mycoses Study Group (EORTC/MSG) Consensus Group," *Clinical Infectious Diseases*, vol. 46, no. 2, pp. 1813–1821, 1813.

12

Cryptococcal Meningitis in a HIV Seronegative Patient: A Rare Complication of Cerebrospinal Fluid Leak Detected with a New Cisternographic Technique

Chukwunonso Chime, Charbel Ishak, Kishore Kumar, Muhammad Kamal, Srinivasan Krishna, Paul Kelly, and Sridhar Chilimuri

BronxCare Health System–A Clinical Affiliate of Mount Sinai Hospital and Academic Affiliate of the Icahn School of Medicine, New York, NY, USA

Correspondence should be addressed to Chukwunonso Chime; cchime@bronxleb.org

Academic Editor: Larry M. Bush

Immune deficiency is usually the underlying predisposing factor for cryptococcal meningitis, though there have been case reports of immunocompetent patients presenting with same. The portal of entry for *Cryptococcus neoformans* is the respiratory tract, and by hematogenous spread, it causes systemic symptoms. The presence of CSF leak is described to have predisposed our immunocompetent patient to infection by this organism possibly through direct spread. The gold standard for diagnosing CSF leak is by cisternography. In this case, we added a technique where nasal gauze is inserted during the procedure and scanned afterwards for dye, thus increasing the confidence of diagnosis of CSF leak through the nares. Prompt diagnosis and treatment is key to prevent adverse outcomes, and we propose that in patients with cryptococcal meningitis without any identifiable risk factor, evaluation for CSF leak should be considered especially with history of head trauma.

1. Introduction

Cryptococcosis, an infection caused by the encapsulated yeast *Cryptococcus neoformans* is commonly associated with immunodeficiency states, both human immunodeficiency virus (HIV) and non-HIV related. Cerebrospinal fluid (CSF) leak, although rare, is a well-recognized cause of headache with annual incidence of spontaneous CSF leak estimated to be 5/100,000 [1]. CSF leak occurs as a result of varying etiologies, one of which is trauma, and presence of compromised dura bacteria from the respiratory tract has been known to cause meningitis through a direct spread. Although the respiratory tract is the known portal of entry for *Cryptococcus neoformans*, the organism has not been reported to cause central nervous system (CNS) infections through direct spread. We report to the best of our knowledge, the first known case of CSF leak detected with our new cisternographic technique, predisposing a patient to cryptococcal meningitis in the absence of another immune compromise.

2. Case Report

A 50-year-old Hispanic female presented to the emergency room (ER) with complaint of severe headache for 1 day. The headache was described as throbbing with associated photophobia and multiple episodes of nonbloody vomiting. She reported a remote history of closed head trauma and intermittent rhinorrhea, especially on leaning forward, with spontaneous resolution a few months prior to this presentation. Her medical history was significant for intermittent "migraine" and coronary artery disease. Physical examination was notable for photophobia, otherwise no nuchal rigidity or focal motor or sensory neurological deficits; the rest of the examination and vital signs were unremarkable. Laboratory parameters revealed hemoglobin

11.6 g/dl, white cell count (WBC) $13.1 \times 10^9/l$ (84.7% neutrophils), serum sodium 138 mEq/l, potassium 4.1 mEq/l, and creatinine 0.7 mg/dl; all liver function tests were within normal limits.

She was admitted to the medical floor where a lumbar puncture was performed with an opening pressure of 35 cm H_2O, CSF fluid analysis with WBC 1850 cells/uL (segmental 70%), red blood cells 5, protein 175 mg/dl (normal 15–45), glucose 40 mg/dl (normal 40–70), cryptococcal CSF antigen detected with a titer of 1 : 1024 (normal < 1 : 2 titer), negative bacterial antigen, and no growth on bacterial CSF culture. Patient also had a negative HIV serology confirmed by nondetectable HIV ribonucleic acid (RNA) and an absolute CD4 count of 1168.

With the patient's history suspicious for traumatic CSF leak, she had a magnetic resonance imaging (MRI) of the head and sinus that were both unrevealing. Given the low sensitivity of a regular MRI in CSF leak diagnosis, a computed tomography (CT) cisternogram was performed. It revealed evidence of leakage of intrathecally injected contrast into the right nasal cavity via the right olfalctory fossa, between the anterior ethmoidal cells and the crista galli bone (Figure 1). This was also confirmed by scanning the gauzes inserted intentionally into both right and left nares by the author (C.I.) during real-time CT cisternogram (Figure 2). This first-time-used innovative, inexpensive, and efficient CT technique confirmed without any doubt the presence of leaked contrast from the opacified CSF in the right nostril gauze when compared to contralateral side; this could have a tremendous role in the preoperative planning, intraoperative performance, and postoperative outcomes.

She was initially started on antimicrobial treatment for presumptive bacterial meningitis and later transitioned to induction therapy for cryptococcal meningitis with liposomal amphotericin B and flucytosine (5-fluorocytosine) after preliminary results of her CSF analysis were obtained. Patient subsequently had an endoscopic-assisted transnasal repair of CSF leak with abdominal fat graft using brainlab navigation system by combined neurosurgical and ear, nose, and throat (ENT) teams. With completion of 2 weeks of induction therapy with liposomal amphotericin B and flucytosine, she demonstrated clinical improvement, and two repeat lumbar punctures during the course of admission showed normalized opening pressure and negative cryptococcal antigen. Fluconazole was then started for consolidation, and she was followed-up on discharge in the outpatient clinic until completion of an 8-week course of fluconazole. Patient has remained symptom free two years after completion of treatment.

3. Discussion

Immune compromise is a common underlying predisposition for infection by *Cryptococcus neoformans*, the causative organism of cryptococcosis, with the following immunodeficiency states described in literature: HIV infection, organ transplantation, chronic steroid use, and sarcoidosis [2]. There have been case reports of cryptococcal meningitis in the immunocompetent population and among HIV-negative patients with cryptococcosis; studies have shown no apparent immune deficiency in 10–40% [3]. Immunodeficient states described in HIV-negative cases include nephrotic syndrome, cirrhosis, diabetes, malignancies, and autoimmune diseases [4]. Abbas et al. described a case of cryptococcosis in a HIV-negative patient with history of splenectomy [5]. CSF leak as a predisposing factor for cryptococcal meningitis in a HIV-negative patient has not been described in literature, and for this reason, we feel compelled to present this rare case.

Cryptococcal infections have a wide range of clinical presentations varying from asymptomatic respiratory tract colonization to disseminated infection [6]. Various organs have been described to be affected by cryptococcosis infection, but the most common site is the central nervous system [7]. The respiratory tract is the usual portal of entry of the fungus into the host; following entry, there is a hematogenous spread of the organism to the central nervous system [8]. Unlike other respiratory tract bacteria that have been described in literature to cause direct CNS involvement in the presence of a compromised brain dura, this is the first report of *Cryptococcus neoformans* causing meningitis through this route in an immunocompetent patient. With CNS involvement and meningitis, elevated intracranial pressure, defined as opening pressure of >20 cm H_2O measured in a reclining position, is present in more than 50% of patients regardless of HIV status [9] and is generally associated with a high CSF yeast burden [10]. Clinical manifestation of cryptococcal meningitis includes fever, nausea, vomiting, and headache; there could also be signs of spinal root irritation in only one-third of patients, commonly the immunocompetent [11]. Other clinical variations exist when comparison is made between this meningitis in HIV and non-HIV infected patients, with the former having much less inflammatory response and shorter duration of symptoms but generally higher burden of organisms [9].

In patients with persistent CSF leakage, meningitis poses a considerable risk and carries a 10% mortality [12] with *Haemophilus influenzae* and *Streptococcus pneumoniae* being the most common pathogens [13]. We are unaware of any published case reports describing *Cryptococcus neoformans* as a causative organism for meningitis in a patient with CSF leak.

For the routine detection of cryptococcal antigens in CSF, certain modalities are available and include historical staining with Indian ink and observation under light microscopy. With almost 100% sensitivity and 98% specificity, newer latex agglutination tests are currently recommended. Definitive diagnosis is made by growing the yeast in CSF culture [14]. We suspect in our case that given the patient was HIV negative and had ongoing drainage of the CSF, the burden of organism may have been low, explaining lack of subsequent growth on CSF culture. Negative CSF culture also raised our concern for possible false-positive CSF cryptococcal antigen latex agglutination test. A few causes have been identified in the literature as potential etiology of false positivity and include cross reaction with *Trichosporon* species infection or disinfectants, soap, or starch [15]. In our index case, there was no clinical evidence of white piedra

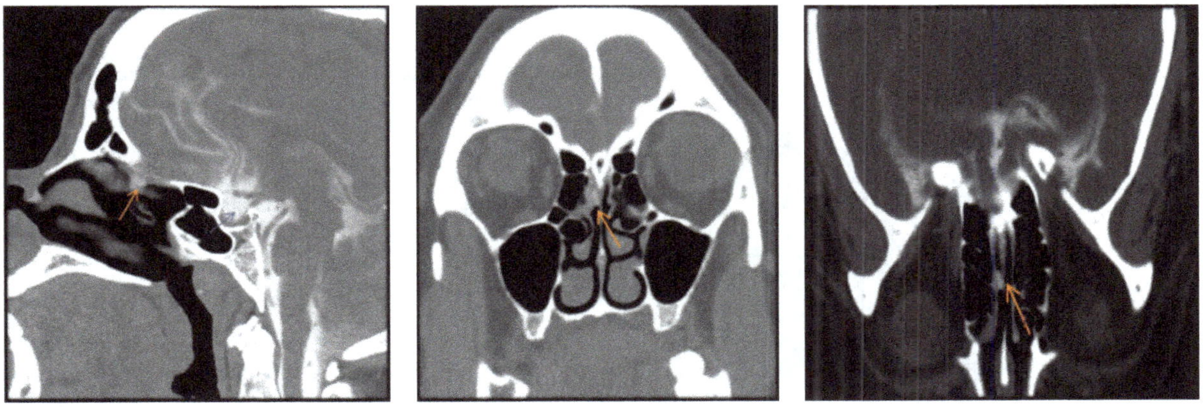

(a) (b) (c)

Figure 1: Sagittal (a), axial (b), and coronal (c) images in prone position with scanning during sneezing maneuver. CT cisternogram demonstrated leakage of intrathecally injected contrast (red arrow) noted in the right nasal cavity, along the right aspect of the perpendicular plate of nasal septum, just below the right cribriform plate. Empty sella filled with intrathecally injected contrast (blue arrow).

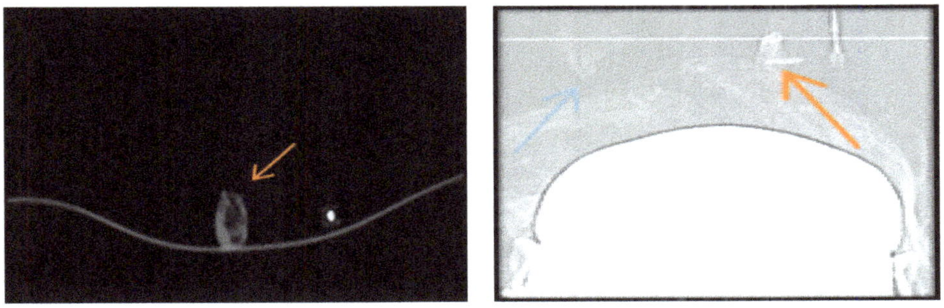

(a) (b)

Figure 2: Axial CT scan (a) and scout (b) of gauzes removed from both right (red arrow) and left (blue arrow) nostrils, after being inserted intentionally by the author (C.I.) during real-time cisternogram. This technique confirmed without doubt the presence of leaky contrast in the right nostril, compatible with CSF leakage.

caused by *Trichosporon species* and no other underling immunocompromise that would predispose her to trichosporonosis; also, no contamination with disinfectants/soap and interference with hydroxyethyl starch were encountered. As part of the initial workup to assess immune status, HIV infection was excluded with negative HIV serologic and RNA testing. Her normal CD4 count also excluded idiopathic T-cell deficiency. Peculiar to our case is a previously unrecognized risk factor for cryptococcal meningitis, a CSF leak, and given her history of traumatic rhinorrhea with postural headache, this was further worked up with a cisternogram to confirm diagnosis and necessitate repair.

Postural headache is an important feature of CSF leak [16]; however, postural headache by itself lacks sensitivity or specificity without a history of head trauma/surgery. Postural headache with rhinorrhea should prompt search for a traumatic CSF leak, as this can lead to life threatening complications in 25–50% of cases including meningitis [16]. In general, the diagnosis of CSF leak would include plain films of the facial bones and skull, CT or MRI cisternography, and high resolution CT. CT cisternography remains the gold standard for diagnosing CSF leak [17]. A history of head trauma and the presence of unusual meningitis could be a result of CSF leak, and we have proposed an algorithm for further diagnostic evaluation (see Figure 3).

Prompt recognition and treatment is required as cryptococcal meningitis is fatal without treatment [18]. The host's immune system and anatomic site of involvement would determine the choice of treatment [19], and with current recommendations, induction therapy is primarily focused at rapid fungicidal activity to achieve sterilization of the CNS [21]. Successful induction regimen evidenced by sterile CSF culture at 2 weeks after initiation of therapy has been linked to favorable outcomes [22]. Regardless of HIV status, an acceptable therapy is induction with amphotericin B and flucytosine for at least 2 weeks, followed by a minimum of 8 weeks of fluconazole for consolidation, but there can be other variations to this regimen [20].

The impact of aggressive management of intracranial pressure in HIV-negative patients is unclear and has not been consistently employed [19]; the same cannot be said for HIV-positive patients. When reduction in intracranial pressure is required, the principal intervention is by lumbar drainage, either by lumbar puncture or use of a lumbar drain [9]. When these options fail to control symptoms of elevated pressure or neurological deficits progress, a ventriculoperitoneal shunt is

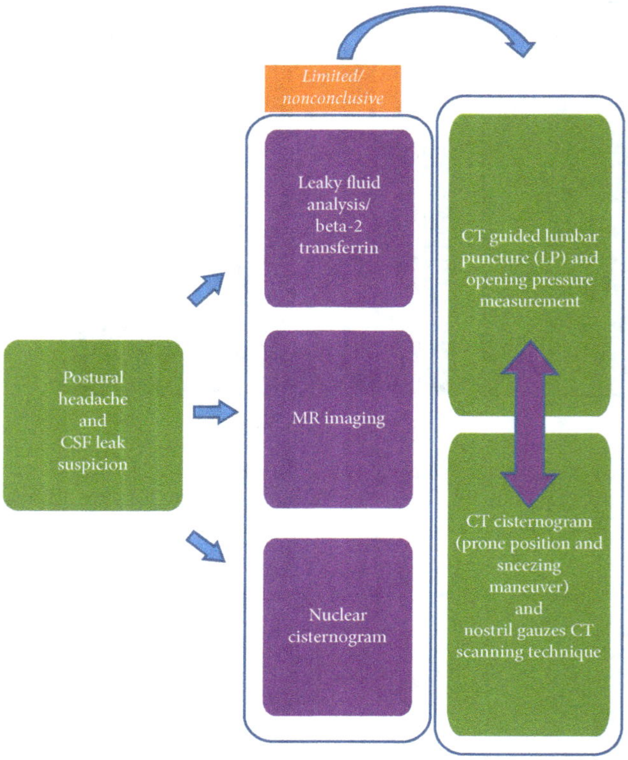

Figure 3

indicated [9]. CSF leaks are mostly treated either surgically or conservatively; the surgical approach involves transnasal endoscopic, intracranial, and extracranial methods [13]. As cisternogram showed leakage into the right nasal cavity in our patient, she was managed with the transnasal approach by a combined ENT and neurosurgical team. Her symptoms improved with antifungal therapy before discharge and she remained asymptomatic in subsequent clinic follow-up.

4. Conclusion

Cryptococcal meningitis is known to be fatal without treatment; prompt recognition is key with regards to changing the clinical course outcome of this deadly disease. Though immune deficiency including HIV has been known as a predisposing factor, there have been reported cases of immunocompetent patients presenting with cryptococcal meningitis. Both spontaneous and head trauma-related CSF leaks are rare conditions, however, when unrecognized, could lead to life-threatening complications. Early recognition is key and could lead to interventions resulting in excellent outcomes. Postural headache, history of trauma/surgery (recent and remote), and the presence of unusual causes of meningitis should prompt workup for CSF leak. CT cisternography remains the gold standard for diagnosing CSF leak, and we propose adding the gauze scanning technique, which is innovative, inexpensive, and efficient.

References

[1] W. Schievink, "Spontaneous spinal cerebrospinal fluid leaks," *Cephalalgia*, vol. 28, no. 12, pp. 1345–1356, 2008.

[2] P. G. Pappas, J. R. Perfect, G. A. Cloud et al., "Cryptococcosis in human immunodeficiency virus-negative patients in the era of effective azole therapy," *Clinical Infectious Diseases*, vol. 33, no. 5, pp. 690–699, 2001.

[3] R. U. Sorensen, K. D. Boehm, D. Kaplan, and M. Berger, "Cryptococcal osteomyelitis and cellular immunodeficiency associated with interleukin-2 deficiency," *The Journal of Pediatrics*, vol. 121, no. 6, pp. 873–879, 1992.

[4] Y.-M. Chuang, Y.-C. Ho, H.-T. Chang, C.-J. Yu, P.-C. Yang, and P.-R. Hsueh, "Disseminated cryptococcosis in HIV-uninfected patients," *European Journal of Clinical Microbiology and Infectious Diseases*, vol. 27, no. 4, pp. 307–310, 2007.

[5] H. Abbas, A. CiFuentes Kottkamp, N. Abbas, R. Cindrich, and M. Singh, "A rare presentation of cryptococcal meningitis and cerebellitis in an asplenic patient, seronegative for human immunodeficiency virus (HIV)," *American Journal of Case Reports*, vol. 19, pp. 183–186, 2018.

[6] A. Desalermos, T. K. Kourkoumpetis, and E. Mylonakis, "Update on the epidemiology and management of cryptococcal meningitis," *Expert Opinion on Pharmacotherapy*, vol. 13, no. 6, pp. 783–789, 2012.

[7] I. S. Kourbeti, A. F. Vakis, J. A. Papadakis et al., "Infections in traumatic brain injury patients," *Clinical Microbiology and Infection*, vol. 18, no. 4, pp. 359–364, 2012.

[8] M. Mitha, P. Naicker, and P. Mahida, "Disseminated Cryptococcosis in an HIV-negative patient in South Africa: the elusive differential diagnosis," *Journal of infection in developing countries*, vol. 4, no. 8, pp. 526–529, 2010.

[9] J. R. Graybill, J. Sobel, M. Saag et al., "Diagnosis and management of increased intracranial pressure in patients with AIDS and cryptococcal meningitis," *Clinical Infectious Diseases*, vol. 30, no. 1, pp. 47–54, 2000.

[10] T. Bicanic, A. E. Brouwer, G. Meintjes et al., "Relationship of cerebrospinal fluid pressure, fungal burden and outcome in patients with cryptococcal meningitis undergoing serial lumbar punctures," *AIDS*, vol. 23, no. 6, pp. 701–706, 2009.

[11] F. A. Lasso, T. O. Zamora Bastidas, J. A. Potosi Garcia, and B. Diaz Idrobo, "Cryptococcal cerebellitis in no-VIH patient," *Colombia Medica*, vol. 48, no. 2, pp. 94–97, 2017.

[12] D. Choi and R. Spann, "Traumatic cerebrospinal fluid leakage: risk factors and the use of prophylactic antibiotics," *British Journal of Neurosurgery*, vol. 10, no. 6, pp. 571–576, 2009.

[13] J.-W. Oh, S.-H. Kim, and K. Whang, "Traumatic cerebrospinal fluid leak: diagnosis and management," *Korean Journal of Neurotrauma*, vol. 13, no. 2, pp. 63–67, 2017.

[14] A. Kambugu, D. B. Meya, J. Rhein et al., "Outcomes of cryptococcal meningitis in Uganda before and after the availability of highly active antiretroviral therapy," *Clinical Infectious Diseases*, vol. 46, no. 11, pp. 1694–1701, 2008.

[15] D. A. Wilson, M. Sholtis, S. Parshall, G. S. Hall, and G. W. Procop, "False-positive cryptococcal antigen test associated with use of BBL Port-a-Cul transport vials," *Journal of Clinical Microbiology*, vol. 49, no. 2, pp. 702-703, 2010.

[16] H. A. Brodie and T. C. Thompson, "Management of complications from 820 temporal bone fractures," *American Journal of Otolaryngology*, vol. 18, no. 2, pp. 188–197, 1997.

[17] W. I. Schievink, "Spontaneous spinal cerebrospinal fluid leaks and intracranial hypotension," *JAMA*, vol. 295, no. 19, pp. 2286–2296, 2006.

[18] S. J. Lee, H. K. Choi, J. Son, K. H. Kim, and S. H. Lee, "Cryptococcal meningitis in patients with or without human immunodeficiency virus: experience in a tertiary hospital," *Yonsei Medical Journal*, vol. 52, no. 3, pp. 482–487, 2011.
[19] M. S. Saag, R. J. Graybill, R. A. Larsen et al., "Practice guidelines for the management of cryptococcal disease," *Clinical Infectious Diseases*, vol. 30, no. 4, pp. 710–718, 2000.
[20] J. R. Perfect, W. E. Dismukes, F. Dromer et al., "Clinical practice guidelines for the management of cryptococcal disease: 2010 update by the infectious diseases society of America," *Clinical Infectious Diseases*, vol. 50, no. 3, pp. 291–322, 2010.
[21] T. Bicanic, G. Meintjes, R. Wood et al., "Fungal burden, early fungicidal activity, and outcome in cryptococcal meningitis in antiretroviral-naive or antiretroviral-experienced patients treated with amphotericin B or fluconazole," *Clinical Infectious Diseases*, vol. 45, no. 1, pp. 76–80, 2007.
[22] C. M. van der Horst, M. S. Saag, G. A. Cloud et al., "Treatment of cryptococcal meningitis associated with the acquired immunodeficiency syndrome," *New England Journal of Medicine*, vol. 337, no. 1, pp. 15–21, 1997.

13

From Bilateral Periorbital Necrotic Wound to Fungal Brain Abscess: A Complicated Case of COVID-19-Associated Mucormycosis

Bahram Eshraghi,[1] **Nastaran-Sadat Hosseini**,[2] **Rasoul Mohammadi**,[3] **Seyed Hamid Reza Abtahi**,[4] **Alireza Ramezani-Majd**,[1] **Roya Azad**,[5] **and Mohsen Pourazizi**[1]

[1]*Isfahan Eye Research Center, Department of Ophthalmology, Isfahan University of Medical Sciences, Isfahan, Iran*
[2]*School of Medicine, Isfahan University of Medical Sciences, Isfahan, Iran*
[3]*Department of Medical Parasitology and Mycology, School of Medicine, Infectious Diseases and Tropical Medicine Research Center, Isfahan University of Medical Sciences, Isfahan, Iran*
[4]*Department of Otolaryngology, Isfahan University of Medical Sciences, Isfahan, Iran*
[5]*Department of Radiology, Faculty of Medicine, Isfahan University of Medical Sciences, Isfahan, Iran*

Correspondence should be addressed to Mohsen Pourazizi; m.pourazizi@yahoo.com

Academic Editor: Annac Skiada

COVID-19-associated mucormycosis (CAM) is categorized as rhinocerebral-orbital (RCOM), pulmonary, gastrointestinal, cutaneous, and disseminated mucormycosis. An alarming surge in morbidity and mortality attributed to mucormycosis concurrent with coronavirus disease 2019 (COVID-19) has emerged as a cause for concern during the current outbreak of COVID-19. The global incidence of CAM has been attributed to environmental, host, and iatrogenic factors. Further, *Mucorales* interacting with epithelial cells followed by endothelium invasion are pivotal in developing mucormycosis in patients with COVID-19. In essence, CAM is an emerging condition that requires increased vigilance in all COVID-19 patients, including those who have recovered. In this case report, we describe a rare case of CAM in a 33-year-old immunocompetent man who developed bilateral periocular pain and a small area of cutaneous necrosis in both medial canthi associated with impaired vision, which progressed into a fungal brain abscess formation in the post-COVID period. Furthermore, this case aims to illustrate the potential underlying risk factors of CAM other than known risk factors, especially in immunocompetent individuals.

1. Introduction

Coronavirus disease 2019 (COVID-19) pandemic has led to a surge in invasive fungal infections, particularly among critically ill patients [1]. Mucormycosis is an invasive fungal infection caused by order *Mucorales*. The causal agents are thermotolerant, rapid-growing fungi belonging to the order *Mucorales* [2]. The capacity of these fungi to infect immunocompetent hosts is uncommon, despite their widespread occurrence in the environment. Patients, in the majority of instances, have underlying health issues [2]. Since the high prevalence is temporally associated with COVID-19, the entity is called COVID-19-associated mucormycosis (CAM). Although an exact causative relationship between COVID-19 and mucormycosis has not been proved, various factors were linked to the development of mucormycosis in COVID-19 patients, including (a) an unexpected increase in the circulating levels of proinflammatory cytokines, particularly interleukin-6 (IL-6) and tumor necrosis factor-α (TNF-α), (b) acute hyperglycemic state, (c) metabolic acidosis, (d) inappropriate immune system response, (e) specific environmental conditions

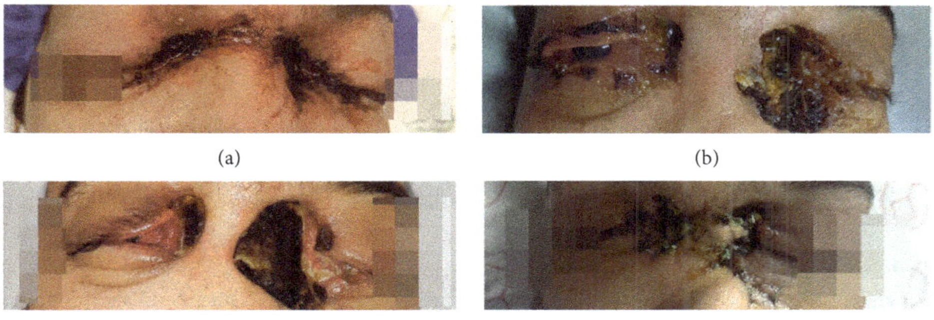

FIGURE 1: The clinical course of COVID-19-associated mucormycosis: (a) cutaneous manifestation of bilateral periorbital mucormycosis. The small area of skin necrosis on bilateral sides; (b) the necrotic epidermal lesion with ill-defined raised margins and a necrotic base significantly worsened and expanded from the medial canthi, eyelids, and periorbital area; (c) progressive cutaneous necrosis associated with the midfacial defect; (d) repaired cutaneous lesions after medical and surgical treatment.

contributed to high spore burden, (f) altered iron metabolism, (g) endotheliitis and microvasculopathy, (h) upregulation of GRP-78, (i) iatrogenic factors (e.g., adverse events associated with corticosteroids, IL-6 inhibitors, etc.), and (j) comorbid conditions, such as diabetes mellitus and obesity [1, 3–6].

Rhinocerebral-orbital mucormycosis (RCOM) is the most frequent clinical kind with the highest mortality rate, followed by pulmonary illness. About three-fourths of them had diabetes as predisposing comorbidity and were treated for COVID-19 with corticosteroids [3]. The involvement of brain tissue may manifest as altered awareness, headache, unsteady gait, stroke, or seizures [7, 8]. Once *Mucorales* first established in the nasal cavity and destroy the adjacent bone and soft tissues in this area, it proceeds to the maxillary and ethmoid sinuses, orbits, cavernous sinuses, meninges, and finally, the brain in terms of its angioinvasive propensity. Mucormycosis can spread to the intracranial cavity via the perivascular channels from the paranasal sinuses or via the cribriform plate into the anterior cranial fossa [9].

Hence, we report a rare case of a complicated case of CAM with a catastrophic course with a fungal brain abscess in a 33-year-old male with no remarkable past medical history.

2. Case Presentation

A 33-year-old previously healthy male with no history of COVID-19 vaccination was diagnosed with a positive reverse transcription-polymerase chain reaction (RT-PCR) for severe acute respiratory syndrome coronavirus-2 (SARS-CoV-2). He had no history of diabetes, immunosuppressive disorders, or cancer. After a diagnosis of moderate to severe COVID-19 pneumonia, the patient was administered remdesivir and methylprednisolone. After 10 days of hospitalization, he was released in a relatively good condition. Five days after discharge, he developed bilateral periocular pain, blurred vision, and a small area of cutaneous necrosis in both medial cantus. On examination, mild facial edema, periorbital edema, and facial paresthesia were apparent (Figure 1(a)).

Moreover, the patient reported a decrease in visual acuity. There was no evidence of a lesion inside the mouth. During the course of the study, hyperglycemia was identified (a random blood sugar of about 400). All paranasal sinuses had mucosal thickening and partial opacification, which was linked to orbital involvement with retrobulbar invasion. During the ocular evaluation, ptosis, proptosis, and chemosis, concomitant ophthalmoplegia and bilateral loss of vision were discovered (the identified visual acuity, using the semiquantitative scale, was light perception (LP) in both eyes). The patient was put on intravenous liposomal amphotericin B at 5 mg/kg/day after a clinical diagnosis of mucormycosis.

Extensive erosion of the nasal septum, bilateral middle and inferior turbinates, and anterior and severe necrosis of the posterior ethmoidal mucosal membrane and lamina papyracea were all seen during the initial endoscopic sinus surgery (ESS). The debridement of the base of the skull was conducted, as well as the complete removal of the nasal septum in the middle and posterior portions and the turbinectomy on both sides. The lamina papyracea and preorbital fat were debrided to the point of apparent necrosis.

The patient's cutaneous lesions deteriorated on the second day of his admission in terms of the disease's rapid progression (Figure 1(b)). The patient's visual acuity varied to a state of no light perception (NLP). Liposomal amphotericin B 3.5 mg/mL was administered to the patient via retrobulbar injection.

Following substantial midfacial bone erosion and skin necrosis, the second surgery was performed (Figure 1(c)). In the second surgery, intraoperative results indicated a necrotic lesion extending from the inferior border of the left orbit to both sides of the nasal bones, which was debrided. The skin in the midface area had a considerable defect, which was reconstructed using advancement flaps following maximal debridement of the bone and skin (Figure 1(d)). Patients reported persistent headaches and fever on the seventh day despite continued antifungal treatment.

A contrast-enhanced brain and orbital magnetic resonance imaging (MRI) revealed the destruction of sinuses walls and intraorbital and intracranial extension with

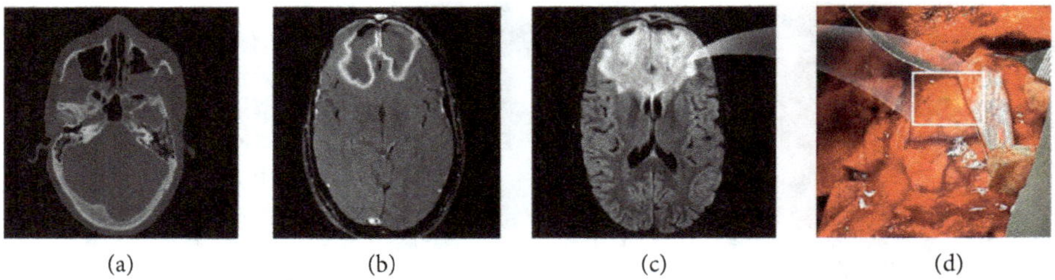

FIGURE 2: Radiologic characteristics of COVID-19-associated mucormycosis: (a) axial bone window CT scan demonstrated partial opacification of bilateral maxillary and sphenoid sinuses. (b) Axial postcontrast T1 weighted image revealed smooth ring enhancement in bilateral frontal lobes mass; (c) axial fluid-attenuated inversion recovery MRI showed a hyperintense mass containing air bubbles with perilesional vasogenic edema in bilateral frontal lobes; (d) drainage of the yellow brain abscess material using craniotomy.

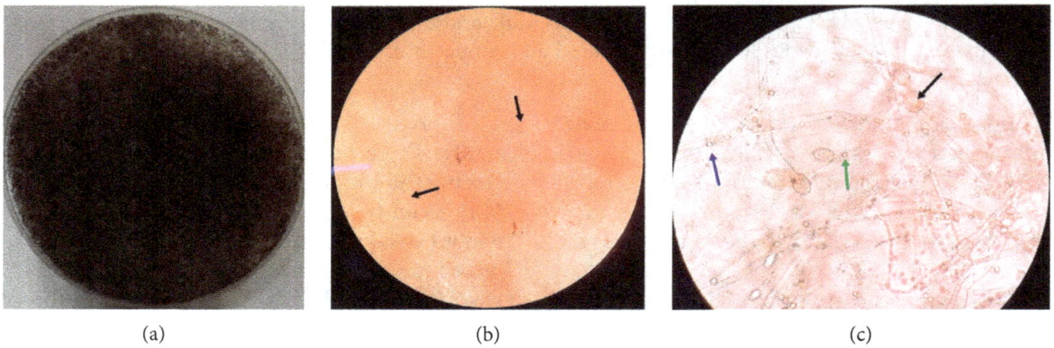

FIGURE 3: Mycology confirmation and detection of fungal elements by phenotypic methods: (a) grayish brown colony of Rhizopus spp. on Sabouraud dextrose agar with chloramphenicol; (b) direct microscopy with potassium hydroxide 10% (KOH 10%) shows broad and aseptate hyphae of Rhizopus spp. in necrotic tissue (black arrows), ×40; (c) reproductive structures of *Rhizopus* spp. sporangium (black arrow), sporangiophore (blue arrow), and sporangiospores (green arrow), ×40.

bilateral frontal and right temporal lobe abscess formation and intraconal and extraconal fat edema and thickening and hyperintensity of extraocular muscles in both orbits, consistent with invasive fungal sinusitis.

The patient's condition had worsened to the point that he was confused. As a result of a mass lesion in the frontal lobe, he underwent craniotomy (Figure 2).

Direct examination of the biopsy of involved tissue in the fungal abscess with potassium hydroxide 10% (KOH 10%) showed aseptate hyphae in necrotic tissues compatible with mucormycosis. A three-day-old culture on Sabouraud dextrose agar (Merck, USA) with chloramphenicol revealed a greyish-brown colony of *Rhizopus* spp. and broad sporangiophores with sporangia and round sporangiospores under the microscope. Biopsy reports from the affected sinuses were in agreement with this conclusion (Figure 3).

After a few weeks, the patient was released with bilateral blindness. Despite this, there was no evidence of disease recurrence during the four-month follow-up.

3. Discussion

It is extremely rare for an immunocompetent patient to present with bilateral orbital mucormycosis accompanied by a brain abscess in the post-COVID-19 phase. The clinical importance of our report was its bilateral presentation and CNS progress, so it is important to consider cerebral CAM in any patient with an altered level of consciousness in the setting of CAM.

In general, mucormycosis is an opportunistic and life-threatening infection usually associated with certain predisposing conditions, such as uncontrolled diabetes, use of corticosteroids, immunosuppressive therapy, immunodeficiency state, malignancies, transplantation, iron overload, intravenous drug use, chronic alcoholism, and malnutrition [10]. In particular, diabetes mellitus, particularly with ketoacidosis, is the most commonly reported risk factor in non-COVID-19 mucormycosis, for 54–76% of such cases in India, Iran, and Mexico [11].

During the COVID-19 pandemic, the clinicoepidemiological pattern of mucormycosis changed, with typical risk factors such as diabetes, transplantation, and hematological malignancies being absent. The development of CAM can probably be attributed to acute hyperglycemia. Thus, using glucocorticoids in mild COVID-19 cases (without hypoxemia) or using higher doses of glucocorticoids should be avoided [12].

Mucorales spores are widely distributed in soil, decaying organic material, and animal feces. Our patient's susceptibility to mucormycosis infection and germination and multiplication of the fungus spores may have been increased as a result of his history of smoking Anbarnesa, a traditional Iranian medicine, or using unclean humidifiers and oxygen delivery masks [3, 6, 13]. The inhalation of Anbarnesa smoke is used to cure a variety of illnesses, including viral infections. Anbarnesa has a considerable impact on the rapid healing of various types of ulcers, notably burn wounds. It has the most potent antioxidant property in higher doses [14].

In our patient, one of the primary signs and symptoms of CAM was secondary cutaneous mucormycosis in the periorbital area. Secondary cutaneous mucormycosis usually develops as a result of disseminated or rhinocerebral infection. Tissue infarction may occur quickly, resulting in the appearance of a black eschar with central ulceration [15]. During infection, the mentioned patient develops progressively spreading cutaneous necrosis. Although the relationship between facial cutaneous necrosis and poor prognosis was statistically insignificant, it appears to be clinically meaningful [15, 16].

Due to the continuous spread of the paranasal sinuses and orbits, CNS involvement is regarded as a significant and unusual consequence of CAM [1, 7]. Possible pathway for brain involvement during ROCM includes (a) nasopharyngeal mucosa penetration and spreading to the brain via blood or lymphatic vessels, (b) proliferation in the internal elastic lamina, entering the endothelium and subsequently obstructing the cerebral vascular lumen, (c) hematogenous transmission via perforating branches of the middle cerebral artery, and finally, (d) host innate immune cells impairment and decrease in antifungal drugs access to Mucorales in terms of the hemorrhagic necrosis and infarction of the brain [17, 18].

Because antifungals cannot reach necrotic tissues, vigorous surgical debridement of necrotic tissues should be explored as soon as a diagnosis of any type of CAM is suspected. Debridement is often disfiguring in instances of rhinocerebral infection, requiring the removal of the palate, nasal cartilage, and orbit. Recent evidence suggests that endoscopic debridement can be accomplished with minimal tissue loss [19, 20]. The treatment of choice for initial antifungal therapy in CAM is intravenous amphotericin B. Patients who do not respond to or cannot tolerate amphotericin B may even receive posaconazole or isavuconazole as salvage or alternative therapy [19]. There are no randomized studies to manage the neurological complications associated with CAM; most of the recommendations are essentially based on expert's opinions.

Decompressive craniectomy may be done in space-occupying lesions to reduce intracranial pressure (ICP) [19]. The management of septic cerebral venous disease, including cavernous sinus thrombosis, in patients with CAM, is challenging. On the one hand, thrombosis formation in CNS is associated with known CNS complications, and on the other hand, thrombosis can prevent the spread of infection, there is a risk of intracranial haemorrhage due to the angioinvasive nature of the fungus. As a result, no firm conclusions can be drawn about the use of systemic anticoagulants in the management of septic cerebral venous thrombosis in the context of CAM [8, 21]. Routine use of antibiotics and prophylactic use of antiepileptic medication are not recommended [19].

4. Conclusion

Mucormycosis should be included in the differential diagnosis when there is no obvious explanation for a worsening clinical course in COVID-19 area. Clinicians should be aware of the potential factors related to CAM and the critical role of optimal glycemic control. A multidisciplinary team approach to addressing fungal infections is essential since it involves early identification, surgical removal of contaminated tissue, optimum antifungal medication, and follow-up care. They should boost their clinical knowledge of the mucocutaneous, ocular, and central nervous system involvement of CAM and educate their patients about these warning signs to provide prompt diagnosis and timely medicinal or surgical management to have a promising outcome.

Consent

A signed statement of informed consent to publish patient data was obtained from the patient.

References

[1] F. Yasmin, H. Najeeb, A. Naeem et al., "COVID-19 associated mucormycosis: a systematic review from diagnostic challenges to management," *Diseases*, vol. 9, no. 4, p. 65, 2021.

[2] O. A. Cornely, A. Alastruey-Izquierdo, D. Arenz et al., "Global guideline for the diagnosis and management of mucormycosis: an initiative of the European confederation of medical mycology in cooperation with the mycoses study group education and research consortium," *The Lancet Infectious Diseases*, vol. 19, 2019.

[3] J. Mathew, A. M. Id, H. Ibrahim, A. Razack, and T. Mathew, "COVID-19—associated mucormycosis: Evidence-based critical review of an emerging infection burden during the pandemic's second wave in India," *PLoS neglected tropical diseases*, vol. 15, Article ID e0009921, 2021.

[4] J. A. Al-Tawfiq, S. Alhumaid, A. N. Alshukairi et al., "COVID-19 and mucormycosis superinfection: the perfect storm," *Infection*, vol. 49, no. 5, pp. 833–853, 2021.

[5] K. Ramphul, R. Verma, N. Kumar, Y. Ramphul, S. Mejias, and P. Lohana, "Rising concerns of mucormycosis (Zygomycosis) among covid-19 patients; an analysis and review based on case reports in literature," *Acta BioMedica: Atenei Parmensis*, vol. 92, no. 4, 2021.

[6] M. Pourazizi, R. Mohammadi, and B. Abtahi-Naeini, "COVID-19 associated mucormycosis and anbarnesa: concerning about important source of spores," *Iranian Journal of Public Health*, vol. 51, no. 1, pp. 223–225, 2022.

[7] G. Singh and V. Y. Vishnu, "Neurological manifestations of rhino-oculo-cerebral mucormycosis in the COVID-19 era," *Nature Reviews Neurology*, vol. 17, no. 11, pp. 657-658, 2021.

[8] M. Dinkin, A. Patsalides, and M. Ertel, "Diagnosis and management of cerebral venous diseases in neuro-ophthalmology: ongoing controversies," *Asia-Pacific journal of ophthalmology (Philadelphia, Pa.)*, vol. 8, no. 1, pp. 73–85, 2019.

[9] M. S. Bae, E. J. Kim, K. M. Lee, and W. S. Choi, "Rapidly progressive rhino-orbito-cerebral mucormycosis complicated with unilateral internal carotid artery occlusion: a case report," *Neurointervention*, vol. 7, no. 1, p. 45, 2012.
[10] I. Mahalaxmi, K. Jayaramayya, and D. Venkatesan, *Elsevier Has Created a COVID-19 Resource Centre with Free Information in English and Mandarin on the Novel Coronavirus COVID- 19. The COVID-19 Resource Centre Is Hosted*, Elsevier Connect, the company's public news and information, Amsterdam, Netherlands, 2020.
[11] J. Stemler, K. Hamed, J. Salmanton-García et al., "Mucormycosis in the Middle East and north africa: analysis of the FungiScope® registry and cases from the literature," *Mycoses*, vol. 63, no. 10, 2020.
[12] L. M. Kimmig, D. Wu, M. Gold, N. N. Pettit, D. Pitrak, and J. Mueller, "IL-6 inhibition in critically ill COVID-19 patients is associated with increased secondary infections," *Frontiers in Medicine*, vol. 7, 2020.
[13] M. Bhatia, "The rise of mucormycosis in Covid-19 patients in India," *Expert Review of Anti-infective Therapy*, vol. 20, no. 2, pp. 137-138, 2021.
[14] S. A. Moghadam, F. R. Charati, R. Akbari, E. G. Alamdari, and B. Behmanesh, "Consideration antimicrobial and antioxidant properties of anbarnesa smoke ointment," *Journal of Medicinal and Chemical Sciences*, vol. 3, no. 3, pp. 245–253, 2020.
[15] A. D. Castrejón-pérez, I. Miranda, and O. Welsh, "Cutaneous Mucormycosis," *Anais Brasileiros De Dermatologia*, vol. 92, pp. 304–311, 2017.
[16] B. E. Shields, M. Rosenbach, Z. Brown-Joel, A. P. Berger, B. A. Ford, and K. A. Wanat, "Angioinvasive fungal infections impacting the skin: background, epidemiology, and clinical presentation," *Journal of the American Academy of Dermatology*, vol. 80, no. 4, 2019.
[17] G. J. Zhang, S. K. Zhang, Z. Wang et al., "Fatal and rapid progressive isolated cerebral mucormycosis involving the bilateral basal ganglia: a case report," *Frontiers in Neurology*, vol. 11, pp. 295-296, 2020.
[18] A. Chikley, R. Ben-Ami, and D. P. Kontoyiannis, "Mucormycosis of the central nervous system," *Journal of Fungi*, vol. 5, no. 3, pp. 59–20, 2019.
[19] H. S. Malhotra, P. Gupta, D. Mehrotra et al., "COVID-19 associated mucormycosis: staging and management recommendations (Report of a multi-disciplinary expert committee)," *Journal of Oral Biology and Craniofacial Research*, vol. 11, no. 4, pp. 569–580, 2021.
[20] L. Ponce-Rosas, J. Gonzales-Zamora, N. Diaz-Reyes, O. Alarco-Cadillo, and J. Alave-Rosas, "Rhino-orbital-cerebral mucormycosis in a post-COVID-19 patient from Peru," *Case Reports in Infectious Diseases*, vol. 2022, Article ID 2537186, 6 pages, 2022.
[21] I. A. Khatri and M. Wasay, "Septic cerebral venous sinus thrombosis," *Journal of the Neurological Sciences*, vol. 362, pp. 221–227, 2016.

14

Disseminated Cryptococcosis in a Non-HIV Patient in Singapore

Jonathan See, Kok Choon Raymond Fong, and Humaira Shafi

Department of Infectious Disease, Changi General Hospital, 2 Simei Street 3, Singapore 529889

Correspondence should be addressed to Jonathan See; jonathansee@outlook.sg

Academic Editor: George N. Dalekos

We present a case of disseminated cryptococcosis (DC) in a 71-year-old gentleman with systemic lupus erythematosus (SLE) on long-term corticosteroids. He initially presented with right arm cellulitis in a tertiary hospital in Singapore and was subsequently diagnosed with DC involving skin, meninges, blood, and possibly pulmonary involvement. He eventually succumbed to the disease despite prolonged antifungal therapy. Through this case, we wish to highlight an atypical clinical presentation of an uncommon infection and hope to share the importance of considering DC in the differential diagnosis of nonresolving cellulitis among immunocompromised individuals. Mortality and morbidity rates for this condition remain high despite appropriate treatment. Early diagnosis and treatment are crucial for improved outcomes. More research is needed to improve the therapeutic modalities for treatment of DC and to improve the clinical outcomes for this life-threatening condition.

1. Introduction

Cryptococcosis is a disease caused by a basidiomycetous encapsulated yeast-like fungal organism [1]. Two pathogenic species of cryptococcus are known to cause disease in humans. *Cryptococcus gattii* is most commonly responsible for cryptococcosis in immunocompetent individuals, while *Cryptococcus neoformans* (CN) being more common in immunocompromised patients, which include HIV-positive patients, patients with systemic lupus erythematosus (SLE), patients on prolonged immunosuppression therapy, and transplant recipients [1–3].

Cryptococcus neoformans can be found in the natural environment and is often associated with dust, soil, contaminated food, plants, and bird faeces [1, 2]. Clinical manifestation can range from asymptomatic pulmonary colonisation to life-threatening meningitis and disseminated infection [4, 5] with pulmonary and central nervous system (CNS) being the most common sites reported for patients with disseminated cryptococcosis (DC) [3, 6]. Skin involvement is generally rare in cryptococcosis, and it occurs in 10–20% of patients. Cutaneous cryptococcosis typically presents with different clinical morphologies including acneiform papules, ulcers, subcutaneous nodules, and, rarely, as cellulitis [7, 8]. Cryptococcal cellulitis, in particular, is usually indistinguishable from bacterial forms, and its delayed diagnosis usually predicts a worse outcome [7, 9, 10].

In Southeast Asia, cryptococcosis is common amongst HIV-infected individuals, with an estimated 120 cases per 1000 HIV-infected individuals per year [11]. SLE patients represent an important group who are susceptible to infection because of disease-related immunological defects and concurrent immunosuppression [12]. The growing size of the immunocompromised patient population from chemotherapy and biological agents further contributes to the medical importance of cryptococcosis [13].

2. Case Presentation

A 71-year-old male patient with a past medical history of SLE and lupus nephritis, who had been on prednisolone for 20 years, was referred to our hospital by his general practitioner after presenting with right arm swelling and erythema of 5 days duration that did not improve despite oral amoxicillin/clavulinic acid. A review of system was unremarkable for headaches, confusion, cough, sputum, shortness of breath, and fever. He had not been exposed to any bird excrement.

On admission he was afebrile, his blood pressure was 122/88 mmHg, pulse rate was 82/min, and respiratory rate

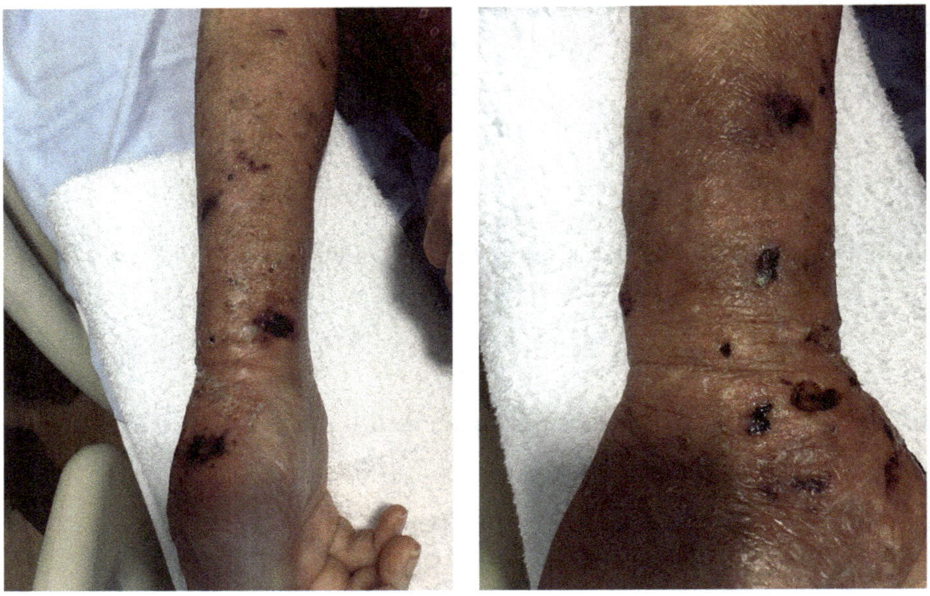

(a) (b)

FIGURE 1: Patient's right forearm cellulitic skin changes and bullae on admission.

TABLE 1: Investigations on day 1 of admission.

Test	Findings
C-reactive protein (CRP)	112.6 mg/L
Procalcitonin	0.44 μg/L
White blood cell count	5.3×10^9/L
Neutrophil count	4.5×10^9/L
Lymphocyte count	0.3×10^9/L
HIV screen	Nonreactive
Chest X-ray	No confluent consolidation is detected. Linear atelectasis of the left lower zone is noted with a stable left pleural effusion

was 18/min and was saturating at 98% on room air. He was noted to have left basal crepitation and bipedal edema. Skin examination (Figure 1) showed diffuse right upper limb pitting edema and erythema, with multiple 1-2 cm hemorrhagic tender bullae scattered over the forearm.

On day 1 of admission, blood cultures were taken, investigations were done (Table 1), and intravenous (IV) cefazolin was started. On day 3, antibiotics were escalated to IV piperacillin-tazobactam because of the temperature of 37.7°C, persistent swelling, and erythema.

Blood culture yielded CN on day 6 of admission and amphotericin-B was commenced. Lumbar puncture was performed which isolated CN on cultures. Antifungal therapy was optimized to liposomal IV amphotericin-B (AmBisome based on 4-5 mg/kg) and oral flucytosine 1 g Q12H (based on 25 mg/kg).

After further investigations (Table 2), clinical impression was for DC involving blood, CNS, lung, and skin involvement. Modest improvement in the skin infection was noted after starting antifungal therapy (Figure 2). Biochemically, CRP also downtrended (Table 3).

Blood culture was sterilised after 8 days of starting antifungals, but CSF culture remained positive for CN at day 10 of treatment (Table 4).

Prednisolone 15 mg/day was lowered to 10 mg/day after discussion with rheumatologist. Further hospital course was complicated by acute on chronic thrombocytopenia secondary to flucytosine, which led to discontinuation of flucytosine after 19 days of administration. He also developed worsening of chronic kidney disease (CKD), fluid overload, haemorrhoidal bleeding, and worsening of anemia. AmBisome was discontinued after 22 days, and the patient was terminally discharged to home in keeping with his wishes. He demised 30 days after initial presentation.

3. Discussion

Cryptococcosis is a serious infection that predominantly affects immunocompromised patients. In this case, the patient was on long-term corticosteroids for 20 years for SLE. He did not receive disease modifying agents. Our patient also had CKD-3 secondary to lupus nephritis. As reported in multiple studies, patients with higher mortality

Table 2: Further investigations (day 7–10) leading to diagnosis of disseminated cryptococcosis.

Test	Findings
Serum cryptococcal antigen (CRAG)	Titer ≥ 1 : 2560
Blood fungal culture	CN
Computed tomography (CT) thorax scan	Patchy areas of consolidation in the left perihilar region and right lower lobe along with scattered subcentimeter pulmonary nodules which suggested infective changes of pulmonary cryptococcosis on a background of fluid overload contributed by congestive cardiac failure and worsening renal function
CT brain scan	No space occupying lesion, no mass effect, and no intracranial hemorrhage or territorial infarcts
Lumbar puncture	
Opening pressure	10.0 cm water
Cerebrospinal fluid (CSF) gram stain	Encapsulated blasticonidia (yeasts)
CSF fungal microscopy	Encapsulated blasticonidia seen, morphology suggestive of *Cryptococcus*
CSF CRAG	Titer ≥ 1 : 2560
CSF fungal culture	CN
CSF aerobic culture	CN
Skin swab taken from blisters	
Skin fungal culture	CN
Skin aerobic culture	CN

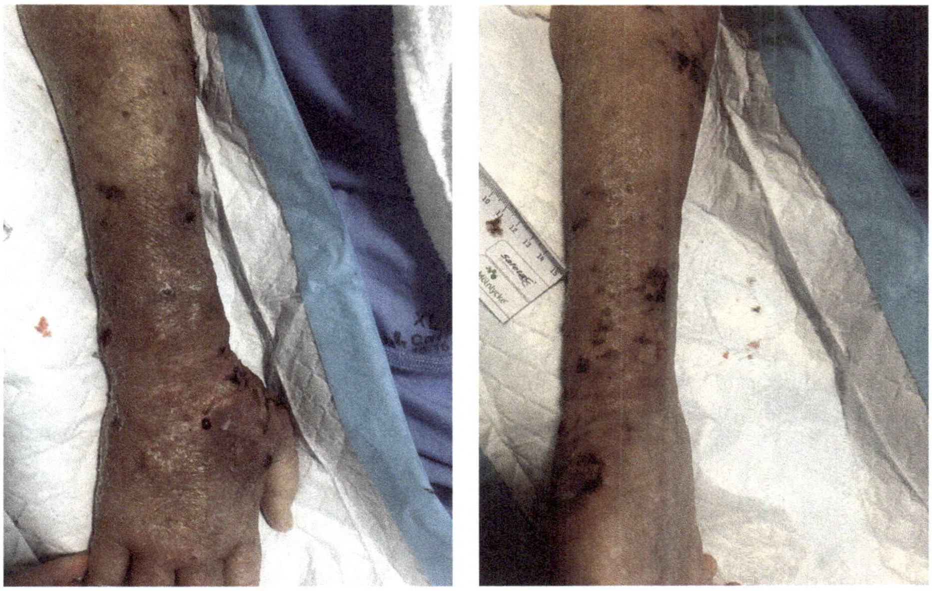

(a) (b)

Figure 2: Patient's right forearm improvement 10 days after appropriate antifungal therapy.

Table 3: C-reactive protein trend in response to antifungal therapy.

CRP (mg/L) on day 6	CRP (mg/L) on day 10	CRP (mg/L) on day 14
117.2	41.7	33.6

risk in cryptococcosis have baseline renal impairment, disseminated disease, and HIV-negative; all 3 factors are present for our patient [14–16].

Cryptococcosis presenting with skin infection/cellulitis is atypical. International literature has shown that skin involvement occurs in only 10–20% of patients [7, 8]. In a large retrospective Singapore study in 2014, only 6 out of 62 patients (9.7%) with cryptococcosis had skin findings [17, 18]. Presenting symptoms were fever (79%), headache (71%), and cough (45%), all of which were absent in our patient during initial presentation. Furthermore, cryptococcosis occurring in HIV-negative patients is relatively rare

Table 4: Repeated microbiological investigations after 10 days of treatment.

Test	Findings
Serum CRAG	Titer ≥ 1 : 2560
Blood fungal culture	Negative after 8 days of starting combination antifungals
Lumbar puncture	
Opening pressure	15.0 cm water
CSF gram stain	Encapsulated blasticonidia (yeasts)
CSF fungal microscopy	Encapsulated blasticonidia seen, morphology suggestive of *Cryptococcus*
CSF CRAG	Titer ≥ 1 : 2560
CSF fungal culture	CN
CSF aerobic culture	CN

as well; only 19% of patients (12 out of 62) in the same study reported cryptococcosis in HIV-negative.

An atypical presentation coupled with atypical risk-group contributed to a delayed diagnosis in our reported case. This corresponds to the study by Chan et al. which revealed that delay in treatment significantly increased in HIV-negative patients ($p = 0.03$) [17, 18]. Prognosis of non-HIV patients with DC is relatively poor compared to HIV patients; studies have reported 1-month mortality rates of 63%, with 81% of deaths occurring within 2 weeks of diagnosis [16]. Delayed diagnosis leading to delay in appropriate treatment is likely to contribute to increased mortality in non-HIV patients.

This case highlights several important points. Firstly, clinicians need to recognise cryptococcosis as a severe systemic infection as it can yield unfavorable outcomes despite treatment, more so in the setting of late diagnosis and initiation of treatment. Secondly, inflammatory skin changes should be promptly investigated for differential diagnoses other than bacterial in immunocompromised hosts and when not responding to conventional antimicrobial treatment as in our case. Thirdly, this case also illustrates how cryptococcosis is known to masquerade conditions like bacterial cellulitis, panniculitis, papules, pustules, nodules, abscesses, edema, ulcers, and mollusum contagiousum-like lesions [19]. Such a wide range of skin presentations makes clinching the diagnosis challenging; in our case, initial dermatology consult suspected the presentation to be due to edema blisters. The need to consider a broader differential diagnosis early in the setting of atypical skin infections in the immunocompromised population cannot be overemphasized through this case.

Lastly, this case also highlights the present challenges with treatment of cryptococcosis. Current recommendations for anticryptoccocal treatment include amphotericin-B (L-AMB as a substitute for amphotericin-B in cases of intolerance) with flucytosine, in non-HIV, nontransplant hosts [20]. Antifungals have side effects and complications, including hematological cell line suppression and renal toxicity. This may prevent efficacious antifungal treatment in patients with comorbid conditions. Furthermore, in autoimmune conditions, antifungal treatment can be further complicated by the complexity of the primary disease. Reduction in immunosuppression has to be balanced against risk of flare, leaving physicians with a delicate balance to thread upon. This is in contrast with HIV patients with cryptococcosis, whereby stronger antiretroviral therapy only serves to aid in the management of both cryptococcosis and HIV, allowing physicians with less management dilemma.

Additional Points

Learning Points. (1) Cryptococcal and atypical mycobacterial skin infections should be reasoned in immunocompromised patients including non-HIV patients because delay in diagnosis and treatment corresponds with increased mortality and morbidity. Skin manifestation of DC, while rare, should be considered when lack of response is observed with conventional antimicrobial therapy for skin and soft tissue infections. (2) Recognising the difficulties in management of cryptococcosis with concurrent autoimmune conditions—multidisciplinary teams may be consulted early to strike a fine balance between adequate immunosuppression and promoting a stronger immune response against the ongoing infection. (3) Mortality remains substantial. Antifungal treatment for cryptococcosis—despite extensive knowledge of cryptococcosis in recent years, our treatment modalities remain limited. Serious side effects limit the efficacy of treatment. Safer and potent antifungal treatment modalities are needed with viable second-line and even third-line alternatives to fall back upon, should first-line treatment be contraindicated due to side effects.

Consent

Informed consent has been obtained from the patient's relative for the writing and submission of this case report. Consent was obtained from patient's relatives as the patient is deceased.

References

[1] C. Probst, G. Pongratz, S. Capellino et al., "Cryptococcosis mimicking cutaneous cellulitis in a patient suffering from rheumatoid arthritis:a case report," *BMC Infectious Diseases*, vol. 10, no. 1, p. 239, 2010.

[2] G. N. Srivastava, R. Tilak, J. Yadav, and M. Bansal, "Cutaneous cryptococcus: marker for disseminated infection," *BMJ Case Reports*, vol. 2015, 2015.
[3] E. S. Valente, M. C. Lazzarin, B. L. Koech et al., "Disseminated cryptococcosis presenting as cutaneous cellulitis in an adolescent with systemic lupus erythematosus," *Infectious Disease Reports*, vol. 7, no. 2, p. 5743, 2015.
[4] J. R. Perfect, D. T. Durack, and H. A. Gallis, "Cryptococcemia," *Medicine*, vol. 62, no. 2, pp. 98–109, 1983.
[5] S. M. Levitz, "The ecology of Cryptococcus neoformans and the epidemiology of cryptococcosis," *Clinical Infectious Diseases*, vol. 13, no. 6, pp. 1163-1169, 1991.
[6] N. Singh, F. Dromer, J. R. Perfect, and O. Lortholary, "Immunocompromised hosts: cryptococcosis in solid organ transplant recipients: current state of the science," *Clinical Infectious Diseases*, vol. 47, no. 10, pp. 1321–1327, 2008.
[7] J. C. Hall, J. H. Brewer, T. T. Crouch, and K. R. Watson, "Cryptococcal cellulitis with multiple sites of involvement," *Journal of the American Academy of Dermatology*, vol. 17, no. 2, pp. 329–332, 1987.
[8] R. Chaya, S. Padmanabhan, V. Anandaswamy, and A. Moin, "Disseminated cryptococcosis presenting as cellulitis in a renal transplant recipient," *The Journal of Infection in Developing Countries*, vol. 7, no. 1, pp. 60–63, 2013.
[9] H.-C. Lu, Y.-Y. Yang, Y.-L. Huang et al., "Disseminated cryptococcosis initially presenting as cellulitis in a rheumatoid arthritis patient," *Journal of the Chinese Medical Association*, vol. 70, no. 6, pp. 249–252, 2007.
[10] W. Ni, Q. Huang, and J. Cui, "Disseminated cryptococcosis initially presenting as cellulitis in a patient suffering from nephrotic syndrome," *BMC Nephrology*, vol. 14, no. 1, p. 20, 2013.
[11] B. J. Park, K. A. Wannemuehler, B. J. Marston, N. Govender, P. G. Pappas, and T. M. Chiller, "Estimation of the current global burden of cryptococcal meningitis among persons living with HIV/AIDS," *AIDS*, vol. 23, no. 4, pp. 525–530, 2009.
[12] T. Caza, Z. Oaks, and A. Perl, "Interplay of infections, autoimmunity, and immunosuppression in systemic lupus erythematosus," *International Reviews of Immunology*, vol. 33, no. 4, pp. 330–363, 2014.
[13] P. G. Pappas, J. R. Perfect, G. A. Cloud et al., "Cryptococcosis in human immunodeficiency virus-negative patients in the era of effective azole therapy," *Clinical Infectious Diseases*, vol. 33, no. 5, pp. 690–699, 2001.
[14] E. Galanis, L. Macdougall, S. Kidd, M. Morshed, and British Columbia Cryptococcus gattii Working Group, "Epidemiology of Cryptococcus gattii, British Columbia, Canada, 1999–2007," *Emerging Infectious Diseases*, vol. 16, no. 2, pp. 251–257, 2010.
[15] R. A. Seaton, S. Naraqi, J. P. Wembri, and D. A. Warrell, "Predictors of outcome in Cryptococcus neoformans var. gattii meningitis," *QJM*, vol. 89, no. 6, pp. 423–428, 1996.
[16] Y.-M. Chuang, Y.-C. Ho, H.-T. Chang, C.-J. Yu, P.-C. Yang, and P.-R. Hsueh, "Disseminated cryptococcosis in HIV-uninfected patients," *European Journal of Clinical Microbiology and Infectious Diseases*, vol. 27, no. 4, pp. 307–310, 2008.
[17] M. Chan, D. Lye, K. W. Mar, A. Chow, and T. Barkham, "Clinical and microbiological characteristics of cryptococcosis in Singapore: predominance of Cryptococcus neoformans compared with Cryptococcus gattii," *International Journal of Infectious Diseases*, vol. 26, pp. 110–115, 2014.
[18] B. Speed and D. Dunt, "Clinical and host differences between infections with the two varieties of Cryptococcus neoformans," *Clinical Infectious Diseases*, vol. 21, no. 1, pp. 28–34, 1995.
[19] N. Kikuchi, T. Hiraiwa, M. Ishikawa et al., "Cutaneous cryptococcosis mimicking pyoderma gangrenosum: a report of four cases," *Acta Dermato Venereologica*, vol. 96, no. 1, pp. 116-117, 2016.
[20] J. R. Perfect, W. E. Dismukes, F. Dromer et al., "Clinical practice guidelines for the management of Cryptococcal disease: 2010 update by the Infectious Diseases Society of America," *Clinical Infectious Diseases*, vol. 50, no. 3, pp. 291–322, 2010.

15

Candida Empyema as a Red Flag for Esophageal Rupture: A Case Report and Literature Review

Naureen Ali and Getahun Abate

Division of Infectious Diseases, Allergy and Immunology, Saint Louis University, St. Louis, USA

Correspondence should be addressed to Naureen Ali; naureen.ali@health.slu.edu

Academic Editor: Gloria Taliani

Background. *Candida* empyema is a rare entity with an extremely high mortality rate.We present a case of multi species *Candida* empyema in an immunocompetent female patient with Boerhaave syndrome secondary to retching and vomiting after heroin withdrawal. This case highlights an unusual presentation of a common infection but stresses on the fact that a high index of suspicion is necessary for early identification, prompt initiation of antifungal therapy, and drainage with surgical repair to improve overall survival and outcomes.

1. Background

Candida empyema is a rare entity with a crude mortality rate as high as 62% [1]. Patients with underlying malignancies such as esophageal, gastric, and breast cancer are more susceptible to this condition. Other risk factors include recent contiguous surgery including lung and heart transplants [2]. Our patient was a 30-year-old immunocompetent female who developed *Candida* empyema secondary to Boerhaave syndrome.

2. Case Report

Our patient was a 30-year-old Caucasian female with a past medical history of bipolar disorder, depression, generalized anxiety disorder, intravenous heroin use, and migraines who presented to an outside hospital emergency department with acute onset shortness of breath and vomiting. Her symptoms started 2 days prior to presentation after she abruptly stopped using heroin in an attempt to quit. The patient had an extensive history of intravenous drug use. She started using intravenous drugs at 14 years of age, initially using only benzodiazepines and then intravenous heroin. She injected heroin in the large veins of her arms, legs, and neck. She however denied sharing needles. She had been in rehabilitation facilities multiple times in the past and had received methadone for her heroin dependence intermittently during the 4-5 years prior to presentation.

The patient has been having vomiting more than 5 times a day with associated retching. The vomitus was bilious. She was also having shortness of breath which was worsening. In the emergency department, she was afebrile with oral temperature of 98°F but was found to be tachypneic with respiratory rate of 24 breaths per minute and hypoxic with oxygen saturation of 87% on 15 L of oxygen via non-rebreather mask. She was subsequently placed on Bilevel Positive Airway Pressure (BiPAP) for her respiratory distress. Physical examination was only remarkable for bilateral diffuse wheezing and rhonchi.

Initial laboratory workup showed a lactic acid level of 3.05 mmol/L and white blood cell count of $23.0 \times 10^3/\mu L$. A urine drug screen was positive for opiates. Given the concern for sepsis and aspiration pneumonia, blood cultures were obtained and patient was empirically started on intravenous vancomycin (with a goal trough of 15–20 mg/L) and extended infusion piperacillin tazobactam (3.375 mg every 6 hours). Her initial chest X-ray was normal. Treatment for opiate withdrawal at this time was also initiated. After admission to the hospital, she developed a new severe upper back pain and continued to require BiPAP.

A repeat chest X-ray performed on day 2 of her admission at the outside hospital showed a 2.7 cm right-sided pneumothorax (measured from the anterior chest wall) and bilateral small pleural effusions. Another chest X-ray about 3 hours later showed that the pneumothorax was persistent, and therefore a right-sided chest tube was placed with approximately 700 mL of fluid removed. Pleural fluid was cloudy in color, with WBC count of 20,200 × 10E6/L (94% Neutrophils), pH 6.00, LDH 837 U/L, glucose 28 mg/dL, and protein 2.5 g/dL. Serum protein resulted as 9.7 g/dL. The findings were consistent with an exudative effusion or empyema.

On day 3, she developed dysphagia and had increased oral secretions, and had to be intubated for air way protection. Postintubation chest X-ray showed increased width of right-sided pneumothorax to 6.65 cm and a kinked chest tube. The chest tube was manipulated, and it drained another 1.0 L of pleural fluid. Overnight, the patient's oxygen requirement increased, necessitating FiO_2 change to 90% and positive end expiratory pressure (PEEP) of 10 cmH_2O. The patient was subsequently transferred to a tertiary care hospital for further management.

At our hospital, a repeat chest X-ray was obtained which showed that the chest tube and endotracheal tube were in place. There was now a left-sided pleural effusion, but the right-sided pneumothorax and effusion had apparently resolved. Antibiotics were switched to ampicillin-sulbactam (3 g intravenous every 6 hours) for suspected aspiration pneumonia. Other laboratory tests indicated that patient was negative for human immunodeficiency virus and positive for hepatitis C.

On day 2 of admission to our hospital (i.e., day 4 since presentation), the patient's condition improved. She was extubated and oxygen nasal cannula was placed. Pleural fluid obtained at the outside hospital grew *Candida albicans*, and therefore intravenous micafungin (100 mg daily) was initiated. At this point, the Infectious Diseases team was consulted for possible *Candida* empyema. It was found that patient's main initial problem soon after she stopped using heroin was severe retching. She was unable to sleep because of retching. She subsequently developed worsening shortness of breath. On examination, she was noted to have a whitish coating on the tongue and oral mucosa suggestive of oral thrush. A CT of the chest was obtained which showed a right apical chest tube within a large loculated appearing right pleural effusion containing locules of gas, likely representing empyema and a moderate to large loculated right pneumothorax anteriorly with mediastinal shift to the left (Figure 1). The patient was having fever with a maximum oral temperature of 102.7°F. The chest tube remained in place during this time. Antibiotics were changed to intravenous meropenem 1 gram every 8 hours and intravenous fluconazole (400 mg daily). Because of history of sever retching, oral thrush, pneumothorax and *Candida* empyema, esophageal perforation was suspected. An esophagogram with water soluble contrast was obtained and confirmed esophageal perforation with contrast extravasation at the level of gastroesophageal junction (Figure 2).

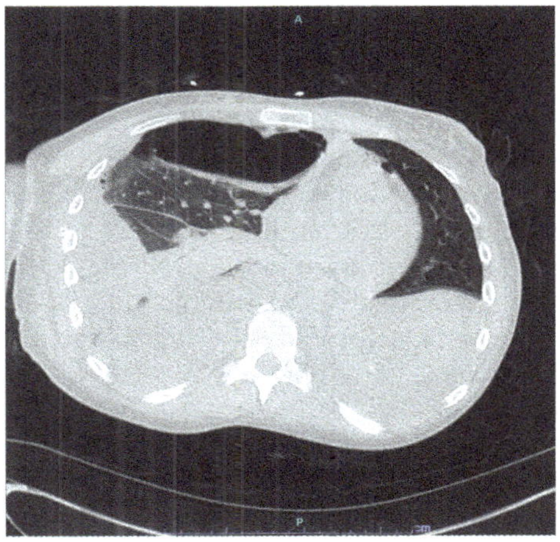

Figure 1: Computed tomography (CT) of the chest without contrast: moderate-large loculated right pneumothorax anteriorly with mediastinal shift to the left suggesting tension component and small volume pneumomediastinum.

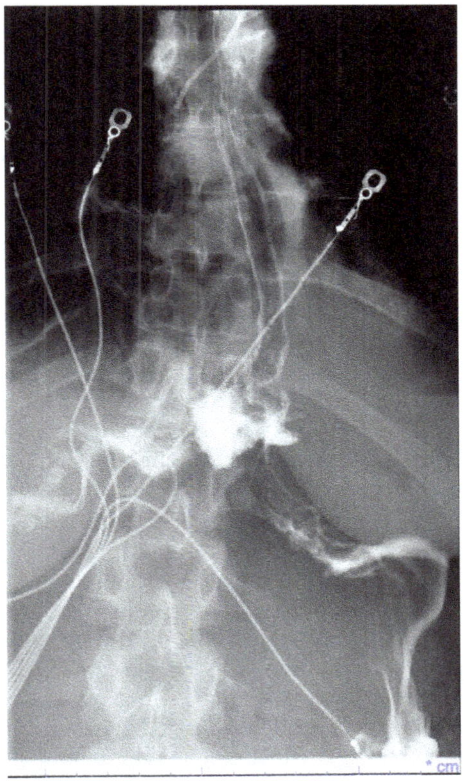

Figure 2: Esophagogram: esophageal perforation with contrast extravasation at the approximate level of the gastroesophageal junction.

On day 4 at our hospital (i.e., day 6 since presentation), the patient underwent a right thoracotomy with decortication and repair of esophageal perforation about 3–5 centimeters above the hiatus. Gross pus and gelatinous material were found in the pleural cavity which were evacuated and sent for culture.

On day 6 at our hospital (i.e., day 8 since presentation), the results of pleural fluid culture obtained at the outside hospital were updated and reported to grow *Candida albicans, Candida dubliniensis, Candida glabrata, and Bacillus* species (not cereus or anthracis). *Candida albicans* was susceptible to anidulafungin, caspofungin, fluconazole with minimum inhibitory concentration (MIC) of 0.25 μg/mL, micafungin, and voriconazole. There were no established Clinical and Laboratory Standards Institute (CLSI) breakpoints to interpret susceptibility of *Candida dubliniensis,* but MICs for the above drugs were <0.08–0.5 which were in susceptible range if CLSI standards for *Candida albicans* were used. *Candida glabrata* was susceptible to anidulafungin, caspofungin, fluconazole (MIC 16), and micafungin. *Bacillus* species was sensitive to meropenem, levofloxacin, trimethoprim sulfamethoxazole, vancomycin, and gentamycin and resistant to penicillin and clindamycin.

Surgical samples obtained during the decortication grew *Candida albicans, Candida dubliniensis,* and *Streptococcus viridans* group (sensitivity testing was not done). Multiple routine blood and blood fungal cultures obtained throughout the admission remained negative. A transthoracic echocardiogram (TTE) was performed and was negative for cardiac valvular vegetations. Therefore, because of negative blood cultures and a negative TTE, endocarditis was considered less likely. A transesophageal echocardiogram could not be performed because of esophageal perforation.

In the following days, the patient's condition improved, and she was switched to intravenous vancomycin (with a goal trough of 15–20 μg/mL), intravenous ampicillin-sulbactam (3 g every 6 hours) and intravenous micafungin (100 mg daily) to complete 3 weeks of therapy from initiation of appropriate antifungal agent (a total of 4 weeks of therapy). A repeat chest CT scan prior to completion of antibiotic therapy demonstrated pleural-based scarring in the lung bases on the right with minimal atelectatic changes. There was no evidence of pneumomediastinum, pneumothorax, or recurrent rupture of the esophagus.

3. Discussion

Here we present a case of *Candida* empyema in a patient with history of severe retching, oral thrush, and esophageal rupture. Our patient was an otherwise healthy female who developed persistent vomiting and retching while attempting to quit heroin use at home. *Candida* empyema is extremely rare and has been reported to occur due to inoculation of the pleural space by *Candida* species secondary to esophageal perforation, extension of abdominal or pulmonary infections, thoracic or abdominal surgical interventions, or from repeated thoracentesis procedures. [1].

In our case, we became concerned about possible esophageal rupture due to history of severe retching, worsening shortness of breath, persistent inability to swallow, oral thrush, and *Candida* empyema. Given the significant oral thrush on examination and pleural fluid cultures also growing *Candida,* our suspicion for a possible perforation was high which prompted us to pursue an esophagogram, resulting in the eventual diagnosis.

Culture results of *Candida* typically take several days, particularly to report sensitivities. Our patient had multiple *Candida* species isolated from her pleural fluid including *Candida albicans, Candida dubliniensis,* and *Candida glabrata* which is extremely rare [3]. Only a handful of cases have been reported in literature with esophageal or gastric ulcer perforation as the cause of *Candida* empyema [4].

Patients with fungal empyema generally benefit from surgery and systemic antifungal therapy. There is an increased risk of morbidity and mortality in immunocompromised patients particularly those with respiratory failure [5], hence early identification, initiation of antifungal therapy, drainage, and surgical repair is necessary to improve overall morbidity and mortality. Multiple studies have identified *Candida albicans* as the most common isolate [1, 6]. Because *Candida* empyema is rare, there are no randomized controlled trials to guide medical or surgical management of these cases. There are, however, case series and single center experience reports which indicate that 2–4 weeks of antibiotic treatment are usually used [1, 2]. Despite appropriate medical treatment, the mortality can be as high as 54% [1, 2] indicating the need for more aggressive work up and management. Physicians should have a high index of suspicion for esophageal perforation in patients presenting with pneumothorax in a setting of recent severe retching. Esophago or gastropleural fistulas should be considered as possible causes of *Candida* empyema. In some cases, patients may have bacterial superinfection of the empyema as seen here with *Bacillus* and *Streptococcus viridans* group isolated from patient's pleural fluid.

4. Conclusion

In summary, our case demonstrates that *Candida* empyema is a rare but serious complication of Boerhaave syndrome. High risk and immunocompromised patients have a greater predisposition to fungal infections and are more susceptible to this entity.

References

[1] K.-H. Lin, Y.-M. Liu, P.-C. Lin et al., "Report of a 63-case series of *Candida* empyema thoracis: 9-year experience of two medical centers in central Taiwan," *Journal of Microbiology, Immunology and Infection*, vol. 47, no. 1, pp. 36–41, 2014.

[2] J. Williams, O. A. Lanfranco, J. Lemos-Ramirez, P. Bhargava, G. Alangaden, and M. Ramesh, "Epidemiology, risk factors and outcomes of *Candida* empyema: a 5-year single-centered experience," *Open Forum Infectious Diseases*, vol. 4, no. 1, p. S88, 2017.

[3] V. Chandrasekaran, B. A. El-Shiekh, and C. A. Karaffa, "Candida (torulopsis) glabrate: a new pathogen found in an empyema," *Clinical Infectious Diseases*, vol. 28, no. 4, pp. 922-923, 1999.

[4] T. Ishiguro, N. Takayanagi, T. Ikeya et al., "Isolation of *Candida* species is an important clue for suspecting gastrointestinal tract perforation as a cause of empyema," *Internal Medicine*, vol. 49, no. 18, pp. 1957–1964, 2010.
[5] S.-C. Ko, K.-Y. Chen, P.-R. Hsueh, K.-T. Luh, and P.-C. Yang, "Fungal empyema thoracis: an emerging clinical entity," *Chest*, vol. 117, no. 6, pp. 1672–1678, 2000.
[6] H.-S. Lin, C.-M. Chao, W.-T. Lin, and C.-C. Lai, "*Candida* empyema thoracis at a hospital in Taiwan," *Surgical Infections*, vol. 15, no. 5, pp. 540–543, 2014.

16

Failed Early Intervention of Pyomyositis in an Immunocompetent Individual

Ranna Al-Dossari[1] and **Sana Zekri**[2]

[1]*University of North Texas Health Science Center, Texas College of Osteopathic Medicine, Fort Worth, TX, USA*
[2]*John Peter Smith Health System, Fort Worth, TX, USA*

Correspondence should be addressed to Ranna Al-Dossari; rga0045@my.unthsc.edu

Academic Editor: Alexandre R. Marra

Pyomyositis is a purulent infection of striated muscle tissue that usually leads to an abscess, commonly due to *S. aureus*. Pyomyositis is typically found in tropic regions, but it is increasingly being recognized in temperate climates, especially in immunocompromised individuals. Patient presentation ranges from afebrile with mildly elevated WBC to frank sepsis. In many reported cases, patients may develop multiple abscesses at different sites. We report a case of a 54-year-old male with a history of chronic obstructive pulmonary disease (COPD) presenting with right pectoral infection. This case demonstrates the possibility that antibiotic therapy in early presentations may not effectively prevent abscess formation, contrary to treatment suggestions found in the literature.

1. Introduction

The first reported case of pyomyositis in temperate climates was in 1971 [1]. Further reported cases demonstrated a predilection in adults with a 3 : 1 male-to-female ratio [1]. The pathophysiology of pyomyositis is unknown but is proposed to be due to hematogenous bacterial spread and seeding in muscle bodies of large skeletal muscles. Pyomyositis cases in tropic regions tend to occur in immunocompetent patients, in contrast to temperate disease presentations, which tend to occur in the immunocompromised individuals [2]. Patients may present with symptoms similar to those seen in necrotizing fasciitis and cellulitis, such as fever, pain, erythema, edema, and induration localized to a particular region [3], thus making diagnosis difficult. Septic shock is a common late-stage presentation [2]. The mortality rate associated with pyomyositis has been estimated to range from 1% to 20% [4].

2. Case Presentation

A 54-year-old Caucasian male with a past medical history of treated rhabdomyolysis, COPD, and occasional methamphetamine use presented to the emergency department for severe right pectoral pain that began 5 days prior. He reported coming to the emergency department 3 days prior to presentation with right pectoral pain and was put on sulfamethoxazole/trimethoprim for suspected cellulitis, but reported worsening of symptoms. Pain radiated from his right pectoral muscle to his right shoulder. He characterized the pain as severe, constant, sharp, and pleuritic.

He reported minor superficial abrasions from steel to his right superior lateral chest while working odd jobs one week prior to onset of symptoms, but denied any blunt trauma, intravenous drug use, recent travel, sick contacts, weight loss, or shortness of breath. He endorsed a fever the night prior to admission, nonproductive chronic cough, and red, swollen skin changes on his right chest.

Upon initial presentation, the patient was febrile and tachycardic, but stable. Patient's right chest was erythematous and tender to palpation along the distal right pectoral insertion and right shoulder, with 4/5 right shoulder strength and sensitivity to light touch along the right arm. His right chest was 3 times the size of his left chest. Nontender induration of the right flank was present. No discrete mass or abscess was palpable; however, a fluid collection was present in the posterior scapula region on the right. Lab results showed elevated levels of procalcitonin, c-reactive protein, and white blood cell count. The creatinine kinase level was not suspicious for rhabdomyolysis.

Chest x-ray was unremarkable. Initial ultrasound of his right pectoral muscle showed an area of skin induration with tiny anechoic areas compatible with cellulitis. Computed tomography (CT) scan of his chest showed fat stranding of the right pectoral, but no abscess (Figure 1).

Upon admission, the patient was placed on piperacillin/tazobactam and vancomycin. However, after ten days on the new antibiotic regimen, his clinical presentation failed to improve. Blood cultures were positive for *S. aureus* that was susceptible to vancomycin. Repeat ultrasonography was performed and showed interval development of abscess in the pectoral muscle body. Surgery was consulted, and they proceeded with incision and drainage. Surgical exploration revealed a large amount of purulent fluid in between the pectoralis minor and major muscles, and the diagnosis of pyomyositis was reached. Wound cultures were consistent with methicillin-resistant *S. aureus* (MRSA). The patient had improvement with serial drainages. In preparation for discharge, the patient's antibiotic regimen was switched to clindamycin for MRSA coverage and a nonparenteral route for administration. The patient was discharged in stable condition on oral clindamycin and a wound vacuum.

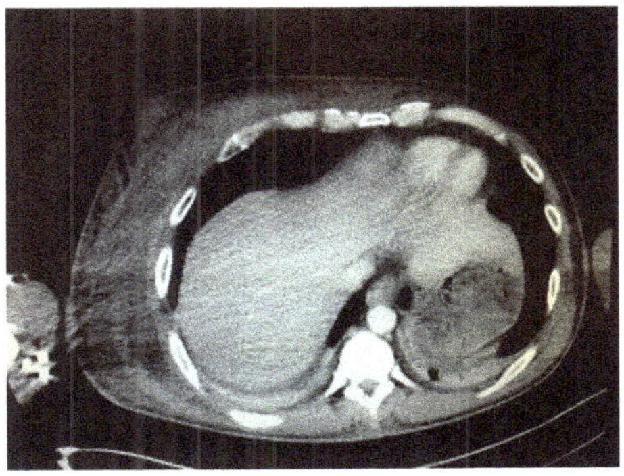

FIGURE 1: CT scan of chest with contrast at the level of the pectoralis muscle.

3. Literature Review

Temperate adult pyomyositis has an increased incidence in immunocompromised individuals. Immunocompromised states and common comorbidities include those with human immunodeficiency virus (HIV), diabetes mellitus, malignancy, cirrhosis, renal insufficiency, and use of immunosuppressive drugs. Other predisposing risk factors include trauma, IV drug abuse, and concurrent infections [5]. Pyomyositis cases in the United States have been commonly reported in patients with HIV infections, which may be linked to increased colonization of *S. aureus* in that population [3]. Furthermore, HIV patients taking antiretroviral therapy can have myopathies due to medication side effects, which renders the muscles prone to infection [3]. Additionally, trauma is an important predisposing factor, as it is reported in about 25–50% of pyomyositis cases [6]. Trauma leads to more iron flow in the muscle bed, providing a ripe environment for bacterial growth [6]. For example, athletes who perform vigorous activity develop minor muscle damage, suggesting that the pathophysiology of the infection in muscle tissue seen in pyomyositis may be due to hematoma formation or increased muscle perfusion from trauma [6].

The clinical course of pyomyositis can be broken down into three stages [7]. Stage 1 is considered the "invasive stage," consisting of local myalgia, low-grade fever, pain, and edema. A deep abscess may not be palpable, but the area may be described as "rubbery quality" [2]. No purulent material will be present when attempting to aspirate muscle. Stage 2 is referred to as the "purulent stage" [2], occurring 10 to 21 days after the initial onset of symptoms and patients present with fever, severe muscle tenderness, and increased edema. A frank abscess may be clinically present [4]. Ninety percent of patients present to the hospital with stage 2 pyomyositis [7]. Stage 3 is a state of systemic toxicity with complications of *S. aureus* bacteremia [4]. Staging is important to delineate in assessing pyomyositis in order to choose the appropriate treatment. As mentioned above, early clinical stages may present similarly to necrotizing fasciitis and may be difficult to distinguish. Necrotizing fasciitis is a rapidly progressing infection that is often fulminant with a mortality rate of 25% to 75% [8]. It involves the superficial and deep fascia with necrosis and fluid collections [9]. Pyomyositis and necrotizing fasciitis may even coexist in tropical climates and in immunocompromised individuals in temperate regions [9]. Although swelling, erythema, and disproportionately severe pain can also be present in necrotizing fasciitis, the presence of blisters, bullae, and skin crepitus is strongly an indicative of necrotizing fasciitis [10].

Ultrasound and CT scan of the symptomatic region are often the first radiographic techniques used to evaluate for abscess formation, as plain radiographs are usually normal [8]. CT scans can be used to visualize diffuse muscle enlargement with heterogeneous attenuation on imaging due to fluid collections. Most commonly in pyomyositis cases, CT scans tend to show muscle enlargement with heterogeneous attenuation and focal rim enhancement in the inflamed muscle region [11]. Ultrasound is useful for image-guided abscess aspiration during the suppurative phase [8]. MRI is the most sensitive imaging modality to assess muscle inflammation, even in the early stages of pyomyositis before a frank abscess forms [9]. T2-weighted MRI often shows diffuse muscle enlargement and intramuscular abscesses [2]. MRI can also be used to distinguish pyomyositis and necrotizing fasciitis [2]. MRI can reveal areas of inflammation along the fascial plains and distinguish spread of infection into compartments and surrounding soft tissue structures [8].

Treatment for pyomyositis is based on staging. Stage 1 pyomyositis is treated with antibiotics in the hopes of preventing abscess formation. Stages 2 and 3 pyomyositis require percutaneous drainage or surgery of abscesses, as well as antibiotics. Antibiotics typically used include those with gram-positive and gram-negative bacteria coverage empirically, with narrowing of spectrum as appropriate [12]. In addition, anaerobic coverage should also be added early in treatment for immunocompromised patients [13]. Repeat drainage is commonly required. Antibiotics should be continued until clinical and radiographic improvement is confirmed [12]. Typically, patients recover after three to four weeks of parenteral antibiotic regimens. However, patients with poorly drained or multiple infections may require a longer duration antibiotic regimen [2].

4. Conclusion

The present case highlights the difficulty of detecting pyomyositis in its early stages without strong clinical suspicion and also points to a possibility that broad-spectrum antibiotics may not effectively treat stage I pyomyositis before abscess formation is achieved. The patient in the case report presented clinically in stage 1 pyomyositis. Surgical intervention is not recommended in the early stages of disease. As in the presented case, the recommended therapy of broad-spectrum antibiotics did not prevent abscess formation at the primary site. The role of antibiotics in early tropical pyomyositis may be to prevent continued hematogenous spread and subsequent appearance of further lesions; however, anecdotal experience from expert tropical medicine physicians indicates that antibiotics often do not prevent the formation of further abscesses. Surgery may be indicated in most cases at the primary site of infection with eventual abscess formation, regardless of initial antibiotic use. Although pyomyositis is relatively rare in temperate climates, this case demonstrates the importance of awareness of this tropical disease. In this case, the patient did not present as immunocompromised, which further adds to the difficulty of detecting the disease without high suspicion.

References

[1] J. J. Gomez-Reino, J. J. Aznar, J. L. Pablos, F. Diaz-Gonzalez, and A. Laffon, "Nontropical pyomyositis in adults," *Seminars in Arthritis and Rheumatism*, vol. 23, no. 6, pp. 396–405, 1994.

[2] L. N. Small and J. J. Ross, "Tropical and temperate pyomyositis," *Infectious Disease Clinics of North America*, vol. 19, no. 4, pp. 981–989, 2005.

[3] C. A. Widrow, S. M. Kellie, B. R. Saltzman, and U. Mathur-Wagh, "Pyomyositis in patients with the human immunodeficiency virus: an unusual form of disseminated bacterial infection," *American Journal of Medicine*, vol. 91, no. 2, pp. 129–136, 1991.

[4] A. Sharma, S. Kumar, A. Wanchu et al., "Clinical characteristics and predictors of mortality in 67 patients with primary pyomyositis: a study from North India," *Clinical Rheumatology*, vol. 29, no. 1, pp. 45–51, 2010.

[5] N. F. Crum, "Bacterial pyomyositis in the United States," *American Journal of Medicine*, vol. 117, no. 6, pp. 420–428, 2004.

[6] R. K. Gibson, S. J. Rosenthal, and B. P. Lukert, "Pyomyositis. Increasing recognition in temperate climates," *American Journal of Medicine*, vol. 77, no. 4, pp. 768–772, 1984.

[7] L. C. Chiedozi, "Pyomyositis. Review of 205 cases in 112 patients," *American Journal of Surgery*, vol. 137, no. 2, pp. 255–259, 1979.

[8] D. E. Low and A. Norrby-Teglund, "Myositis, pyomyositis, and necrotising fasciitis," in *Principles and Practice of Pediatric Infectious Diseases*, Elsevier, Amsterdam, Netherlands, 2012.

[9] H. Chou, H. E. L Teo, N. Dubey, and W. C. G. Peh, "Tropical pyomyositis and necrotizing fasciitis," *Seminars in Musculoskeletal Radiology*, vol. 15, no. 5, pp. 489–505, 2011.

[10] K. Saeed, S. Esposito, I. Gould et al., "Hot topics in necrotising skin and soft tissue infections," *International Journal of Antimicrobial Agents*, vol. 52, no. 1, pp. 1–10, 2018.

[11] B. A. Gordon, S. Martinez, and A. J. Collins, "Pyomyositis: characteristics at CT and MR imaging," *Radiology*, vol. 197, no. 1, pp. 279–286, 1995.

[12] Y. G. Kwak, S. H. Choi, T. Kim et al., "Clinical guidelines for the antibiotic treatment for community-acquired skin and soft tissue infection," *Infection & Chemotherapy*, vol. 49, no. 4, pp. 301–325, 2017.

[13] D. L. Stevens, A. L. Bisno, H. F. Chambers et al., "Practice guidelines for the diagnosis and management of skin and soft tissue infections: 2014 update by the Infectious Diseases Society of America," *Clinical Infectious Diseases*, vol. 59, no. 2, pp. e10–e52, 2014.

17

The Forgotten Disease: A Case of Lemierre's Syndrome with Distal Extremity Involvement

John Gaskill and Michael Aronson

Lewis-Gale Hospital Montgomery, 3700 South Main St., Blacksburg, VA 24060, USA

Correspondence should be addressed to John Gaskill; jgaskill@vcom.vt.edu

Academic Editor: Peter Olumese

Once coined the "Forgotten Disease," Lemierre's syndrome is a rare condition that results from oropharyngeal infection with the gram-negative, anaerobic *Fusobacterium necrophorum*. The typical progression of illness involves spread to adjacent structures such as the internal jugular vein with resulting thrombophlebitis. Septic emboli to distant sites are also a common sequela. Here, we present a case of Lemierre's syndrome in a 20-year-old, otherwise healthy, male. The patient presented with fever, sore throat, and dysphagia. Imaging revealed peritonsillar multiloculated fluid collections and necrotizing pneumonia with multiple pulmonary abscesses. The patient's hospital course was complicated by the development of necrotizing fasciitis in his right lower leg, which required incision and drainage with surgical washout. In addition to systemic intravenous antibiotics and anticoagulation, he underwent multiple thoracentesis procedures. The patient was ultimately transferred to a tertiary care center due to persistent fevers and lung abscesses. This case highlights the challenges of initial diagnosis, as well as the treatment choices faced by the attending physicians.

1. Introduction

In 1936, the French bacteriologist Andre Lemierre published a report detailing the link between septicemia and pharyngitis that he had observed while working at the Claude Bernard Hospital in Paris [1]. The postanginal septicemia which now bears his name is most often precipitated by a suppurative oropharyngeal infection. The infection is typically caused by the gram-negative, anaerobic *Fusobacterium necrophorum*. Fusobacteria can be found as normal flora in the upper respiratory tract of humans [2]. Other anaerobic bacteria have been identified as sources of infection, but these are atypical [3]. The disease mostly affects young, otherwise healthy adults. The first symptom is typically a sore throat secondary to exudative tonsillitis or peritonsillar abscess. The infection then spreads into adjacent structures, such as the internal jugular vein and carotid artery. Thrombophlebitis of the neck veins can cause pain, swelling, and dysphagia. Sepsis with complicating metastatic spread of septic microemboli is the typical progression of illness [4]. The most common site of metastatic spread is the lungs, with 85% of cases demonstrating pulmonary infiltrates [5]. Other feared complications include spread of infection along the carotid sheath and into the mediastinum [4]. Mortality rate before advent of antibiotics was extremely high, with 18 of Andre Lemierre's 20 identified patients succumbing to their disease [1]. In the modern era of medicine, mortality rates range from 6.4 to 17% [6, 7].

2. Case Presentation

AT is a 20-year-old Caucasian male who was seen in the emergency department for evaluation of fever, chills, sore throat, and some difficulty swallowing. He was also complaining of mid-back pain, made worse with deep inspiration, and tender swollen glands in his neck. He denied any recent dental procedures or tooth infections. He was seen at his university health center for evaluation five days prior and was diagnosed with viral pharyngitis. He was prescribed a course of prednisone, which he had completed one day prior to presenting to the emergency department. His temperature in the emergency department was 106° Fahrenheit, and his heart rate was 150 beats per minute (bpm). He also complained of some pain in his right calf that he attributed to "slipping and hyperextending his ankle" several days prior. A computed tomography with contrast of his neck was obtained that showed an inflammatory and infectious process of the soft tissue posterior to the oral cavity and extending into the prevertebral soft tissue in the midline. The patient was then transferred to a nearby facility that had otorhinolaryngology coverage for further evaluation. He was admitted to the intensive care unit under sepsis protocol, where he continued to complain of a sore throat in addition to a cough productive of purulent sputum.

Physical examination at the time of admission revealed a swollen neck with fullness and tenderness in the anterior and posterior cervical lymph nodes bilaterally. He was unable to open his mouth more than 1.5–2 inches due to pain and swelling. His oropharynx appeared erythematous. He was breathing fast and shallow due to pain with deep inspiration, but he was still able to complete full sentences. He had decreased breath sounds at the bases bilaterally without wheezes or crackles. His right calf was moderately swollen compared to the left and was tender. He had good pulses in both dorsalis pedis and posterior tibialis in both legs in addition to full range of motion in his ankles. Initial lab results showed an elevated white count of 14.1 with 19% bands. His hemoglobin was 15.4, and platelet count was low at 46,000. Creatinine was 1.33, glucose 105, albumin low at 2.6, potassium 3.7, and calcium 8.5. Other lab values of note included alkaline phosphatase 151, aspartate aminotransferase (AST) 46, alanine aminotransferase (ALT) 30, lactate 2.1, and bilirubin 2.6.

The treatment plan involved broad-spectrum coverage with administration of intravenous vancomycin and piperacillin/tazobactam, in addition to aggressive IV fluid repletion. The patient was started on low-molecular-weight heparin 40 mg subcutaneous daily for deep vein thrombosis prophylaxis. The chest computed tomography (CT) with contrast showed multifocal areas of necrotizing pneumonia with multiple pulmonary abscesses. A multiloculated effusion was also identified on the left side with a smaller free flowing effusion on the right side. A repeat neck computed tomography (CT) with contrast (Figure 1) showed persistent retropharyngeal and bilateral peritonsillar multiloculated enhancing fluid collections. It also showed thrombosis of the left retromandibular vein and punctate foci within the left internal jugular vein, which was thought to represent partial thrombosis. On the day of admission, the patient underwent computed tomography (CT) guided empyema drainage with placement of left-sided chest tube (Figure 2). The following day, a second chest tube was placed on the left side and a right-sided chest tube was placed on the third day of hospitalization.

On the first day of admission, a right lower extremity ultrasound was ordered due to the pain and swelling in his right calf. This study was negative for deep vein thrombosis. The following day, a magnetic resonance imaging (MRI) of the right lower leg, with and without contrast (Figure 3),

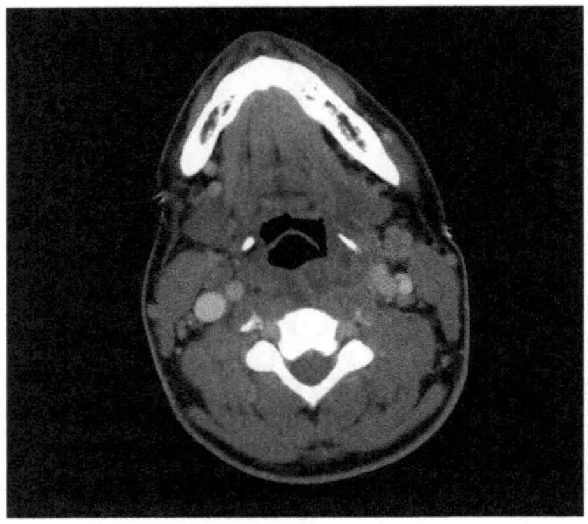

Figure 1: Horizontal section of neck computed tomography (CT) with contrast showing retropharyngeal and bilateral peritonsillar multiloculated enhancing fluid collections in addition to thrombosis of the left retromandibular vein and punctate foci within the left internal jugular vein.

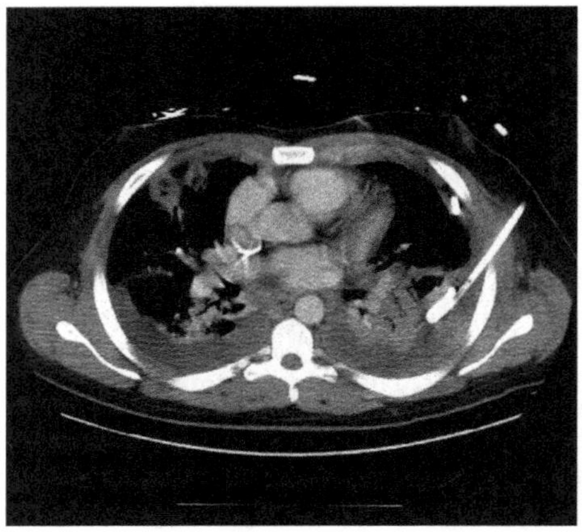

Figure 2: Horizontal section of chest computed tomography (CT) with contrast showing left-sided, multiloculated pleural effusion, status postplacement of pigtail catheter. Multifocal areas of necrotizing pneumonia and multiple pulmonary abscesses with smaller right-sided pleural effusion are also shown.

showed edema within the fascial compartments between the gastrocnemius and soleus muscles, as well as in the superficial fascia. A crescent-shaped subfascial fluid collection was also noted over the medial head of the gastrocnemius muscle, indicative of right lower leg fasciitis. The decision was made to proceed with incision and drainage of the fluid collection, in addition to a debridement of the right leg necrotizing fasciitis. Abscess drainage resulted in approximately 500 ml of purulent foul-smelling fluid, some of which was sent for gram stain and culture. A wash out of the right lower extremity wounds would be performed several days later with subsequent placement of negative pressure wound dressing.

Infectious disease was consulted on the second day of admission. At this time, the patient was being treated with IV cancomycin and piperacillin/tazobactam. The decision was made to add clindamycin to help with possible toxin production and doxycycline due to concern for Brucella and

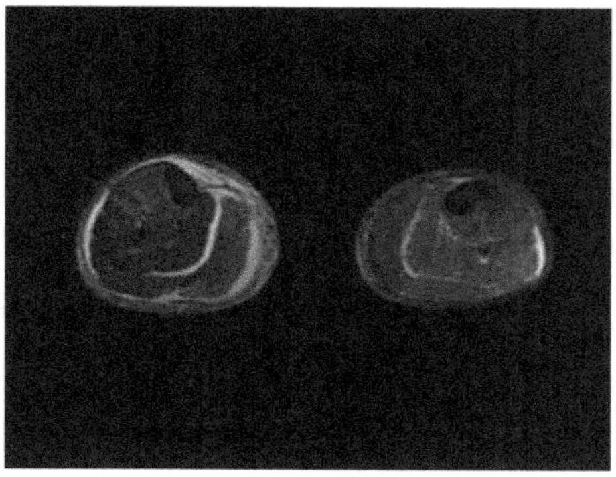

FIGURE 3: Horizontal section of magnetic resonance imaging (MRI) of lower extremities, with and without contrast, showing edema within the fascial compartments between the right gastrocnemius and right soleus muscles, as well as in the superficial fascia. A crescent-shaped subfascial fluid collection was also noted over the medial head of the right gastrocnemius muscle, indicative of fasciitis.

Coxiella. Initial blood cultures had been negative; however, gram-negative anaerobic bacteria were isolated from the fluid sample taken off the right leg abscess. This was later identified to be *Fusobacterium necrophorum*. On the seventh day of admission, antibiotics were deescalated to meropenem based on susceptibilities. The patient had improved clinically since his admission, but he continued to spike fevers. A follow-up chest CT showed persistence of numerous lung abscesses in the subpleural area with risk of bronchopleural fistula evolution. Due to concern over persistent fevers and empyema, despite multiple chest tube placements, the patient was transferred to a tertiary care center for further evaluation.

The patient remained in the ICU at the tertiary care center for another week where he had two more surgeries on his right leg. He also underwent a lung decortication surgery. The patient reported that in his mind, the lung decortication was a turning point in his recovery. He was transferred to a step-down unit and then discharged to home on a four-week course of oral clindamycin. He also underwent outpatient physical therapy. He has since made a complete recovery and was able to continue his undergraduate education.

3. Discussion

The increased use of antibiotics to treat pharyngitis has led to a decreased occurrence of Lemierre's Syndrome, earning it the moniker "the forgotten disease." One source states incidence in the early 1990s was as low as 0.8–1.5 per million persons per year [8]. However, there have been an increased number of cases reported over the last 20 years [9]. There have been several proposed reasons for this increase in incidence. One possible cause is a decreased use of antibiotics to treat uncomplicated pharyngitis. Routine use of antibiotics to treat pharyngitis has been discouraged over recent years, which could be contributing to the progression of *Fusobacterium* infection into Lemierre's syndrome. Another postulate is that improved anaerobic culturing techniques have led to increased detection of *Fusobacterium* infection. In this case, the increased number of cases would be due to more sensitive testing rather than an actual increase in incidence. Yet another theory is that the increased number of cases is due to emerging antibiotic resistance amongst *Fusobacterium* species. A recent study showed the resistance rate to erythromycin was as high as 15% amongst strains of *Fusobacterium necrophorum* [10]. Penicillin resistance has also been reported due to production of beta-lactamase by some strains of *Fusobacterium necrophorum* [11]. Appropriate antibiotic selection is discussed later in the section.

Regardless of the cause of the increasing incidence, a high level of clinical suspicion is required to make the diagnosis of Lemierre's syndrome. The disease is often initially misdiagnosed as a viral pharyngitis, especially mononucleosis [2]. Several clinical clues can be helpful in distinguishing Lemierre's syndrome from mononucleosis. For instance, mononucleosis typically presents with more generalized lymphadenopathy in contrast to the more localized cervical lymphadenopathy of Lemierre's syndrome. Another clue, and one of the most typical findings of a Lemierre's syndrome, is the presence of lung infiltrates. In young patients with pharyngitis, the presence of concurrent lung lesions should raise the clinical suspicion for Lemierre's syndrome. Critical to the diagnosis of Lemierre's syndrome is the prompt collection of blood cultures and the culturing of any fluid drained from abscesses that may be present. However, *Fusobacterium necrophorum* takes at least 48 hours to grow in culture and sometimes as long as seven days [2], so clinicians may find it necessary to treat empirically while awaiting culture results. There are also multiple case reports of atypical presentations of Lemierre's syndrome, including with ARDS and septic shock [12], further adding to the diagnostic challenge that the disease presents.

Once Lemierre's syndrome is suspected, administration of IV antibiotics should begin immediately. However, the optimal antibiotic regimen is not agreed upon. Most reports have recommended use of high-dose beta-lactamase-resistant beta-lactam antibiotic in conjunction with metrondizole. However, use of clindamycin alone has also been shown to be effective [7]. Of note is the slow response time of Lemierre's syndrome to antibiotics. Time from antibiotic administration to resolution of fever can last upwards of 8–12 days [2]. The slow response time is thought to result from sequestration of the infection with resulting poor penetration of antibiotics. Another point of controversy is whether to administer anticoagulants in treatment of Lemierre's syndrome due to the propensity for thrombus formation. Some reports have supported use of anticoagulants in addition to systemic antibiotics, but no clear guidelines exist [13]. A retrospective study has shown that use of anticoagulants did not affect thrombus outcome in cases of Lemierre's syndrome, with thrombus resolution occurring in all 24 cases regardless of anticoagulant use [14]. However, anticoagulants may be indicated for high-risk patients, such as those with extensive internal jugular thrombosis, or those who have not responded to antimicrobial therapy [13].

While Lemierre's syndrome remains a rare condition, it nonetheless is associated with considerable morbidity and mortality. With an increased awareness of the condition, physicians will be more likely to consider it in a differential diagnosis. Prompt recognition by the treating physician and the timely administration of systemic antibiotics are key to successful outcomes. However, the use of anticoagulants remains controversial. Physicians would benefit from using a case-by-case approach when making a decision regarding the use of anticoagulation. These patients are also more likely to develop complications secondary to septic embolic phenomenon. Transfer to a larger hospital center with greater surgical capabilities may be a prudent decision.

Additional Points

Learning Points. (1) Lemierre's syndrome is a relatively rare disease process that results from oropharyngeal infection involving *Fusobacterium necrophorum*; however, increasing prevalence has been reported. Local invasion into the internal jugular vein with metastatic spread of septic microemboli is the typical progression of illness. (2) The diagnosis should be considered in young, otherwise healthy patients who present with pharyngitis and lung abscess concurrently. However, it can also present more atypically, as with the lower extremity necrotizing fasciitis seen in our patient. (3) Treatment is centered around early antibiotic administration and infection source control. Antimicrobial resistance to erythromycin and penicillin has been documented and should be taken into consideration when selecting initial antibiotics.

Consent

Consent for publication was obtained from patient prior to submission.

References

[1] A. Lemierre, "On certain septicæmias due to anaerobic organisms," *The Lancet*, vol. 227, no. 5874, pp. 701–703, 1936.

[2] T. Riordan and M. Wilson, "Lemierre's syndrome: more than a historical curiosa," *Postgraduate Medical Journal*, vol. 80, no. 944, pp. 328–334, 2004.

[3] C. M. Leugers and R. Clover, "Lemierre syndrome: postanginal sepsis," *The Journal of the American Board of Family Practice*, vol. 8, pp. 384–391, 1995.

[4] D. L. Kasper, A. S. Fauci, S. L. Hauser, D. L. L. Longo, J. L. Jameson, and J. Loscalzo, *Harrison's Principles of Internal Medicine*, McGraw Hill Education, New York, NY, USA, 19th edition, 2015.

[5] S. Moreno, J. G. Altozano, B. Pinilla et al., "Lemierre's disease: postanginal bacteremia and pulmonary involvement caused by *Fusobacterium necrophorum*," *Clinical Infectious Diseases*, vol. 11, no. 2, pp. 319–324, 1989.

[6] J. A. Chirinos, D. M. Lichtstein, J. Garcia, and L. J. Tamariz, "The evolution of Lemierre syndrome: report of 2 cases and review of the literature," *Medicine*, vol. 81, no. 6, pp. 458–465, 2002.

[7] L. H. Kristensen and J. Prag, "Human necrobacillosis, with emphasis on Lemierre's syndrome," *Clinical Infectious Diseases*, vol. 31, no. 2, pp. 524–532, 2000.

[8] L. H. Hagelskjær, J. Prag, J. Malczynski, and J. H. Kristensen, "Incidence and clinical epidemiology of necrobacillosis, including Lemierre's syndrome, in Denmark 1990–1995," *European Journal of Clinical Microbiology and Infectious Diseases*, vol. 17, no. 8, pp. 561–565, 1998.

[9] P. D. Karkos, S. Asrani, C. D. Karkos et al., "Lemierre's syndrome: a systematic review," *The Laryngoscope*, vol. 119, no. 8, pp. 1552–1559, 2009.

[10] J. S. Brazier, B. I. Duerden, E. Yusuf, and V. Hall, "*Fusobacterium necrophorum* infections in England and Wales 1990–2000," *Journal of Medical Microbiology*, vol. 51, no. 3, pp. 269–272, 2002.

[11] B. Itzhak, "Infections caused by beta-lactamase-producing Fusobacterium spp. in children," *Pediatric Infectious Disease Journal*, vol. 12, no. 6, pp. 532-533, 1993.

[12] D. R. Nemakayala, M. P. Rai, S. Kavuturu, and S. Rayamajhi, "Atypical presentation of Lemierre's syndrome causing septic shock and acute respiratory distress syndrome," *Case Reports in Infectious Diseases*, vol. 2018, Article ID 5469053, 4 pages, 2018.

[13] C. K. Phua, V. M. Chadachan, and R. Acharya, "Lemierre syndrome-should we anticoagulate? A case report and review of the literature," *International Journal of Angiology*, vol. 22, no. 02, pp. 137–142, 2013.

[14] M. C. Cupit, A. NageswaraRao, D. M. Warad, S. Khan, and V. Rodriguez, "Lemierre's syndrome: role of anticoagulation and thrombosis outcomes, a retrospective study," *Blood*, vol. 126, no. 23, p. 2296, 2015.

18

Burkholderia cepacia Complex Lumbar Spondylodiscitis: A Rare Nosocomial Infection

Rachel Subramanian[1] **and Lynn Fitzgibbons**[2]

[1]*Department of Medical Education, Santa Barbara Cottage Hospital, Santa Barbara, CA, USA*
[2]*Department of Infectious Diseases, Santa Barbara Cottage Hospital, Santa Barbara, CA, USA*

Correspondence should be addressed to Rachel Subramanian; rsubramanianmd@gmail.com

Academic Editor: Larry M. Bush

Pyogenic spondylodiscitis is rarely caused by *Burkholderia cepacia* complex. *B. cepacia* is widespread in the environment and recognized as an opportunistic pathogen for patients with cystic fibrosis and immune disorders. A female in her mid-30s with underlying hyperthyroidism, but otherwise immunocompetent, was admitted to the hospital with persistent lower back pain after elective bariatric surgery in Mexico. Lumbar MRI showed L2/L3 osteomyelitis and discitis. Culture of disk aspiration grew *Burkholderia cepacia* complex sensitive to cefepime, ceftazidime, ciprofloxacin, gentamicin, imipenem, levofloxacin, and trimethoprim-sulfamethoxazole. The infection failed to respond to cefepime; however, she was successfully treated with levofloxacin monotherapy.

1. Introduction

Pyogenic spondylodiscitis is an infection of the intervertebral discs and/or adjacent vertebrae. It occurs by hematogenous seeding of bacteria, direct spread from a nearby infection, or from direct inoculation during spinal surgery [1].

The most common pathogen identified is *Staphylococcus aureus*, followed by Gram-negative rods, coagulase-negative staphylococci, streptococci, enterococci, and anaerobes. In many cases, an organism is not identified. The diagnosis is based on clinical, radiological, and microbiological findings [2].

The diagnosis of pyogenic spinal infection is often delayed because of its insidious presentation and nonspecific signs and symptoms. While the most common initial complaint is back or neck pain in 90% of cases, fever and neurological involvement are rarely present [1]. Diagnostic delay is common, especially in a patient without risk factors, but prompt diagnosis and treatment are critical because pyogenic spondylodiscitis can lead to spinal instability and neurologic complications [2].

Burkholderia cepacia complex *(B. cepacia)* is a Gram-negative bacillus known to infect immunocompromised patients. This microorganism is notoriously hard to target because of its multidrug-resistant nature [3]. Here, we report a case of *Burkholderia cepacia* complex lumbar pyogenic spondylodiscitis after bariatric surgery in an otherwise healthy patient. She failed treatment with cefepime but achieved clinical remission with levofloxacin monotherapy.

2. Case Presentation

A 34-year-old female with a past medical history of obesity (body mass index: 33) and Graves' disease presented to the emergency room with progressive lower back pain and difficulty walking. The pain initially started four days after an elective laparoscopic sleeve gastrectomy performed in Tijuana, Mexico. The patient was seen in the emergency department one day after pain onset for significant lower back pain radiating to her right leg. She was diagnosed with musculoskeletal pain and sciatica and then discharged on oral morphine. Ten days later, she visited her primary care provider for the same lower back pain and was started on gabapentin. A lumbosacral X-ray and lumbar magnetic resonance imaging (MRI) were ordered, but never completed.

She returned to the emergency room within one week of her primary care visit for worsening back pain, paresthesia affecting the anterior thighs, and impaired gait. Vital signs were blood pressure 149/97 mmHg, heart rate 132 beats per minute, temperature 36°C, respiratory rate 18 breaths per minute, and oxygen saturation 100% on room air. Physical examination was notable for point tenderness over the lumbar spine region. Neurological exam was otherwise normal. Laboratory results demonstrated white blood cell count 6,300/μL (normal: 4,000–11,000/μL), C-reactive protein (CRP) 36 mg/L (normal: <10 mg/L), erythrocyte sedimentation rate (ESR) 90 mm/Hr (normal: <20 mm/Hr), and procalcitonin 1.6 ng/mL (normal: <0.5 ng/mL), compatible with infection. She denied postoperative complications, intravenous drug use, or immunosuppressive medications. She was prescribed methimazole for hyperthyroidism but had not taken it since undergoing surgery. Her HIV test was negative. Spinal MRI with contrast showed L2/L3 early discitis and osteomyelitis without a fluid collection or abscess (Figure 1).

A fluoroscopically guided aspiration of the L2/L3 disk was performed by injecting a 1 cc sterile saline wash which was aspirated and sent for culture. *Burkholderia cepacia* complex grew on chocolate agar and was identified using matrix-assisted laser desorption/isolation time-of-flight mass spectroscopy (MALDI-TOF MS). The sensitivities were determined with the VITEK system, which showed resistance to piperacillin-tazobactam and susceptibility to cefepime, ceftazidime, ciprofloxacin, gentamicin, imipenem, levofloxacin, and trimethoprim-sulfamethoxazole. Cytology showed mild to moderate neutrophils. Blood and urine cultures remained negative.

She was treated initially with vancomycin and ceftriaxone awaiting culture results and then switched to six weeks of cefepime 2 g every 12 hours via a peripherally inserted central catheter. Four weeks later, the patient returned to the hospital for unrelenting lower back pain and increasing inflammatory markers. Spinal survey MRI showed worsening L2/L3 osteomyelitis. A repeat intervertebral aspiration grew *Burkholderia cepacia* complex susceptible to levofloxacin. Levofloxacin 750 mg IV was given for six weeks; ESR normalized, and CRP decreased to 11 mg/L. Lumbar spine MRI was repeated after completion of antibiotics. Imaging showed improvement of discitis and osteomyelitis at L2/L3 and no drainable fluid collection. The patient reported intermittent lower back pain which could be explained by the interval development of subacute mild compression fractures of the superior endplates of L1, L4, and L5.

3. Discussion

Originally described in 1950 by an American microbiologist William Burkholder as the causative agent of onion rot, *Burkholderia cepacia* complex is a motile, catalase-producing, and nonlactose-fermenting aerobic Gram-negative bacillus. This bacterium is found ubiquitously in the environment, dwelling in water, soil, and various plants, where it thrives in moisture [3]. *B. cepacia* is known for infecting the respiratory tracts of patients with cystic fibrosis (CF) and chronic granulomatous disease, resulting in a wide range of clinical manifestations from chronic asymptomatic colonization to bacteremia and necrotizing pneumonia [4, 5].

Our patient developed osteomyelitis within one month postoperatively after bariatric surgery in Mexico. While the source of the patient's infection remains unknown, the development of symptoms soon after surgery raises suspicion for an infection of nosocomial origin. In recent years, immunocompetent patients have become infected with *Burkholderia cepacia* complex in healthcare settings [4]. There are reports of intensive care unit outbreaks of this pathogen after exposure to contaminated antiseptics, disinfectants, dextrose solutions, nebulizer solution, sublingual probes, nasal spray, mouthwash, chlorhexidine, tap water, enteral feeding, and ultrasound gel [3]. As a result, infections such as meningitis, pneumonia, endocarditis, septic arthritis, peritonitis, osteomyelitis, and bacteremia have been reported in the literature [6].

B. cepacia bacteria cause such significant morbidity and mortality in patients because of their various resistance mechanisms to overcome the action of antimicrobials. These include beta-lactam resistance, efflux pump-mediated multidrug resistance, outer membrane permeability barrier, and alterations in drug targets. Such mechanisms lead to innate resistance to antipseudomonal penicillins, polymyxin B, and aminoglycosides [7]. The recommended first-line therapy is trimethoprim and sulfamethoxazole, but meropenem, ceftazidime, fluoroquinolones, chloramphenicol, piperacillin, and minocycline, alone or in combination, are considered appropriate antimicrobial treatments [8].

Cefepime given intravenously twice daily was chosen because it distributes widely in most body tissues and fluids. Twice daily dosing is also more feasible than three times per day as an outpatient. The pharmacokinetic profile of two grams of cefepime demonstrates excellent cortical and cancellous bone penetration [9]. Intravenous as opposed to oral antibiotics were selected because of the concern for unpredictable bioavailability of beta-lactams and fluoroquinolones after bariatric surgery [10]. For the minority of patients who do not respond to antibiotics alone, the next step in treatment may be spinal stabilization or surgical debridement. Indications for surgery include the development of neurological deficits or spinal cord compression, spinal instability, presence of epidural or paravertebral abscesses, or evidence of progression despite appropriate antimicrobial therapy [11]. In our case, *B. cepacia* did not respond to cephalosporins (despite being sensitive); however, the infection was eliminated with levofloxacin.

Pyogenic spondylodiscitis caused by *Burkholderia cepacia* complex is a very uncommon entity; few cases are reported in the literature. Our patient is unique because she had no predisposing risk factors for pyogenic spondylodiscitis but developed osteomyelitis and discitis at L2/L3. Among patients with Graves' disease, there is no established increased susceptibility to *B. cepacia* infections. The risks of

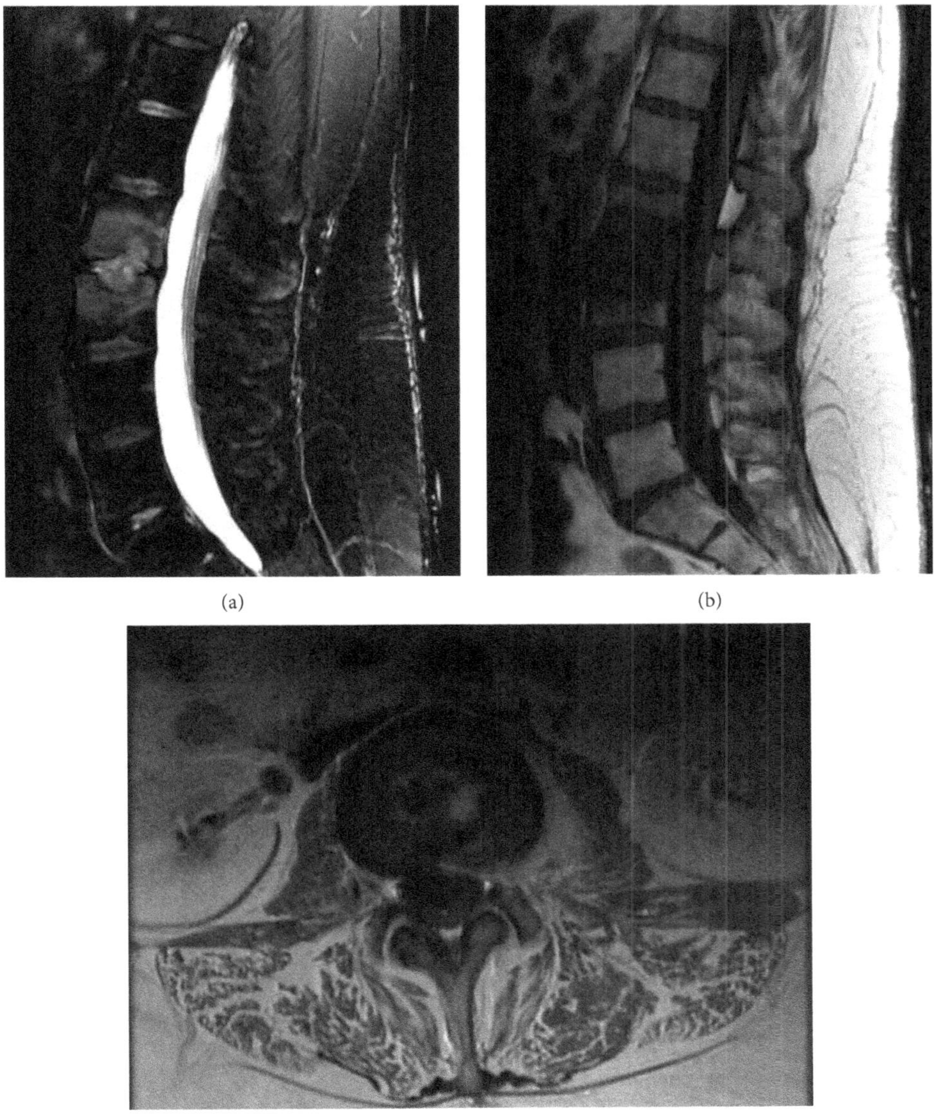

(a) (b) (c)

Figure 1: Sagittal T2-weighted (a), T1-weighted (b), and axial T1-weighted postcontrast (c) images demonstrating signal abnormality within the L2 and L3 vertebral bodies adjacent to the intervertebral disk space, consistent with osteomyelitis and discitis, with an extension to the left psoas muscle and epidural space.

osteomyelitis include chronic kidney disease, malnutrition, substance abuse, HIV, diabetes mellitus, long-term steroid use, liver cirrhosis, and malignancy [1]. This case is also remarkable because *B. cepacia* rarely causes osteomyelitis and discitis. Most cases are related to spinal surgery, trauma, intravenous drug use, or postoperative complications [4, 12–16]. One case-control study of non-CF patients found recent abdominal surgery to be an independent risk factor for *Burkholderia cepacia* bacteremia [17].

In summary, *Burkholderia cepacia* complex is an underrecognized, but important cause of pyogenic spondylodiscitis in immunocompetent patients. Due to the debilitating nature of this disease and multidrug resistance of this bacterium, a swift diagnosis and determination of susceptibility are paramount for treatment. If left untreated or treated with an inappropriate antibiotic, spinal infections may spread to adjacent structures in the spinal canal and cause abscess formation in the epidural space and in soft tissues and muscles. This can lead to destruction of the intervertebral disk and vertebral bodies, ultimately causing spinal cord compression, paralysis, and death [2].

4. Conclusion

Pyogenic spondylodiscitis is rarely caused by *Burkholderia cepacia* complex. Our case reports a patient with *B. cepacia* lumbar osteomyelitis and discitis after bariatric surgery. This case highlights how critical it is to obtain a Gram stain and culture with sensitivities when selecting antibiotics, especially for microorganisms with inherent resistance mechanisms.

Although uncommon in immunocompetent patients, *B. cepacia* is an important emerging nosocomial pathogen which should be considered in the differential for osteomyelitis after surgery.

References

[1] W. Y. Cheung and K. D. K. Luk, "Pyogenic spondylitis," *International Orthopaedics*, vol. 36, no. 2, pp. 397–404, 2012.

[2] J. Widdrington, I. Emmerson, M. Cullinan et al., "Pyogenic spondylodiscitis: risk factors for adverse clinical outcome in routine clinical practice," *Medical Science*, vol. 6, no. 4, p. 96, 2018.

[3] V. Gautam, L. Singhal, and P. Ray, "Burkholderia cepacia complex: beyond pseudomonas and acinetobacter," *Indian Journal of Medical Microbiology*, vol. 29, no. 1, pp. 4–12, 2011.

[4] D. Jaafar, M. Rizkallah, F. Atallah et al., "Lumbar spondylodiscitis caused by Burkholderia cepacia in a previously healthy patient," *Case reports in orthopedics*, vol. 2017, Article ID 1396950, 3 pages, 2017.

[5] J. M. Courtney, K. E. A. Dunbar, A. McDowell et al., "Clinical outcome of Burkholderia cepacia complex infection in cystic fibrosis adults," *Journal of Cystic Fibrosis*, vol. 3, no. 2, pp. 93–98, 2004.

[6] M. Dizbay, O. G. Tunccan, B. E. Sezer, F. Aktas, and D. Arman, "Nosocomial Burkholderia cepacia infections in a Turkish university hospital: a five-year surveillance," *Journal of infection in developing countries*, vol. 3, no. 4, pp. 273–277, 2009.

[7] K. A. Rhodes and H. P. Schweizer, "Antibiotic resistance in Burkholderia species," *Drug Resistance Updates*, vol. 28, pp. 82–90, 2016.

[8] S. G. Avgeri, D. K. Matthaiou, G. Dimopoulos, A. P. Grammatikos, and M. E. Falagas, "Therapeutic options for Burkholderia cepacia infections beyond co-trimoxazole: a systematic review of the clinical evidence," *International Journal of Antimicrobial Agents*, vol. 33, no. 5, pp. 394–404, 2009.

[9] D. Breilh, E. Boselli, J. C. Bel, D. Chassard, M. C. Saux, and B. Allaouchiche, "Diffusion of cefepime into cancellous and cortical bone tissue," *Journal of Chemotherapy*, vol. 15, no. 2, pp. 134–138, 2003.

[10] S. Anvari, Y. Lee, M. Lam, A. G. Doumouras, and D. Hong, "The effect of bariatric surgery on oral antibiotic absorption: a systematic review," *Obesity Surgery*, vol. 30, no. 8, pp. 2883–2892, 2020.

[11] E. F. Berbari, S. S. Kanj, T. J. Kowalski et al., "2015 infectious diseases society of America (IDSA) clinical practice guidelines for the diagnosis and treatment of native vertebral osteomyelitis in adultsa," *Clinical Infectious Diseases*, vol. 61, no. 6, pp. e26–e46, 2015.

[12] S. K. Li and W. B. Messer, "Burkholderia cepacia complex cervical osteomyelitis in an intravenous drug user," *Case reports in infectious diseases*, vol. 2018, Article ID 7638639, 3 pages, 2018.

[13] M. Hammoud, Y. Fares, R. Atoui, and B. Dabboucy, "Burkholderia cepacia as a cause of pyogenic spondylodiscitis in immunocompetent patients: a single-institution case series and literature review," *Journal of Spine Surgery*, vol. 5, no. 3, pp. 372–377, 2019.

[14] M. Rodriguez, M. Nelson, J. E. Kelly, A. Elward, and S. C. Morley, "Successful use of temocillin as salvage therapy for cervical osteomyelitis secondary to multidrug-resistant Burkholderia cepacia," *Journal of the Pediatric Infectious Diseases Society*, vol. 3, no. 1, pp. 77–80, 2014.

[15] L. Weinstein, C. A. Knowlton, and M. A. Smith, "Cervical osteomyelitis caused by Burkholderia cepacia after rhinoplasty," *Journal of Infection in Developing Countries*, vol. 2, no. 1, pp. 76-77, 2008.

[16] R. Ghimire, J. Hussain, A. Abubaker, T. Henderson, and P. Cook, "Vertebral osteomyelitis due to an unusual pathogen: a case report," *European Journal of Medical Case Reports*, vol. 3, no. 2, pp. 65–67, 2019.

[17] A. M. Bressler, K. S. Kaye, J. J. LiPuma et al., "Risk factors for Burkholderia and cepacia complex bacteremia among intensive care unit patients without cystic fibrosis: a case-control study," *Infection Control & Hospital Epidemiology*, vol. 28, no. 8, pp. 951–958, 2007.

19

A Case of *Fusobacterium necrophorum* without Lemierre's Syndrome Mimicking Acute Leptospirosis

Ryo Yasuhara,[1] **Shunichi Shibazaki**,[2] **and Takayoshi Yamanouchi**[3]

[1]*Tokyo Medical and Dental University Hospital Faculty of Medicine, Tokyo, Japan*
[2]*Department of Emergency and General Internal Medicine, Hitachinaka General Hospital, Hitachinaka, Japan*
[3]*Department of Cardiology, Hitachinaka General Hospital, Hitachinaka, Japan*

Correspondence should be addressed to Ryo Yasuhara; yasuhara.ryo@gmail.com

Academic Editor: George N. Dalekos

Jaundice, conjunctival hyperemia, and acute kidney injury (AKI) are the characteristics of leptospirosis. However, it is not well known that *Fusobacterium necrophorum* infection can have a clinical picture similar to that of leptospirosis. A 38-year-old man was admitted with jaundice, conjunctival hyperemia, and AKI for 7 days. Chest CT scan showed multiple pulmonary nodules, atypical for leptospirosis. We started treatment with IV piperacillin-tazobactam and minocycline. He became anuric and was urgently started on hemodialysis on the second hospital day. Later on, blood cultures grew *Fusobacterium necrophorum* and other anaerobic bacteria. Antibody and PCR assays for *Leptospira* were negative. We narrowed the antibiotics to IV ceftriaxone and metronidazole. He responded well to the treatment and was discharged on the 18th hospital day. *F. necrophorum* infection is known to cause mixed infection with other anaerobic bacteria. The resistance of many anaerobic bacteria continues to progress, and *F. necrophorum* itself sometimes produces β-lactamase. This case highlights the potential risks of using penicillin before diagnosis of leptospirosis.

1. Introduction

Jaundice, conjunctival hyperemia, and acute kidney injury (AKI) are the characteristics of leptospirosis [1, 2], which can be treated with penicillin [3]. However, *Fusobacterium necrophorum* infection may mimic leptospirosis [4–6], which is not well known. *F. necrophorum* often causes mixed infections with other anaerobic bacteria. In addition, the antimicrobial resistance of anaerobic bacteria is serious, and sometimes *F. necrophorum* itself also produces β-lactamase [7]. We present a case of *F. necrophorum* mixed-infection mimicking leptospirosis that might have treatment failure with penicillin.

2. Case Summary

A 38-year-old man presented with a seven-day history of fatigue, fever, and jaundice. He initially went to a nearby clinic as symptoms worsened. Subsequently, he was also diagnosed with AKI and transferred to our hospital. He had no contact with rats and did not do field work. He had no prior medical history.

Vital signs at the time of visit were as follows: blood pressure 116/73 mmHg, pulse 110/min, body temperature 37.4°C, and respiration rate 18/min. His ocular conjunctivae wereyellow-tinged and congested. His oral cavity was not swollen or reddish; however, he complained of a sore throat.

Blood tests revealed a white blood cell count of 18900/μL. His hemoglobin was 10.8 g/dL and platelet count was $2.6 \times 10^4/\mu$L, and no schizocytes were observed. Aspartate aminotransferase was 31 U/L, alanine aminotransferase 18 U/L, lactate dehydrogenase 234 U/L, alkaline phosphatase 340 U/L, γ-glutamyltransferase 41 U/L, total bilirubin 12.4 mg/dL, and direct bilirubin 10.5 mg/dL, which is above the threshold for hyperbilirubinemia. Blood urea nitrogen was 85.6 mg/dL, creatinine was 8.3 mg/dL, and C-reactive protein was elevated to 29.26 mg/dL (normal range 0.0–0.3 mg/dL). In urine qualitative assays, positive results were observed for proteins, urobilinogen, bilirubin, and occult blood. In addition, urine sugar was positive despite not having diabetes. Chest CT showed multiple nodules in both lungs (Figure 1). Abdominal CT showed no abnormality that could explain the jaundice and kidney failure.

We initially strongly suspected leptospirosis. However, other infectious diseases could not be excluded because the multiple nodules in the lungs were atypical for leptospirosis.

Because there was a possibility of various diseases, we avoided IV penicillin and started IV piperacillin-tazobactam and minocycline instead. He became anuric and was started on urgent hemodialysis on the second hospital day. Later on, antibody and PCR assays for *Leptospira* were negative. *F. necrophorum* was isolated in blood cultures on the second day. Further late, *Streptococcus intermedius* were isolated in blood cultures on the seventh day. We diagnosed his main disease as *F. necrophorum* rather than *S. intermedius* bacteremia based on the past case reports and the speed of positive blood cultures. Since *F. necrophorum* is famous for Lemierre's syndrome, we performed ultrasound in his jugular vein but found no thrombus. In addition, the dentist diagnosed a minor periodontal infection. *F. necrophorum* is thought to spread from periodontal infections. The main pathogen was *F. necrophorum*, but other anaerobic bacteria were also suspected to be involved. In addition, we were not able to test the susceptibility of *F. necrophorum* to penicillin. His treatment was thus de-escalated to IV ceftriaxone (CTRX) 1 g every 24 h and metronidazole (MNZ) 500 mg every 12 h on the 3rd day. Later, MNZ was increased up to 500 mg every 6 h. These treatments were continued up to the 17th day. The multiple lung nodules formed cavities and later disappeared after definitive therapy (Figure 2). He responded well to the treatment, was taken off hemodialysis, and discharged on the 18th hospital day. After discharge, he continued the treatment with amoxicillin and MNZ orally for three weeks (Figure 3). He had no relapse after three months of follow-up.

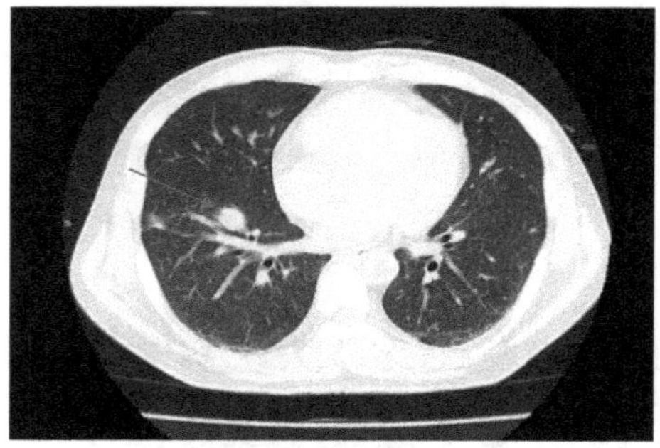

Figure 1: The chest computed tomography on the 1st day showing multiple nodules (red arrow).

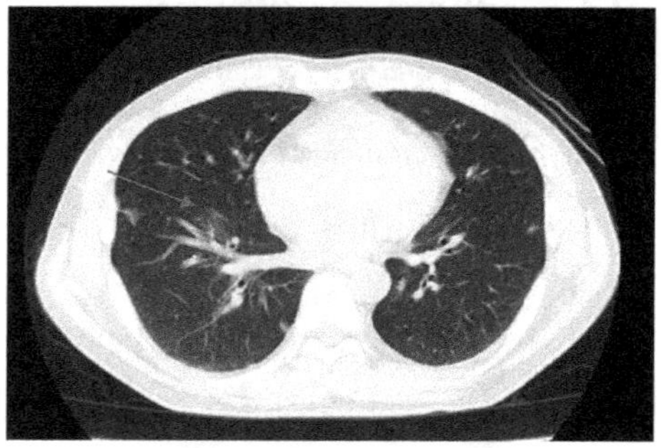

Figure 2: The chest computed tomography on the 38th day showing multiple nodules disappeared (red arrow).

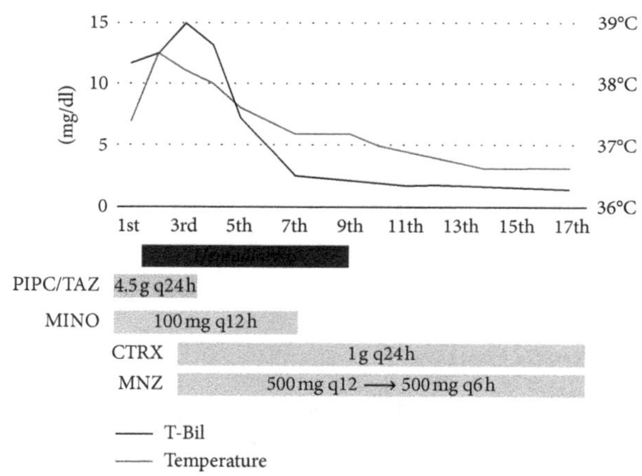

Figure 3: The clinical course. T-Bil: total bilirubin; PIPC/TAZ: piperacillin-tazobactam; MINO: minocycline; CTRX: ceftriaxone; MNZ: metronidazole.

3. Discussion

This was a case of *F. necrophorum* infection without Lemierre's mimicking leptospirosis. Differentiating between these two diseases is important from the viewpoint of early antibacterial drug selection and identification of complications.

Leptospirosis is a zoonosis caused by the pathogenic spirochete *Leptospira* spp. Its occurrence is distributed throughout the world but is especially frequent in tropical areas [8]. The main vectors are rodents. *Leptospira* infects humans via contact of the skin, mucous membranes, and conjunctiva with animal urine and contaminated water and soil. After the incubation period, which is usually ten days, fever, muscle pain, and headache appear in 75–100% of patients [9]. When leptospirosis becomes severe, it complicates with symptoms of jaundice and renal failure [1]. That is also known as Weil's disease. Conjunctival hyperemia has also been observed in 55% of cases and is a symptom useful for differentiation from other infectious diseases [2].

F. necrophorum is an anaerobic Gram-negative bacillus that is resident in the oral cavity [10]. *F. necrophorum* infection decreased after the spread of penicillin [11]; however, *F. necrophorum* infection, and especially pharyngitis, has increased in recent years [12]. In addition, *F. necrophorum* infection has a 5–9% mortality rate even with antibiotics [10].

F. necrophorum infection is sometimes accompanied by jaundice. Especially, most cases of frank jaundice or hyperbilirubinemia due to *F. necrophorum* infection had a thrombus in the internal jugular vein, which progressed to

Lemierre's syndrome [13]. This is a new point from this case: this case had no thrombus in the internal jugular vein. The exact frequency of jaundice by *F. necrophorum* is unknown. Moreover, there are completely different reports: frank jaundice is rare [14] or up to 49% [15]. In addition, the exact mechanism of jaundice by *F. necrophorum* remains unclear. We assume the lipopolysaccharide of *F. necrophorum* may affect jaundice because hyperbilirubinemia in sepsis is due to cholestasis by the lipopolysaccharide of bacteria [16], and the main toxicity of *F. necrophorum* is also from its lipopolysaccharide [17]. In addition, hemophagocytic lymphohistiocytosis can also be a differential diagnosis of jaundice and liver damage. In general, diagnosis of hemophagocytic lymphohistiocytosis in adults is due to multiple findings: fever ≥38.5°C, splenomegaly, pancytopenia, hypertriglyceridemia, and hyperferritinemia [18]. In this case, we did not measure triglyceride and ferritin, nor do a bone marrow puncture; therefore, we cannot deny hemophagocytic lymphohistiocytosis completely.

F. necrophorum sometimes has remote infection sites; in particular, septic embolism in the lung is found in 97% of *F. necrophorum* infections [13]. Septic embolism in the lung is an important feature of *F. necrophorum* infection and is not usually seen in leptospirosis. As the presence or absence of septic embolism can also affect the treatment period, it is important to differentiate between the two diseases. Incidentally, in this case, septic embolism in the lung was observed, and it was thought to be a disease condition close to Lemierre's syndrome, which is a severe clinical disease type of *F. necrophorum* infection characterized by pharyngitis and purulent thrombophlebitis in the jugular vein accompanied with bacteremia. However, thrombophlebitis of the jugular vein was not found by ultrasound or CT scan in this case.

This case showed the potential risks of using penicillin before diagnosis of leptospirosis. Penicillin is common for the treatment of leptospirosis [3]. *F. necrophorum* infection often causes a mixed infection with other anaerobic bacteria. In fact, our case was a mixed infection with *S. intermedius*. Antimicrobial resistance of anaerobic bacteria continues to progress; some anaerobic bacteria is resistance to penicillin. In addition, *F. necrophorum* itself occasionally produce β-lactamase [7]; that is, 2% of *F. necrophorum* is resistance to penicillin [19]. Unfortunately, we did not test susceptibility of *F. necrophorum* to PCG. Therefore, it is not exactly known whether this case has failed with penicillin or not; however, it remains a possibility that it may fail in a case of *F. necrophorum* and mixed infection. *F. necrophorum* is sensitive to CTRX and β-lactamase inhibitor combination drugs [2], and CTRX is equivalent to the penicillin group in the therapeutic effect against *Leptospira* [20, 21]. Therefore, initial treatment with cephalosporin or a β-lactamase inhibitor combination drug may be preferred when the cause of an infection has not been or cannot be distinguished.

We experienced a case of *F. necrophorum* infection mimicking leptospirosis. This case suggests the potential risks of using penicillin before a diagnosis of leptospirosis.

Authors' Contributions

RY and SS were responsible for writing the manuscript and the literature search. TY was involved in reviewing the manuscript and the literature search.

References

[1] S. Schreier, G. Doungchawee, S. Chadsuthi, D. Triampo, and W. Triampo, "Leptospirosis: current situation and trends of specific laboratory tests," *Expert Review of Clinical Immunology*, vol. 9, no. 3, pp. 263–280, 2013.

[2] N. B. Vanasco, M. F. Schmeling, J. Lottersberger, F. Costa, A. I. Ko, and H. D. Tarabla, "Clinical characteristics and risk factors of human leptospirosis in Argentina (1999–2005)," *Acta Tropica*, vol. 107, no. 3, pp. 255–258, 2008.

[3] M. D. Baber and R. D. Stuart, "Leptospirosis canicola a case treated with penicillin," *The Lancet*, vol. 248, no. 6426, pp. 594–596, 1946.

[4] D. Lin, N. Suwantarat, and R. S. Young, "Lemierre's syndrome mimicking leptospirosis," *Hawaii Medical Journal*, vol. 69, no. 7, pp. 161–163, 2010.

[5] T. Wingfield, T. J. Blanchard, and K. M. B. Ajdukiewicz, "Severe pneumonia and jaundice in a young man: an atypical presentation of an uncommon disease," *Journal of Medical Microbiology*, vol. 60, no. 9, pp. 1391–1394, 2011.

[6] Y. W. Han, "Fusobacterium nucleatum: a commensal-turned pathogen," *Current Opinion in Microbiology*, vol. 23, pp. 141–147, 2015.

[7] S. Ahkee, L. Srinath, M. J. Raff, A. Huang, and J. A. Ramirez, "Lemierre's syndrome: postanginal sepsis due to anaerobic oropharyngeal infection," *Annals of Otology, Rhinology & Laryngology*, vol. 103, no. 3, pp. 208–210, 1994.

[8] R. A. Hartskeerl, M. Collares-Pereira, and W. A. Ellis, "Emergence, control and re-emerging leptospirosis: dynamics of infection in the changing world," *Clinical Microbiology and Infection*, vol. 17, no. 4, pp. 494–501, 2011.

[9] A. R. Katz, V. E. Ansdell, P. V. Effler, C. R. Middleton, and D. M. Sasaki, "Assessment of the clinical presentation and treatment of 353 cases of laboratory-confirmed leptospirosis in Hawaii, 1974–1998," *Clinical Infectious Diseases*, vol. 33, no. 11, pp. 1834–1841, 2001.

[10] T. Riordan, "Human infection with *Fusobacterium necrophorum* (necrobacillosis), with a focus on Lemierre's syndrome," *Clinical Microbiology Reviews*, vol. 20, no. 4, pp. 622–659, 2007.

[11] C. L. Weesner and J. E. Cisek, "Lemierre syndrome: the forgotten disease," *Annals of Emergency Medicine*, vol. 22, no. 2, pp. 256–258, 1993

[12] R. M. Centor, "Expand the pharyngitis paradigm for adolescents and young adults," *Annals of Internal Medicine*, vol. 151, no. 11, pp. 812–815, 2009.

[13] C. P. Sinave, G. J. Hardy, and P. W. Fardy, "The Lemierre syndrome: suppurative thrombophlebitis of the internal jugular vein secondary to oropharyngeal infection," *Medicine*, vol. 68, no. 2, pp. 85–94, 1989.

[14] J. A. Chirinos, D. M. Lichtstein, J. Garcia, and L. J. Tamariz, "The evolution of Lemierre syndrome: report of 2 cases and review of the literature," *Medicine*, vol. 81, no. 6, pp. 458–465, 2002.

[15] C. M. Leugers and R. Clover, "Lemierre syndrome: postanginal sepsis," *The Journal of the American Board of Family Practice*, vol. 8, no. 5, pp. 384–391, 1995.

[16] N. Chand and A. J. Sanyal, "Sepsis-induced cholestasis," *Hepatology*, vol. 45, no. 1, pp. 230–241, 2007.
[17] J. S. Brazier, "Human infections with *Fusobacterium necrophorum*," *Anaerobe*, vol. 12, no. 4, pp. 165–172, 2006.
[18] M. B. Jordan, C. E. Allen, S. Weitzman, A. H. Filipovich, and K. L. McClain, "How I treat hemophagocytic lymphohistiocytosis," *Blood*, vol. 118, no. 15, pp. 4041–4052, 2011.
[19] J. S. Brazier, B. I. Duerden, E. Yusuf, and V. Hall, "*Fusobacterium necrophorum* infections in England and Wales 1990-2000," *Journal of Medical Microbiology*, vol. 51, no. 3, pp. 269–272, 2002.
[20] T. Panaphut, S. Domrongkitchaiporn, A. Vibhagool, B. Thinkamrop, and W. Susaengrat, "Ceftriaxone compared with sodium penicillin G for treatment of severe leptospirosis," *Clinical Infectious Diseases*, vol. 36, no. 12, pp. 1507–1513, 2003.
[21] Y. Suputtamongkol, K. Niwattayakul, C. Suttinont et al., "An open, randomized, controlled trial of penicillin, doxycycline, and cefotaxime for patients with severe leptospirosis," *Clinical Infectious Diseases*, vol. 39, no. 10, pp. 1417–1424, 2004.

20

Bilateral Facial Diplegia: A Rare Presenting Symptom of Lyme

John Ashurst and Matthew Perry

Duke Lifepoint Conemaugh Memorial Medical Center, Department of Emergency Medicine, Johnstown, PA, USA

Correspondence should be addressed to John Ashurst; ashurst.john.32.research@gmail.com

Academic Editor: Sinésio Talhari

Lyme disease is a common disease that is faced by the physician but also acts a mimicker of many other disease processes. Facial palsies, especially bilateral, are a relatively rare presenting symptom of Lyme disease and may warrant further investigation. A thorough history and physical examination coupled with precision testing may aid the physician when faced with a patient with the diagnostic dilemma of facial diplegia.

1. Introduction

Lyme disease is the most common tick borne illness in the United States with an estimated 36,000 reported cases annually [1]. Although a large number of cases are reported to the Center for Disease Control, more than 300,000 cases remain unreported each year [1]. The most common sign of the disease is a rash known as erythema migrans, which may occur up to 1 to 2 weeks after infection but has been seen up to 4 weeks later [2]. Unlike the commonality of the "bulls eye rash" of Lyme disease, bilateral facial palsy is a relatively rare presenting symptom of the disease. The authors report a case of Lyme disease that presented with two-week history of facial swelling and facial diplegia.

2. Case

A 21-year-old male presented to the emergency department with a 2-week history of facial swelling and now decreased facial movement for the last several days. He was recently seen by his dentist and placed on clindamycin for a presumed dental infection several days prior to presentation but notes that the symptoms have worsened. Currently, he notes that he has a difficult time opening and closing his mouth but denies any difficulty with mastication. His past medical history was negative and his social history noted that he recently returned from a camping trip in western Pennsylvania.

On physical exam, vital signs were within normal limits. He was able to open and close his mouth but noted that he could not open to the full extent. He had no drooling or changes in phonation. Upon examination of his teeth, he had dental fillings but no evidence of dental abscess, dental discomfort, or gingival abscess. A neurological exam revealed a normal gait and strength. He stated that he had a difficult time raising his eyebrows (Figure 1) and was only able to make a very small smile (Figure 2). He also had subjective sensory loss to light touch over the cheeks bilaterally but this could not be reproduced on examination. Besides the bilateral peripheral nerve palsy, the remainder of his neurological examination was with in normal limits.

Labs revealed a normal complete blood count, basic metabolic panel, and sed rate. Rapid Lyme titers were sent and revealed a positive Lyme IgM and IGG titer (Vidas Lyme IGG II and IgM II, Biomerieux). The patient was started on doxycycline for 21 days and a confirmatory western blot was sent out to a reference lab. The western blot confirmed that the patient was Lyme IgM positive, which was consistent with early infection of *Borrelia burgdorferi*.

3. Discussion

Bilateral facial paralysis (diplegia) is a relatively rare condition and comprises roughly 0.3% to 2% of all facial palsies [3]. In order to be described as a simultaneous facial palsy,

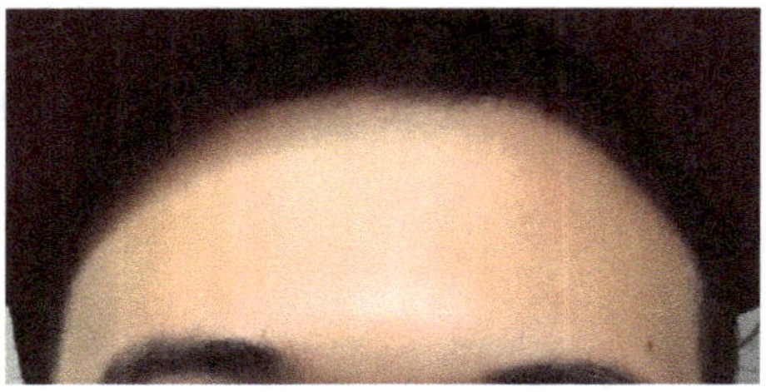

FIGURE 1: Bilateral loss of forehead creases while attempting to elevate the eyebrows.

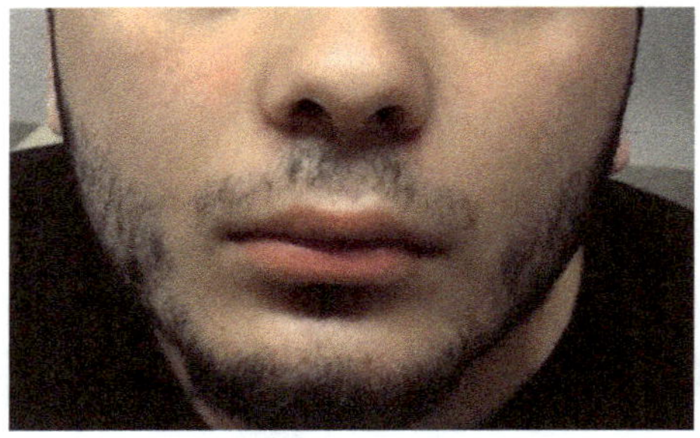

FIGURE 2: Patient attempting to smile with loss of cranial nerve VII bilaterally.

instead of a recurrent unilateral facial palsy, the patient must present with opposite sided facial symptoms within 30 days of the onset of the first side. The differential diagnosis of patients with facial diplegia is broad and should include infection, trauma, metabolic, neoplastic, autoimmune, neurological, and idiopathic causes [4]. However, several studies have noted that Lyme disease is one of the most common causes of facial diplegia [4, 5].

Lyme disease is caused by the spirochete *Borrelia burgdorferi* and is transmitted through the bite of infected *Ixodes ricinus* ticks. Neurological manifestations can occur in up to 15% of patients and the classic triad of lymphocytic meningitis, cranial neuritis, and radiculoneuritis is a hallmark of this level of infection [6]. Cranial neuritis most commonly involves the seventh cranial nerve but can also involve cranial nerves involved in extraocular eye movements, hearing, and sensation of the face [6]. Classically, when cranial nerve VII is involved the patient will present with acute onset of one sided facial weakness, but approximately 25% of cases are now being reported as having bilateral diplegia [6].

The standard of care for diagnosing disseminated Lyme disease is a two-tiered serologic approach that garners approximately 70–100% sensitivity and a specificity of approximately 95% [7]. The first tier involves either enzyme immunoassay (EIA) or an immunofluorescence assay (IFA) measuring the overall antibody response to either IgM or IgG [7]. If either of these results is equivocal or positive, an immunoblot should be used to detect antibodies against *B. burgdorferi* (Figure 3) [7]. The immunoblot detects antibody reactivity to specific preselected *B. burgdorferi* antigens and is considered positive if bands are equal or greater than the intensity of the control [7].

Currently, the Infectious Disease Society of America has published guidelines on the treatment of Lyme disease and is based upon diagnosis. For those with cranial nerve palsies without clinical evidence of meningitis, doxycycline, amoxicillin, and cefuroxime are all considered appropriate treatment modalities [8]. Although doxycycline should be considered first-line therapy due to its penetrance into the central nervous system, the physician should tailor antibiotic choice to the patient's age and allergies [8].

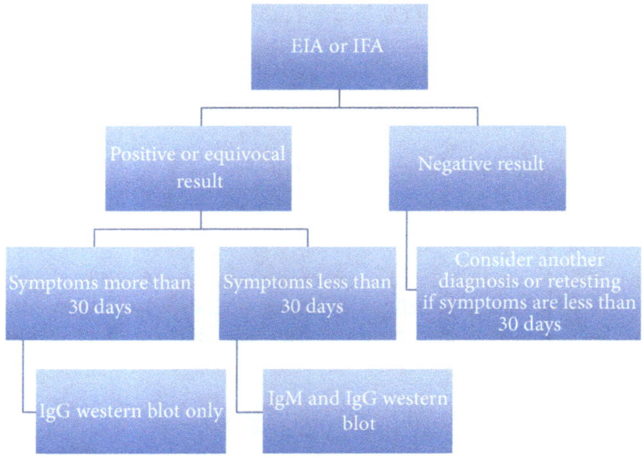

FIGURE 3: A step-wise approach for the diagnosis of *Borrelia* infection in a patient with clinically suspected Lyme disease.

4. Conclusion

In conclusion, those who present to the physician with facial diplegia represent a diagnostic dilemma due to both the relative scarcity of this presenting symptom and the morbidity of the diseases in the differential. However, those who live in endemic areas for Lyme disease should be aware of the correlation between facial diplegia and the disease. A thorough history and physical exam may aid the physician in diagnosis and allow for prompt treatment in order to prevent long term sequelae.

Authors' Contributions

John Ashurst and Matthew Perry contributed equally to this manuscript.

References

[1] P. S. Mead, "Epidemiology of Lyme disease," *Infectious Disease Clinics of North America*, vol. 29, no. 2, pp. 187–210, 2015.

[2] E. D. Shapiro, "Lyme disease," *The New England Journal of Medicine*, vol. 370, no. 18, pp. 1724–1731, 2014.

[3] A. Kamaratos, S. Kokkoris, J. Protopsaltis et al., "Simultaneous bilateral facial palsy in a diabetic patient," *Diabetes Care*, vol. 27, no. 2, pp. 623–624, 2004.

[4] V. Jain, A. Deshmukh, and S. Gollomp, "Bilateral facial paralysis case presentation and discussion of differential diagnosis," *Journal of General Internal Medicine*, vol. 21, no. 7, pp. C7–C10, 2006.

[5] R. A. Baudin, N. Jowett, C. A. Banks, C. J. Knox, and T. A. Hadlock, "Bilateral facial paralysis: a 13 year experience," *Plastic and Reconstructive Surgery*, vol. 138, no. 4, pp. 879–887, 2016.

[6] J. J. Halperin, "Nervous system lyme disease," *Infectious Disease Clinics of North America*, vol. 29, no. 2, pp. 241–253, 2015.

[7] A. Moore, C. Nelson, C. Molins, P. Mead, and M. Schriefer, "Current guidelines, common clinical pitfalls, and future directions for laboratory diagnosis of Lyme disease, United States," *Emerging Infectious Diseases*, vol. 22, no. 7, pp. 1169–1177, 2016.

[8] G. P. Wormser, R. J. Dattwyler, E. D. Shapiro et al., "The clinical assessments treatment, and prevention of lyme disease, human granulocytic anaplasmosis, and babesiosis: clinical practice guidelines by the Infectious Diseases Society of America," *Clinical Infectious Diseases*, vol. 43, no. 9, pp. 1089–1134, 2006.

21

Prepatellar Bursal Infection Caused by *Mycobacterium tuberculosis* with an In Situ Total Knee Arthroplasty: A Case Report and Comprehensive Literature Review

Abdulrahman D. Algarni

Department of Orthopedic Surgery, King Saud University, Riyadh, Saudi Arabia

Correspondence should be addressed to Abdulrahman D. Algarni; abdulrahmanga@gmail.com

Academic Editor: Gernot Walder

Prepatellar bursal infection is a rare occurrence. The incidence of tuberculosis, including musculoskeletal type, is increasing. We present a case of isolated prepatellar bursal swelling associated with a discharging sinus; the condition developed in an elderly patient 4 years after total knee arthroplasty. Aspiration of the bursa revealed acid-fast bacilli on Ziehl–Neelsen staining, typical of *Mycobacterium tuberculosis*; this was confirmed later on culture. The patient was successfully treated with a 6-month course of antituberculous chemotherapy. To the best of our knowledge, only two previous cases of tuberculous prepatellar bursal infection have been reported in English literature. Our case illustrates the importance of considering tuberculous prepatellar bursal infection in the differential diagnosis of anterior knee swelling. All physicians treating patients with musculoskeletal disease should be aware of the possibility of this diagnosis and maintain a high index of suspicion; this is especially true in areas where tuberculosis is still endemic and in high-risk patients, such as the elderly.

1. Introduction

Prepatellar bursitis is common among people involved in occupations that require prolonged kneeling or crawling. Infection of the prepatellar bursa, however, is a rare occurrence. The risk factors for infection include a history of repetitive skin trauma, such as during prolonged kneeling, repeated local steroid injections, immunocompromised status, and previous instances of bursitis [1]. Unlike hematogenous seeding in septic arthritis, local trauma and the direct transcutaneous route is the proposed mechanism of infection for infected bursitis, probably because of the poor blood supply to the bursa [2]. Approximately, 80% of the cases of infected prepatellar bursitis are caused by *Staphylococcus aureus* and 15% by streptococcal species [2]. Rarely, atypical mycobacteria, *Brucella*, and fungi have been isolated as the causative organisms [3–6].

Existing literature suggests that the incidence of tuberculosis is increasing, both in developing and developed countries [7]. This increase is attributed to the rise in the number of immunocompromised patients, including the elderly and those with acquired immunodeficiency syndrome. Musculoskeletal involvement occurs in approximately 1%–5.2% of cases. Bursal tuberculous infection occurs in a small percentage of these cases and is mostly reported to occur in the greater trochanter bursa [8].

In this report, we describe a rare case of isolated prepatellar bursal infection with typical *Mycobacterium tuberculosis* and present a review of previously published cases in the English literature. The patient gave an informed consent that anonymous data and pictures concerning his case would be submitted for publication.

2. Case Presentation

A 74-year-old male patient underwent left total knee arthroplasty (TKA) at our institution for degenerative knee osteoarthrosis. He had an uneventful postoperative course

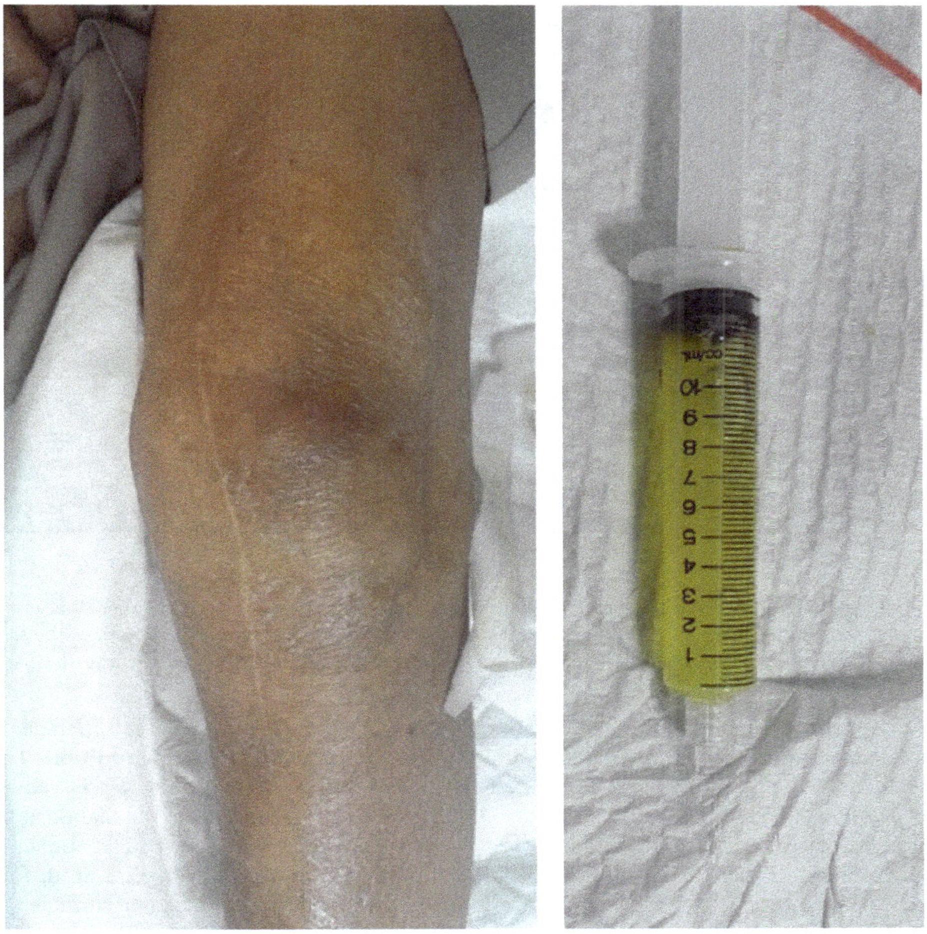

(a) (b)

FIGURE 1: (a) Clinical photograph of the left knee showing the prepatellar swelling and the discharging sinus. (b) A syringe showing the colour of the aspirated fluid.

with no history of delayed wound healing or persistent drainage. Four years later, he presented with a 2-month history of a gradually developing painless swelling over the anterior aspect of the operated knee; the swelling was associated with a small sinus that was extruding a straw-coloured fluid. He had no history of fever, decreased appetite, or weight loss. He had no other musculoskeletal, respiratory, or systemic symptoms of note. He had no history of antecedent trauma, recent travel, or contact with infectious diseases. The patient is a known hypertensive, but the blood pressure was well controlled with treatment, and he is otherwise healthy. He is a retired teacher with no history of involvement in activities requiring excessive kneeling. He is ambulatory in his community and can walk comfortably with the assistance of a cane.

The patient's general physical examination results were within normal limits; positive physical findings were limited to the involved knee. There was an anterior knee swelling involving mainly the prepatellar area, approximately 7 cm in diameter, fluctuant, and not tender to palpation, with minimal surrounding erythema; the erythema was present mainly at the punctum. The punctum was draining a yellowish discharge on pressure (Figure 1(a)). There was no bony tenderness at the patella, distal femur, or proximal tibia. There was no detectable knee effusion, instability, or crepitus. The range of motion was well preserved (5–110°), as it was a prosthetic knee. It was only painful at the end of flexion as this movement compressed the prepatellar bursa.

Plain radiographs of the knee showed a prepatellar soft tissue swelling (Figure 2(a)). There were no obvious bony changes, osteolysis, or loosening at the bone-prosthesis interface. Needle aspiration of the prepatellar bursa yielded 50 mL of slightly turbid straw-coloured yellowish fluid that was sent as per our protocol for cell count determination, microcrystal analysis, Gram staining, and Ziehl–Neelsen (ZN) staining for acid-fast bacilli (Figure 1(b)). Cultures for aerobic and anaerobic bacteria, *Mycobacterium tuberculosis*, *Brucella*, and fungi were requested.

Considering the patient's age, chronic presentation, and the presence of sinus, he was admitted with a diagnosis of infected prepatellar bursitis. The primary aims of admission were wound dressing, awaiting aspiration results, and further work-up. Aspiration results revealed normal cell counts,

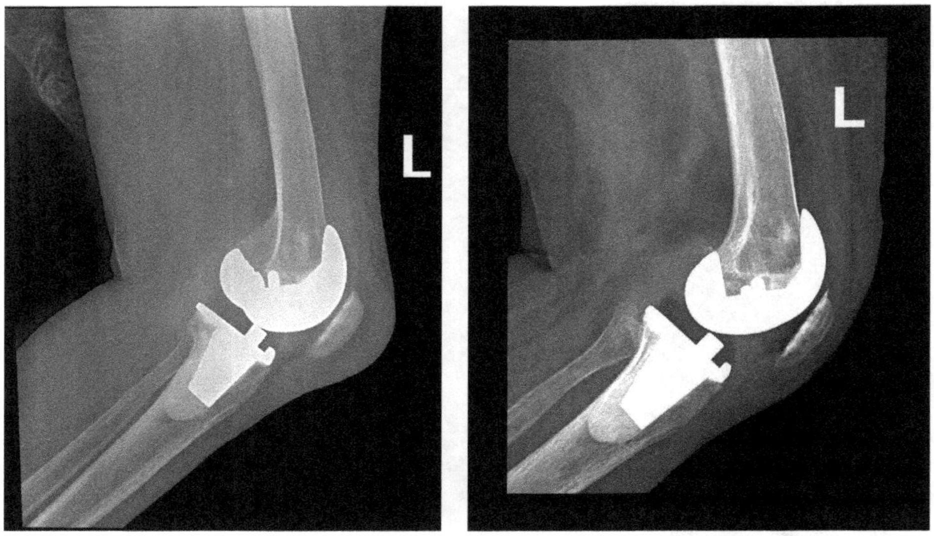

(a) (b)

FIGURE 2: (a) Plain lateral view radiograph of the left knee showing the prepatellar soft tissue swelling and otherwise well-fixed prosthesis with no signs of osteolysis at the bone-prosthesis interface or at the patella. (b) Plain lateral view radiograph of the same knee at the 6-year follow-up showing regression of the swelling and otherwise normal appearance of the prosthetic knee and the patella.

no crystals, and no organisms on Gram stain. To our surprise, ZN stain revealed acid-fast bacilli consistent with typical tuberculous infection; the bacterium was confirmed on culture 6 weeks later as *Mycobacterium tuberculosis*-sensitive to rifampicin, isoniazid, ethambutol, and streptomycin. Cultures for bacteria, *Brucella*, and fungi were negative. Aspiration was repeated and yielded similar results. The blood work-up showed normal total and differential white blood cell count and slight elevation of both erythrocyte sedimentation rate (ESR) (80 mm/hr; normal: 30–70 mm/hr) and C-reactive protein (CRP) (8 mg/L; normal: 0–4 mg/L). Tuberculin skin test revealed a negative result (<5 mm induration at 72 hrs), and further work-up including chest radiograph and echocardiogram revealed no evidence of systemic disease. A triple three-phase bone scan displayed normal uptake both at the bone-prosthesis interface and at the patella. An infectious disease consult was obtained. The patient was started on rifampicin (600 mg/day), isoniazid (300 mg/day), pyrazinamide (1500 mg/day), and ethambutol (800 mg/day) for 2 months and continued on the same dosage of rifampicin and isoniazid to complete a 6-month course.

Three weeks later, the swelling significantly subsided in size and the sinus healed; therefore, the patient was discharged. He was reviewed at 6-week intervals at both the orthopaedic and infectious disease clinics for clinical progression and for any side effects of the medication. At the most recent 6-year follow-up, he was doing well with no evidence of local recurrence or prosthetic loosening (Figure 2(b)).

3. Discussion

The subcutaneous prepatellar bursa is a synovial bursa that lies between the skin and the patella. It is anatomically distinct from the superficial infrapatellar bursa, which lies in front of the patellar tendon and tibial tubercle. Sometimes, the two bursae are collectively referred to as the prepatellar bursa, which is inaccurate [1]. Standard textbooks of human anatomy describe the prepatellar bursa as a unilaminar or bilaminar bursa; however, Dye et al. found in a cadaveric study that the bursa has a trilaminar structure in 93% of knees [9, 10]. The three layers are a superficial subcutaneous layer, which lies between the subcutaneous tissue and an extension of the fascia lata, called the transverse superficial fascia; an intermediate subfascial layer, localized between the transverse superficial fascia and an oblique fascia formed by fascial extension of the vastus lateralis and medialis muscles; and a deep subaponeurotic layer, situated between the intermediate oblique fascia and the deep longitudinal fibres of the rectus femoris tendon [10].

Mycobacterial infection of the prepatellar bursa has been rarely reported. To date, only five cases have been reported in the English literature [4–6, 11, 12]. Of these 5, only 2 showed typical *Mycobacterium tuberculosis* infection, the rest showed atypical mycobacteria. Stewart reported the first case of mycobacterial tuberculous infection of the prepatellar bursa [11]. Schickendantz and Watson described another case of infected prepatellar bursa secondary to *Mycobacterium tuberculosis* infection [12]. Other authors published three similar cases due to infection with atypical mycobacteria; two of them were due to *Mycobacterium marinum (balnei)* and one due to *Mycobacterium fortuitum* [4–6]. In this report, we presented a third case of isolated mycobacterial tuberculous infection of the prepatellar bursa in an elderly patient with an in situ TKA.

The diagnosis of tuberculous prepatellar bursal infection is often difficult and requires a high index of clinical suspicion. Along with clinical assessment for possible intraarticular and/or patellar involvement, sufficient musculoskeletal imaging work-up is important. Owing to the presence of prosthesis and unavailability of prosthesis-compatible magnetic resonance imaging (metal artefact reduction sequence- (MARS-) MRI) at our institution, we were unable to perform an MRI, which would have enabled better delineation of the soft tissues and detect any possible early bony changes. MacLean and Kulkarni reported a case of tuberculous infection of the patella that presented as prepatellar bursitis [13]. There was no evidence of patellar or prosthetic joint involvement in our patient. Aspiration is helpful and is usually required for diagnosis. Unless special staining or polymerase chain reaction (PCR) test reveals the organism, culture requires 6 weeks of incubation to grow; this can further delay the diagnosis and treatment. It was fortunate in the present patient that ZN staining revealed the organism, as PCR testing is not available in most institutions, including ours. If a biopsy tissue is obtained, histopathological examination is nonspecific and demonstrates evidence of chronic inflammation and caseating granulomas [8].

Empiric antituberculous chemotherapy is recommended if the clinical scenario and the work-up are suggestive of this diagnosis, regardless of the diagnostic team's ability to isolate the organism [14]. A general work-up for systemic tuberculous disease is also mandated. In tuberculous infection, as in this case, ESR and CRP are often only mildly elevated or can even be normal. Our patient had no evidence of systemic tuberculosis nor did he have a previous known contact with the disease despite being from a country where tuberculosis is still prevalent. We hypothesised that transcutaneous inoculation of mycobacteria was the probable mechanism for bursal infection, similar to what was reported in previously mentioned cases [4–6, 11, 12].

Multidrug antituberculous chemotherapy is considered the mainstay of treatment; surgical drainage and debridement are performed in case of a pointing abscess [14]. A well-placed incision is recommended; generally, the lateral parapatellar incision is used. Schickendantz and Watson performed a total bursectomy in their Case [12]. Quayle and Robinson proposed a technique in which only the posterior wall is resected, leaving the anterior wall adherent to the subcutaneous tissue; they recommended this to reduce the skin-related complications of total bursectomy, [15]. Our patient was effectively treated only with antituberculous chemotherapy.

4. Conclusion

Although tuberculous prepatellar bursal infection is a rarely reported entity, this case illustrates that it should be considered in the differential diagnosis of anterior knee swelling that does not respond to conventional management. Physicians who treat patients with musculoskeletal disease should be aware of the possibility of this diagnosis and maintain a high index of suspicion, especially in areas where tuberculosis is still endemic as well as in high-risk groups such as elderly patients.

References

[1] D. L. Aaron, A. Patel, S. Kayiaros, and R. Calfee, "Four common types of bursitis: diagnosis and management," *American Academy of Orthopaedic Surgeon*, vol. 19, no. 6, pp. 359–367, 2011.

[2] B. W. Zimmermann, D. J. Mikolich, and G. Ho Jr, "Septic bursitis," *Seminars in Arthritis and Rheumatism*, vol. 24, no. 6, pp. 391–410, 1995.

[3] P. J. Kelley, L. A. Weed, and P R. Lipscomb, "Infection of tendon sheaths, bursae, joints, and soft tissues by acid-fast bacilli other than tubercle bacilli," *Journal of Bone and Joint Surgery*, vol. 45, no. 2, pp. 327–386, 1963.

[4] F. E. Winter and E. H. Runyon, "Prepatellar bursitis caused by mycobacterium marinum (balnei)," *Journal of Bone and Joint Surgery*, vol. 47, no. 2, pp. 375–379, 1965.

[5] P. J. Kelly, A. G. Karlson, L. A. Weed, and P. R. Lipscomb, "Infection of synovial tissues by mycobacteria other than mycobacterium tuberculosis," *Journal of Bone and Joint Surgery*, vol. 49, no. 8, pp. 1521–1530, 1967.

[6] J. C. Wallach, M. V. Delpino, R. Scian, B. Deodato, C. A. Fossati, and P. C. Baldi, "Prepatellar bursitis due to Brucella abortus: case report and analysis of the local immune response," *Journal of Medical Microbiology*, vol. 59, no. 12, pp. 1514–1518, 2010.

[7] A. Jitmuang, V. Yuenyongviwat, K. Charoencholvanich, and M. Chayakulkeeree, "Rapidly-growing mycobacterial infection: a recognized cause of early-onset prosthetic joint infection," *BMC Infect Dis*, vol. 17, no. 1, p. 802, 2017.

[8] M. Crespo, C. Pigrau X. Flores et al., "Tuberculous trochanteric bursitis: report of 5 cases and literature review," *Scandinavian Journal of Infectious Diseases*, vol. 36, no. 8, pp. 552–558, 2009.

[9] F. H. Netter, *Atlas of Human Anatomy*, S. Colacino, Ed., Ciba-Geigy, Summit, NJ, USA, 1989.

[10] S. F. Dye, D. Campagna-pinto, C. C. Dye, S. Shifflett, and T. Eiman, "Soft-tissue anatomy anterior to the human patella," *Journal of Bone and Joint Surgery-American Volume*, vol. 85, no. 6, pp. 1012–1017, 2003.

[11] W. J. Stewart, "Tuberculous bursitis without adjacent joint involvement following trauma," *Journal of Bone and Joint Surgery*, vol. 15, p. 626, 1933.

[12] M. S. Schickendantz and J. T Watson, "Mycobacterial prepatellar bursitis," *Clinical Orthopaedics and Related Research*, vol. 258, pp. 209–12, 1990.

[13] S. MacLean and S. Kulkarni, "Tuberculosis of the patella masquerading as prepatellar bursitis," *Annals of The Royal College of Surgeons of England*, vol. 95, no. 1, pp. e17–9, 2013.

[14] J. I. Hogan, R. M. Hurtado, and S. B. Nelson, "Mycobacterial musculoskeletal infections," *Infectious Disease Clinics of North America*, vol. 31, no. 2, pp. 369–382, 2017.

[15] J. B. Quayle and M. P. Robinson, "An operation for chronic prepatellar bursitis," *Journal of Bone and Joint Surgery*, vol. 58, pp. 504–506, 1978.

22

Neisseria meningitidis Infecting a Prosthetic Knee Joint: A New Case of an Unusual Disease

Berta Becerril Carral,[1] Elvira Alarcón Manoja,[2] Salvador López Cárdenas,[1] and Jesús Canueto Quintero[1]

[1] *Unidad Clínica de Gestión de Enfermedades Infecciosas y Microbiología del Área Sanitaria del Campo de Gibraltar, Cádiz, Spain*
[2] *Unidad Clínica de Gestión de Medicina Interna del Área Sanitaria del Campo de Gibraltar, Cádiz, Spain*

Correspondence should be addressed to Elvira Alarcón Manoja; elviraalarconmanoja@hotmail.com

Academic Editor: Oguz R. Sipahi

Primary meningococcal meningitis is an infrequent but known disease. However, the infection of a prosthetic joint with *Neisseria meningitidis* is rare. We hereby describe the second case of an arthroplasty infected with *Neisseria meningitidis* that responded favourably to prosthesis retention with surgical debridement, in combination with antibiotics treatment.

1. Introduction

Neisseria meningitidis is a Gram-negative, facultative, aerobic, or anaerobic diplococcus. It was isolated for the first time by Anton Weischselbaum in 1887 in the cerebrospinal fluid of a meningitis patient [1]. It is a strict human pathogen with a wide variety of clinical manifestations. *N. meningitidis* can cause extremely severe diseases, such as meningitis and life-threatening sepsis, as well as the asymptomatic colonization of the nasopharynx in approximately 10% of the population during endemic periods of infection [2]. It rarely provokes localized forms, such as septic arthritis, pneumonia, pericarditis, otitis, sinusitis, and urethritis [3]. Primary purulent arthritis caused by *N. meningitidis* is a rare but known disease. However, as far as we know, there is only one published case report of an arthroplasty infected with *Neisseria meningitidis* [4]. We hereby present a new case of this exceptional infection.

The duration and form of administration of antibiotic agents in these infections are based on expert opinions. The traditional recommendation duration of total postdebridement antibiotic treatment of 6 to maximal 12 weeks or the duration of its initial parental part (2–4 weeks) is discussed in favour of an oral antibiotic treatment from the start [5].

2. Case Presentation

A 78-year-old Caucasian female patient with dislipemia, stable ischemic cardiopathology, degenerative aortic and mitral valves, and generalized osteoarthritis arrived at the Emergency Department of Hospital Punta de Europa, Algeciras, Spain, a 328-bed general hospital, with a chief complaint of pain in her left knee. The patient had undergone a total left knee arthroplasty 7 months before due to a severe functional limitation secondary to osteoarthritis. Seven days before admission and while experiencing symptoms of pharyngitis, she had an accident at home and suffered a sprain in her left ankle. The patient complained of pain and swelling in the above joint that radiated towards her left knee. Within days of the accident, the patient reported a gradual reduction in the symptoms in her ankle but an increase of pain in her knee. She started complaining of intense pain, functional impairment, redness, and increase of local temperature but without evidence of skin rash. The presence of intra-articular fluid was confirmed in the operated knee. There were no other affected joints or presence of skin lesions. Main analytical data were as follows: leukocytes: 13.6 × 109/L with 80% granulocytes; haemoglobin: 11.8 g/dL; platelets: 486 × 109/L; immunoglobulin levels in serum were normal. An arthrocentesis was performed and it yielded an amber-coloured fluid with 9.9 × 109/L (67% polymorphonuclear), glucose: 97 mg/dL, proteins: 4.2 g/dL, and LDH: 1866 U/L. No crystals were observed. The joint fluid culture was positive for *N. meningitidis* serogroup B (latex agglutination (Difco™ Neisseria Meningitidis Antiserum, Becton, Dickinson and Company®, Sparks, MD)), with an intermediate sensitivity to penicillin (minimum inhibitory concentration (MIC): 0,25 microg/ml by *E*-test (BioMerieux® Inc, Marcy L'Etoil, France)) and sensitivity to cefotaxime (0,01 microg/ml by *E*-test (BioMerieux Inc, Marcy L'Etoil, France)) and ciprofloxacin (by disk diffusion (Sensi-Disc™, Becton, Dickinson and Company, Sparks, MD) according to the CLSI guidelines [6, 7]. *N. meningitidis* was identified by growth on chocolate agar and blood agar, and by utilization of enriched media (API NH biochemical testing (BioMerieux Inc, Marcy L'Etoil, France)). Blood cultures were negatives (BacT/ALERT® 3D system (BioMerieux Inc, Mercy L'Etoil, France)). The procedure included arthroscopic debridement with implant retention because of individual patient circumstances and acute onset of symptoms in the setting of a well-fixed prosthesis without a sinus tract and antibiotics and 2 grams ceftriaxone administered intravenously every 24 hours over a 3-week period, followed by oral administration of 750 mg ciprofloxacin every 12 hours over the total 12-week study period. No recurrence has been observed during a two-year follow-up. The Department of Preventive Medicine and Public Health was notified of the case and the recommendations on prophylaxis and treatment of possible carriers were followed, and the patient was vaccinated with meningococcal vaccines following this episode [8].

3. Discussion

Infection is the most feared complication after an arthroplasty and has proven to be the cause for a notable rate of morbidity and a nonnegligible rate of mortality [9]. There are two ways of how microorganisms can infect a prosthetic joint, and the most frequent is direct inoculation during surgery. The second one is haematogenous dissemination, responsible for 10% of the cases.

In his article, Aslam et al. [10] include nonsurgical trauma to the implant as a risk factor for the acquisition of a haematogenous prosthetic infection. In the case described, a traumatic event that had happened in the past and that had affected the left ankle and knee could have created an environment allowing the bacteria, which just happened to be in the blood at the time due to a concomitant pharyngitis, to seed the prosthetic joint.

The most frequently isolated bacteria in prosthetic joint infections are: *Staphylococcus aureus*, *Streptococcus* spp., and Gram-negative bacilli, although the proportions vary depending on the series [11].

Three clinical syndromes have been described in association to the bloodstream infection with *Neisseria meningitidis*. The first one, acute meningococcemia, is a severe condition that occurs within the context of a sepsis, a septic shock, or meningitis. Although rarer, bacteraemia adopts a less aggressive clinical course, such as chronic meningococcemia, indistinguishable from chronic gonococcemia, which is a rare infection characterized by intermittent fever episodes, maculopapular rash, and arthralgia; it can also adopt the form of transient meningococcemia, characterized by fever and unspecified rash over a 2–5-day evolution period where presence of *N. meningitidis* in the blood usually comes as an unexpected finding [12].

Besides, the ability of *N meningitidis* to infect prosthetic joints shall depend upon the affinity for the osteoarticular tissue, the type of prosthesis employed, and the residual joint tissue. The frequency of arthritis complicating acute meningococcal disease in adults ranges from 4 to 50%. Schaad [13] describes the following three clinical types of arthritis in meningococcal disease. (1) The most common type is arthritis complicating acute meningococcal disease. Its mechanism is of an immunologic basis and affects larger joints, mainly knees, and, less frequently, the direct invasion of the joint by the bacteria. (2) Chronic meningococcemia is accompanied more often by arthralgia. (3) Primary meningococcal arthritis, which is a rare form of acute septic arthritis, affects large joints almost exclusively and is monoarticular in two-thirds of the cases.

Both the case described by Vikram et al. [4] and the present description should be classified in the third category, where the germ's route of entry is supposedly haematogenous.

Biofilm formation plays a crucial role in the ability of germs to colonize nonbiological surfaces. Both encapsulated and nonencapsulated forms of *N. meningitidis* are capable of producing biofilm. This favours its persistence in the nasopharynx and seems to play an important role in the process of colonization and the carrier status (in this case the pharyngitis seven days before admission was the probable entry site but was not confirmed). Nonetheless, the role of biofilm-forming strains in the different clinical syndromes associated with the meningococcal disease is still to be determined.

To our knowledge, this is the second reported case of primary meningococcal arthritis in a prosthetic joint. The previous case, published in 2001, described the infection of a total knee prosthesis by *N. meningitidis* serogroup Y in an 80-year-old female patient. This patient's prosthesis had been placed 3 years before and as in the case hereby presented, it did not have any distinctive clinical feature. The management included prosthesis retention and a 6-week course of i.v. ceftriaxone.

In both cases, the most likely route of entry for the germ into the joint was the haematogenous route, although the presence of this germ in blood could never be confirmed. The case presented was probably favoured by a minor local trauma. Besides, the infection of other types of nonarticular prosthetic grafts with *N. meningitidis* is very rare and limited to a very reduced number of endocarditis on prosthetic valves [14, 15]. Therefore, *N. meningitidis* is a germ that has low affinity for the joint tissue and, although capable of producing biofilm in order to survive in the surface secretions of the nasopharynx, it has very limited capacity to cause infections in abiotic surfaces, and here lies the exceptional significance of the case hereby presented.

Authors' Contributions

Berta Becerril Carral and Elvira Alarcón Manoja contributed equally to this case report.

References

[1] A. Weichselbaum, "Über die aetiologie der akuten meningitis cerebro-spinalis," *Fortschritte der Medizin*, vol. 5, pp. 573–583, 1887.

[2] S. P. Yazdankhah and D. A. Caugant, "*Neisseria meningitidis*: an overview of the carriage state," *Journal of Medical Microbiology*, vol. 53, no. 9, pp. 821–832, 2004.

[3] A. P. Yung and M. I. McDonald, "Early clinical clues to meningococcaemia," *Medical Journal of Australia*, vol. 178, no. 3, pp. 134–137, 2003.

[4] H. R. Vikram, R. B. Buencamino, and S. I. Aronin, "Primary meningococcal arthritis in a prosthetic knee joint," *Journal of Infection*, vol. 42, no. 4, pp. 279–281, 2001.

[5] L. Deabate, P. Leonardo, and U. İlker, "Modern antibiotic treatment of chronic long bone infections in adults-theory, evidence and practice," *Mediterranean Journal of Infection, Microbes and Antimicrobials*, vol. 3, article 9, 2014.

[6] Clinical and Laboratory Standards Institute, *Methods for Dilution Antimicrobial Susceptibility Tests for Bacteria That Grow Aerobically*, Approved Standard M07-A8, CLSI, Wayne, Pa, USA, 8th edition, 2009.

[7] Clinical and Laboratory Standards Institute, *Performance Standards for Antimicrobial Susceptibility Testing: Twentieth Informational Supplement*, CLSI Document M100-S22, CLSI, Wayne, Pa, USA, 2012.

[8] D. van de Beek, C. Cabellos, O. Dzupova et al., "ESCMID guideline: diagnosis and treatment of acute bacterial meningitis," *Clinical Microbiology and Infection*, vol. 22, pp. S37–S62, 2016.

[9] D. Rodríguez, C. Pigrau, G. Euba et al., "Acute haematogenous prosthetic joint infection: prospective evaluation of medical and surgical management," *Clinical Microbiology and Infection*, vol. 16, no. 12, pp. 1789–1795, 2010.

[10] S. Aslam, C. Reitman, and R. O. Darouiche, "Risk factors for subsequent diagnosis of prosthetic joint infection," *Infection Control and Hospital Epidemiology*, vol. 31, no. 3, pp. 298–301, 2010.

[11] C. J. E. Kaandorp, H. J. Dinant, M. A. F. J. Van De Laar, H. J. Bernelot Moens, A. P. A. Prins, and B. A. C. Dijkmans, "Incidence and sources of native and prosthetic joint infection: a community based prospective survey," *Annals of the Rheumatic Diseases*, vol. 56, no. 8, pp. 470–475, 1997.

[12] D. S. Stephens, B. Greenwood, and P. Brandtzaeg, "Epidemic meningitis, meningococcaemia, and *Neisseria meningitidis*," *Lancet*, vol. 369, no. 9580, pp. 2196–2210, 2007.

[13] U. B. Schaad, "Arthritis in disease due to *Neisseria meningitidis*," *Reviews of Infectious Diseases*, vol. 2, no. 6, pp. 880–888, 1980.

[14] J. Dennis, L. D. Edwards, T. N. Fisher, and L. Makeever, "Endocarditis on a Bjork-Shiley mitral prosthesis due to Neisseria meningitidis," *Scandinavian Journal of Thoracic and Cardiovascular Surgery*, vol. 11, no. 3, pp. 205–209, 1977.

[15] A. E. Jephcott and C. A. Hardisty, "Meningococcal septicaemia in a patient with a prosthetic valve—a sucessfully treated case," *The British Journal of Clinical Practice*, vol. 30, no. 9, pp. 180–185, 1976.

23

Typhoid Fever due to Extended Spectrum β-Lactamase-Producing *Salmonella enterica* Serovar Typhi: A Case Report and Literature Review

Abdul Azeez Ahamed Riyaaz,[1] **Vindya Perera**,[2] **Sabaratnam Sivakumaran**,[1] **and Nelun de Silva**[2]

[1]*Department of Internal Medicine, Dr. Neville Fernando Teaching Hospital, Malabe, Sri Lanka*
[2]*Department of Microbiology, Faculty of Medicine, South Asian Institute of Technology and Medicine, Malabe, Sri Lanka*

Correspondence should be addressed to Vindya Perera; v.perera83@yahoo.com

Academic Editor: Larry M. Bush

Emergence of cephalosporin-resistant strains of *Salmonella enterica* serovar Typhi is a cause of concern in the management of enteric fever. Cephalosporin resistance in *Salmonella* species is mainly due to the production of extended-spectrum β-lactamases (ESBLs). The majority of ESBLs in *Salmonella enterica* serovar Typhi are derivatives of the TEM, SHV, and CTX-M β-lactamase families. Of these, CTX-M appears to be predominant. This paper discusses the detection and molecular characterization of an ESBL-producing *Salmonella enterica* serovar Typhi strain isolated from a patient who was admitted to a private hospital in Sri Lanka. The three main types of β-lactamases such as TEM, SHV, and CTX-M were identified in this isolate. This case report from Sri Lanka contributes to the knowledge of the increasingly reported cases of typhoid fever due to *Salmonella enterica* serovar Typhi resistant to β-lactamase by ESBL production.

1. Introduction

The emergence of resistance to fluoroquinolones had led to the frequent use of azithromycin for empirical treatment of uncomplicated enteric fever and the use of third-generation cephalosporins as the first-line drug for intravenous treatments [1]. However, the recent emergence of cephalosporin-resistant strains of *Salmonella enterica* serovar Typhi is a cause for concern in the management of enteric fever. Cephalosporin resistance in *Salmonella* species is mainly due to the production of extended-spectrum β-lactamases (ESBLs). The majority of ESBLs in *Salmonella* are derivatives of the TEM, SHV, and CTX-M β-lactamase families.

The production of ESBL leads to multidrug resistance in *Salmonella enterica* isolates. Multidrug resistance (MDR) in *Salmonella enterica* has been described around the world and shown to be more common in *Salmonella* Typhi than in *Salmonella* Paratyphi [2, 3]. The geographic variations have been described for MDR *Salmonella* Typhi isolates in Asia. For example, some studies have shown higher prevalence of MDR phenotypes in India, Pakistan, and Vietnam when compared to those in China and Indonesia [4]. In developed countries such as the United States and Germany, *Salmonella* Typhi with MDR has been reported with travel to developing countries [5, 6].

In Sri Lanka, there are no published data on molecular characteristics of ESBL-producing *Salmonella enterica* serovar Typhi. This case reports the detection and molecular characterization of an ESBL-producing *Salmonella enterica* serovar Typhi strain isolated from a patient with typhoid fever who was admitted to a private hospital in Sri Lanka.

2. Case Presentation

An 18-year-old previously healthy male was admitted to our medical unit with a history of fever of 5-day duration. He had high-grade fever associated with generalized aches and frontal headache. He denied any respiratory or urinary symptoms. He mentioned that he had not passed faeces for the last three days but had developed nonbloody diarrhoea on the day of admission without any vomiting or abdominal pain. He denied any recent travel, but he had been eating from various food outlets for the past 2 weeks during his after-school cricket practice sessions.

On examination, he was not ill looking despite his temperature of 40°C. There were no pallor, icterus, lymphadenopathy, and skin rashes. Cardiovascular and respiratory examination was normal. Abdominal examination revealed a soft, nontender abdomen with a 3 cm nontender hepatomegaly and a 2 cm splenomegaly. His blood test showed a haemoglobin count of 14.8 g/dl, a white cell count of 2.8×10^9/l (neutrophils 79% and lymphocytes 14%), and a platelet count of 97×10^9/l. Dengue NS1 antigen and IgM against dengue virus detected by a commercial kit (Standard Diagnostics, Inc., Germany) were negative. C-reactive protein (CRP) was elevated more than 250 mg/dl in two subsequent samples. His liver function tests were normal except elevated liver transaminases (ALT 145 U/l and AST 118 U/l; ALT/AST normal range 8–40 U/L). An ultrasound scan of the abdomen confirmed mild hepatosplenomegaly. On days 2 and 3 of his admission, he continued to have high fever spikes, diarrhoea, and persistent thrombocytopenia with a high CRP.

Intravenous ceftriaxone 2 g daily was commenced. After 48 hours, the patients' clinical condition had not improved and the high fever spikes continued. After antibiotic susceptibility test results, his antibiotic was changed to imipenem 1 g 8 hourly. He showed clinical improvement after 48 hours, but the diarrhoea and fever settled only around the 10th day of treatment. Imipenem was continued for a total duration of 14 days. His platelet count, liver transaminases, and CRP returned to normal. A repeat blood and faeces culture performed on discharge was negative for *Salmonella enterica* serovar Typhi.

3. Laboratory Methods

The blood culture from the patient grew nonlactose fermenting colonies on MacConkey agar which were identified as *Salmonella enterica* serovar Typhi by standard laboratory methods and by the Rapid ID Test Kit (Oxoid).

The antibiotic-susceptibility results of the isolate performed according to CLSI disc diffusion method [2] showed resistance to antibiotics such as ampicillin, chloramphenicol, ciprofloxacin, cotrimoxazole, and co-amoxiclav. The isolate was susceptible to imipenem, meropenem, ertapenem, amikacin, and netilmicin but was resistant to cefotaxime, cefixime, cefepime, and aztreonam (Table 1). The resistance was further confirmed by determining the minimum inhibitory concentrations (MIC in μg/ml) of the antibiotics to the isolate by VITEK® 2 system, and the results were as follows: ciprofloxacin >4, ceftriaxone >64, ceftazidime >64, imipenem <0.25, and ertapenem <0.5 (Table 2).

ESBL production of the isolate was screened according to CLSI breakpoints for cefpodoxime, ceftazidime, aztreonam, cefotaxime, and ceftriaxone. The combined disc test was done using ceftazidime and cefotaxime individually and in combination with clavulanic acid according to the Clinical and Laboratory Standards Institute (CLSI) guidelines to confirm ESBL production [7]. The isolate was further tested phenotypically with the modified double-disc synergy test (MDDST) by using a disc of amoxicillin-clavulanate along with four cephalosporins: cefotaxime, ceftriaxone, cefpodoxime, and cefepime [8]. Suggestive evidence of ESBL production was observed with reduced susceptibility for the five antimicrobial agents used in CLSI screening test. In the confirmatory test, >5 mm increase in zone diameters for the combined discs of ceftazidime and cefotaxime with clavulanic acid versus the zone diameter of the agent when tested alone was observed (Figure 1). In MDDST, a synergy between amoxicillin/clavulanate and four cephalosporins was observed which provided further evidence of ESBL production (Figure 2).

To detect ESBL genes, polymerase chain reaction (PCR) was performed as described previously [9, 10]. PCR results showed that the isolate harbored bla_{TEM} (Figure 3), bla_{SHV} (Figure 4), and $bla_{CTX\text{-}M}$ (Figure 5) gene types.

Table 1: Antimicrobial susceptibility results of the isolate according to CLSI disc diffusion method.

Antimicrobial	CLSI disc diffusion method (interpretation)
Ampicillin	R
Chloramphenicol	R
Ciprofloxacin	R
Cotrimoxazole	R
Co-amoxiclav	R
Cefotaxime	R
Cefixime	R
Cefepime	R
Aztreonam	R
Imipenem	S
Meropenem	S
Ertapenem	S
Amikacin	S
Netilmicin	S

R, resistance; S, susceptible.

Table 2: The minimum inhibitory concentrations (MIC in μg/ml) of the antibiotics to the isolate by VITEK 2 system.

Antimicrobial	MIC (mg/l)	Interpretation
Ciprofloxacin	>4	R
Ceftriaxone	>64	R
Ceftazidime	>64	R
Imipenem	<0.25	S
Ertapenem	<0.5	S

R, resistance; S, susceptible.

4. Discussion

Enteric fever is one of the major health concerns in developing countries. *Salmonella* Typhi enters the lymphatic system after ingestion and then survives and replicates within macrophages, later on disseminating into the reticuloendothelial system. The

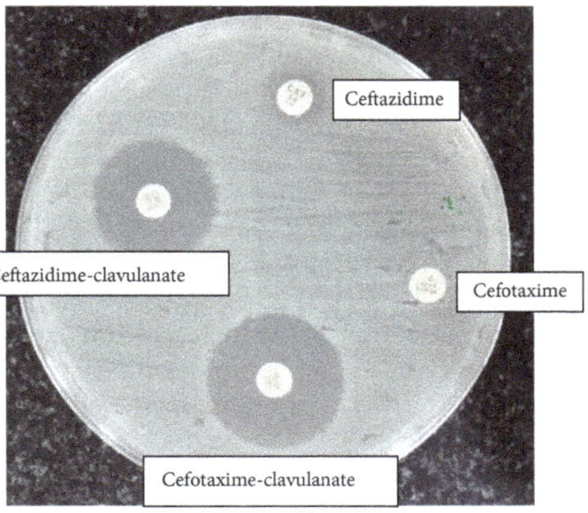

Figure 1: CLSI confirmatory test for ESBL production with >5 mm increase in zone diameters for combined discs of ceftazidime and cefotaxime with clavulanic acid versus the zone diameter of the agent when tested alone.

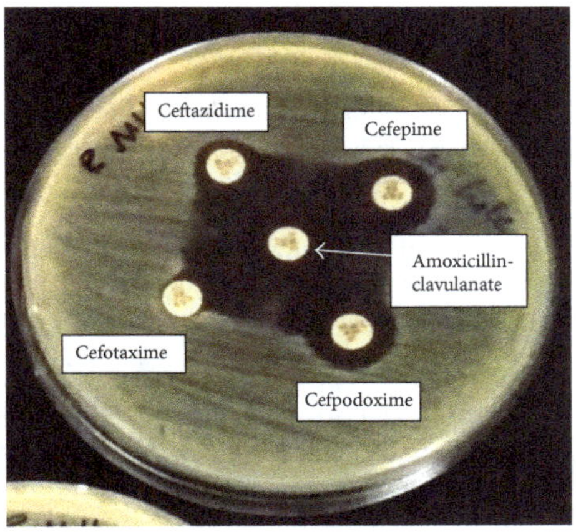

Figure 2: Modified double disc synergy test (MDDST) showing synergy between amoxicillin/clavulanate and four cephalosporins.

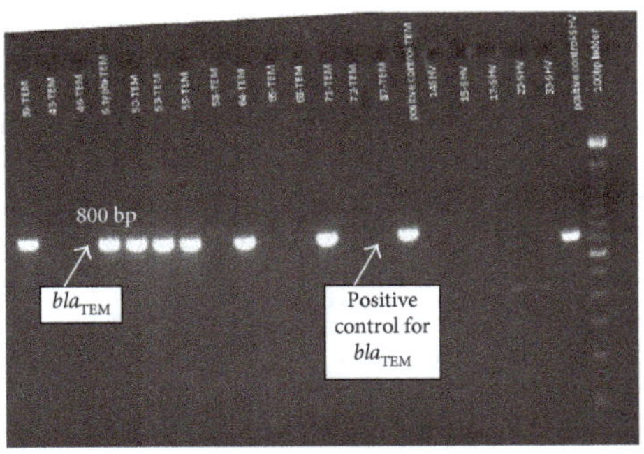

Figure 3: Gel image of PCR product showing bla_{TEM} gene.

common clinical features of enteric fever include fever, chills, abdominal pain, and appearance of rose spots. Leucopenia and anaemia are well-recognised haematological manifestations of enteric fever. Isolated thrombocytopenia is a rare finding in typhoid fever, and there are only few case reports found in the literature [11]. Our patient had both leucopenia and thrombocytopenia at presentation without anaemia,

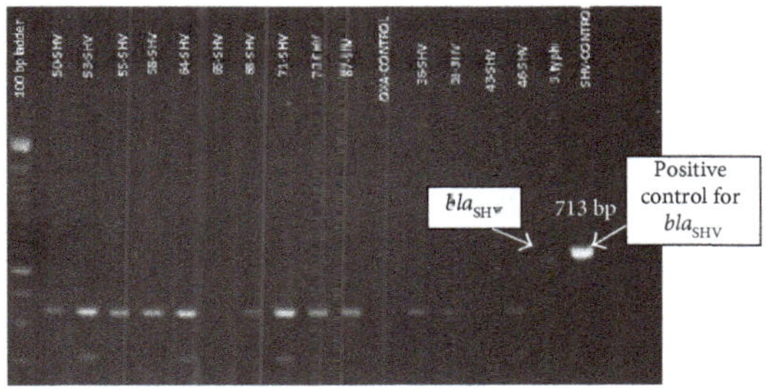

Figure 4: Gel image of the PCR product showing bla_{SHV} gene.

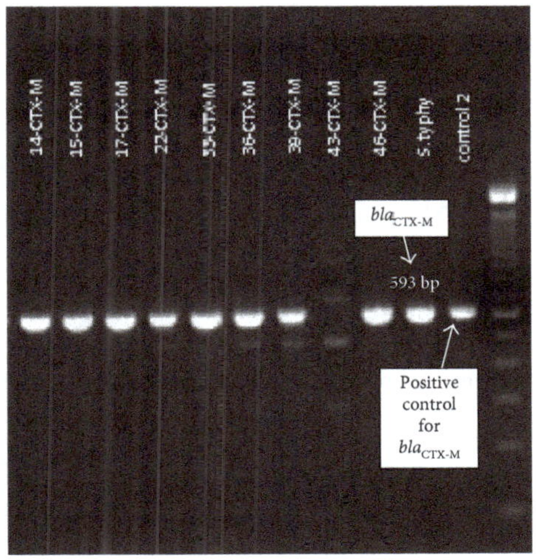

Figure 5: Gel image of the PCR product showing bla_{CTX-M} gene.

which is a common finding in febrile patients due to viral aetiology particularly dengue infection. Our patient presented during a dengue epidemic period where these findings could have been easily overlooked.

According to the literature, multidrug-resistant *Salmonella* Typhi had been documented more than *Salmonella* Paratyphi [12–14]. In our study, the isolate was resistant to all first-line antibiotics (i.e., ampicillin, chloramphenicol, cotrimoxazole, and ciprofloxacin).

The production of β-lactamases is a major factor that makes Gram-negative bacteria resistant to antibiotics [15]. TEM, SHV, and CTX-M are the main types of β-lactamases produced by these organisms that confer resistance to penicillins and cephalosporins. In this case, we identified the gene types responsible for the production of all the three main types of β-lactamases.

The TEM-type β-lactamase is commonly present in Enterobacteriaceae such as *Escherichia coli*, *Klebsiella pneumoniae*, and *Proteus mirabilis*, and SHV types were found to be common in *Klebsiella pneumonia* [16]. The CTX-M-type β-lactamases were found in *E. coli* and *Klebsiella* spp. Salmonella strains were documented to acquire these genes from *E. coli* and *Klebsiella* sp. [17]. Variants of these types of β-lactamases have conferred resistance only to penicillins and early cephalosporins as well as to second-, third-, and fourth-generation cephalosporins [18].

Several cases of *S. enterica* ser. Typhi resistant to β-lactamase by ESBL production have been reported in Asian countries. In the Philippines, a strain that harbors bla_{SHV} gene was identified in 2008 [19]. In Kuwait, the United Arab Emirates, and Bangladesh, there had been reports of ESBL-producing *Salmonella* Typhi with CTX-M genes [20, 21]. A study carried out in India in 2013 identified five multidrug-resistant isolates belonging to serotype *Salmonella* Typhi that were positive to TEM-1-type β-lactamase, but none of these isolates were positive for SHV- or CTX-M-type β-lactamase [22]. In the present case, we found a *S. enterica* serovar Typhi positive all TEM-, SHV-, and CTX-M-type β-lactamases.

The emergence of ESBL-producing *Salmonella* is a result of selective pressure imposed by the misuse of broad-spectrum antibiotics such as third-generation cephalosporins. Increased prevalence of these resistant salmonella will lead to failures of the current treatment practices. Continuous surveillance of the susceptibility profiles and improving infection control measures will help to control the spread of the infection with resistant strains. This case report describes a patient with typhoid fever caused by *Salmonella enterica* serovar Typhi strain that carried three major genes responsible for the production of ESBL that resulted in resistance to cephalosporins. To our knowledge, *Salmonella* Typhi resistant to β-lactamase by ESBL production and the genes encoding this resistance have not been described in Sri Lanka previously.

Acknowledgments

The invaluable technical assistance of Mr. Sirithilak Gamage, Chief Staff Technical Officer in the Department of Microbiology, Faculty of Medicine, University of Colombo, in molecular detection of resistance genes is gratefully acknowledged.

References

[1] R. Hassing, W. Goessens, W. van Pelt et al., "*Salmonella* subtypes with increased MICs for azithromycin in travelers returned to the Netherlands," *Emerging Infectious Diseases*, vol. 20, no. 4, pp. 705–708, 2014.

[2] S. K. Gupta, F. Medalla, M. W. Omondi et al., "Laboratory-based surveillance of paratyphoid fever in the United States: travel and antimicrobial resistance," *Clinical Infectious Diseases*, vol. 46, no. 11, pp. 1656–1663, 2008.

[3] C. M. Parry and E. J. Threlfall, "Antimicrobial resistance in typhoidal and nontyphoidal salmonellae," *Current Opinion in Infectious Diseases*, vol. 21, no. 5, pp. 531–538, 2008.

[4] R. L. Ochiai, C. J. Acosta, M. C. Danovaro-Holliday et al., "A study of typhoid fever in five Asian countries: disease burden and implications for control," *Bulletin of the World Health Organization*, vol. 86, no. 4, pp. 260–268, 2008.

[5] M. F. Lynch, E. M. Blanton, S. Bulens et al., "Typhoid fever in the United States, 1999–2006," *JAMA*, vol. 302, no. 8, pp. 859–865, 2009.

[6] Y. Pfeifer, J. Matten, and W. Rabsch, "*Salmonella enterica* serovar Typhi with CTX-M β-Lactamase, Germany," *Emerging Infectious Diseases*, vol. 15, no. 9, pp. 1533–1535, 2009.

[7] Clinical and Laboratory Standards Institute, *Performance Standards for Antimicrobial Susceptibility Testing; Twenty Second Informational Supplement, CLSI document 100–S22*, Clinical and Laboratory Standards Institute, Wayne, PA, USA, 2012.

[8] J. Kaur, S. Chopra, Sheevani, and G. Mahajan, "Modified double disc synergy test to detect ESBL production in urinary isolates of *Escherichia coli* and *Klebsiella pneumonia*," *Journal of Clinical and Diagnostic Research*, vol. 7, no. 2, pp. 229–233, 2013.

[9] C. Dallenne, A. Da Costa, D. Decré, C. Favier, and G. Arlet, "Development of a set of multiplex PCR assays for the detection of genes encoding important β-lactamases in Enterobacteriaceae," *Journal of Antimicrobial Chemotherapy*, vol. 65, no. 3, pp. 490–495, 2010.

[10] H. Fang, C. Lundberg, B. Olsson-Liljequist et al., "Molecular epidemiological analysis of *Escherichia coli* isolates producing extended-spectrum β-lactamases for identification of nosocomial outbreaks in Stockholm, Sweden," *Journal of Clinical Microbiology*, vol. 42, no. 12, pp. 5917–5920, 2004.

[11] S. Charan, R. Chander, and I. Singh, "Isolated thrombocytopenia a rare presenting feature of enteric fever," *International Journal of Advances in Medicine*, vol. 3, pp. 438-439, 2016.

[12] S. Dutta, D. Sur, B. Manna, S. K. Bhattacharya, J. L. Deen, and J. D. Clemens, "Rollback of *Salmonella enterica* serotype Typhi resistance to chloramphenicol and other antimicrobials in Kolkata, India," *Antimicrobial Agents and Chemotherapy*, vol. 49, no. 4, pp. 1662-1663, 2005.

[13] S. Verma, S. Thakur, A. Kanga, G. Singh, and P. Gupta, "Emerging *Salmonella* Paratyphi A enteric fever and changing trends in antimicrobial resistance pattern of salmonella in Shimla," *Indian Journal of Medical Microbiology*, vol. 28, no. 1, pp. 51–53, 2010.

[14] S. S. Bhattacharya, U. Das, and B. K. Choudhury, "Occurrence & antibiogram of *Salmonella* Typhi & *S.* Paratyphi A isolated from Rourkela, Orissa," *Indian Journal of Medical Research*, vol. 133, pp. 431–433, 2011.

[15] K. Bush, "New β-lactamases in Gram-negative bacteria: diversity and impact on the selection of antimicrobial therapy," *Clinical Infectious Diseases*, vol. 32, no. 7, pp. 1085–1089, 2001.

[16] V. Gupta, "An update on newer β-lactamases," *Indian Journal of Medical Research*, vol. 126, no. 5, pp. 417–427, 2007.

[17] V. O. Rotimi, W. Jamal, T. Pal, A. Sovenned, and M. J. Albert, "Emergence of CTX-M-15 type extended-spectrum β-lactamase-producing *Salmonella* spp. in Kuwait and the United Arab Emirates," *Journal of Medical Microbiology*, vol. 57, no. 7, pp. 881–886, 2008.

[18] M. L. Salverda, J. A. De Visser, and M. Barlow, "Natural evolution of TEM-1 b-lactamase: experimental reconstruction and clinical relevance," *FEMS Microbiology Reviews*, vol. 34, no. 6, pp. 1015–1036, 2010.

[19] N. Al Naiemi, B. Zwart, M. Rijnsburger et al., "Extended-spectrum-β-lactamase production in a *Salmonella enterica* serotype Typhi strain from the Philippines," *Journal of Clinical Microbiology*, vol. 46, no. 8, pp. 2794-2795, 2008.

[20] C. M. Parry, T. T. Hien, G. Dougan, N. J. White, and J. J. Farrar, "Typhoid fever," *New England Journal of Medicine*, vol. 347, no. 22, pp. 1770–1782, 2002.

[21] D. Ahmed, A. Hoque, R. Mazumder, K. Nahar, N. Islam, and S. A. Gazi, "*Salmonella enterica* serovar Typhi strain producing extended-spectrum β-lactamases in Dhaka, Bangladesh," *Journal of Medical Microbiology*, vol. 61, no. 7, pp. 1032-1033, 2012.

[22] E. Sathishkumar, E. M. Muthu, and R. Srivani, "Detection of TEM-, SHV- and CTX-M-type β-lactamase production among clinical isolates of *Salmonella* species," *Journal of Medical Microbiology*, vol. 63, no. 7, pp. 962–967, 2014.

24

All Signs Point to Cancer: A Case of Cryptic Miliary Tuberculosis in the Setting of Concomitant Cancer

Victoria Cress,[1] **Sue Min Sophia Kwon**,[2] **and Michael T. Ulrich**[2,3]

[1]*Loma Linda University School of Medicine, 11175 Campus Street Loma Linda, Loma Linda 92350, CA, USA*
[2]*Loma Linda University Medical Center, Department of Medicine, 1234 Anderson Street Rm. 1503 Loma Linda, Loma Linda 92354, CA, USA*
[3]*Riverside University Health System, Department of Medicine, 26520 Cactus Avenue Moreno Valley, Moreno Valley 92555, CA, USA*

Correspondence should be addressed to Victoria Cress; vcress@students.llu.edu

Academic Editor: Mohd Adnan

Dissemination of tuberculosis (TB) is known as miliary tuberculosis. When miliary tuberculosis lacks classic radiographic and clinical features, it can be labeled cryptic miliary tuberculosis and may mimic metastatic cancer. This unusual presentation of an already atypical form of TB often delays diagnosis. We present a case of a 58-year-old female who presented with presumed metastatic carcinoma, who was ultimately diagnosed with both primary breast cancer and disseminated TB. This case emphasizes the need for a high index of suspicion for miliary tuberculosis in patients with presumed or proven malignancy.

1. Introduction

Cryptic miliary tuberculosis is a rare presentation of tuberculosis (TB) known as disseminated or miliary TB. Miliary TB accounts for just 2–5% of all TB cases and 8–20% of extrapulmonary TB cases in immunocompetent individuals [1–3]. Multiple organ involvement in disseminated TB can mask classic signs and symptoms and even mimic metastatic cancer; this is known as cryptic miliary TB. In these cases, patients (commonly older) may present with absent or mild fever, progressive wasting, and diffuse lymphadenopathy. This unusual presentation of an already atypical form of TB often delays diagnosis. We present a case of a 58-year-old female who presented with presumed metastatic carcinoma, who was ultimately diagnosed with both primary breast cancer and disseminated TB.

2. Case Presentation

A 58-year-old female patient with no pertinent past medical history presented to the emergency department as a transfer from an outside hospital for computerized tomography (CT) findings of retroperitoneal lymphadenopathy with nodularity and stranding of the omental fat, concerning for malignancy/metastatic disease requiring higher level of care for malignancy workup. The patient stated she experienced increasing fatigue, a decrease in appetite, and an unmeasured amount of weight loss over the past month. The patient stated that over the past two weeks, her symptoms had worsened significantly. She endorsed increased thirst, but denied fevers, chills, headache, cough, dyspnea, night sweats, chest pain, or sick contacts. She denied recent travel, stating she had only travelled to Thailand greater than 10 years previously.

On physical exam, the patient was afebrile with stable vital signs. She had clear lung sounds bilaterally, was nontender to abdominal palpation with a negative Murphy's sign, and had an unremarkable cardiac exam. A 2 cm mass in the 4 o'clock position of the left breast was palpated on clinical breast exam.

Laboratory analysis was remarkable for leukocytosis of 13.9x10e9/L, alkaline phosphatase of 310 U/L, and aspartate aminotransferase of 78 U/L. Malignancy workup was obtained: cancer antigen 19–9 and carcinoembryonic antigen were elevated to 301.4 U/mL and 9.0 ng/mL, respectively, with alpha-fetoprotein tumor marker within normal limits. Evaluation for acute and chronic liver pathology was positive solely for hepatitis A, with kidney microsomal antibodies, mitochondrial antibodies, antinuclear antibodies, alpha-1-antitrypsin, and ceruloplasmin all being negative. An iron panel demonstrated findings consistent with anemia of chronic disease (ferritin 2410.3 ng/mL, total iron 47 mcg/dL, and total iron binding capacity 80 mcg/dL). Blood cultures and urine cultures demonstrated no growth. Interferon-gamma release assay (IGRA) for tuberculosis was indeterminate.

The patient received extensive imaging. A CT abdomen/pelvis demonstrated retroperitoneal lymphadenopathy, nodularity and stranding in the omental fat, thickened ring along the periphery of the liver, and cholelithiasis. A CT chest demonstrated mediastinal lymphadenopathy, multiple small nodules scattered in the lungs bilaterally, and a small left pleural effusion. Cardiac bedside ultrasound showed no apparent focal wall motion abnormality and demonstrated adequate systolic left ventricular systolic function with an ejection fraction greater than 60%. Abdominal bedside ultrasound demonstrated multiple gallstones within an enlarged gallbladder measuring approximately 10 cm. Formal right upper quadrant ultrasound demonstrated cholelithiasis with sludge and gallbladder wall thickening as well as a nodular hepatic contour. Magnetic resonance cholangiopancreatography (MRCP) was unable to be obtained due to a history of a bullet wound to the left breast with retained metal fragments. The patient's hepatobiliary iminodiacetic acid (HIDA) scan demonstrated nonvisualization of the bladder supporting cystic duct obstruction and acute cholecystitis. Mammogram showed a 2.5 × 2.7 cm breast mass of the left breast.

The patient was started on Zosyn for cholecystitis and underwent an esophagogastroduodenoscopy (EGD) and colonoscopy which demonstrated nodular gastric mucosa and duodenal erosions. During her hospital course, she underwent multiple biopsies, including an ultrasound-guided core biopsy of her left breast mass, a colon biopsy, a retroperitoneal node biopsy, and a gastric mucosa biopsy. Throughout her hospital course, consultants from hematology/oncology, general surgery, and surgical oncology services informed the patient of the high likelihood of a cancer diagnosis upon pathologic examination of biopsied tissue. However, the patient left the hospital against medical advice before the biopsy results were available.

Upon outpatient hematology/oncology follow-up, the patient received her biopsy results. Her colon biopsy and gastric mucosa biopsy demonstrated no abnormalities. However, her left breast biopsy demonstrated a new diagnosis of cT2N0 grade-2 estrogen receptor-positive, progesterone receptor-positive, and her2-negative invasive carcinoma of no special time with lobular features with a minor component of ductal carcinoma in situ. Her retroperitoneal node biopsy demonstrated lymphoid tissue with necrotizing giant-cell granulomas, positive for mycobacteria on acid-fast bacilli staining. Treatment of the abdominal tuberculosis was to be coordinated by infectious disease and hematology/oncology before undergoing surgical treatment for the breast mass. Upon phone call to confirm an appointment, the patient's husband informed medical staff that the patient had passed away, less than two weeks after her discharge.

3. Discussion

Tuberculosis (TB) is a disease that affects people of all age groups in all countries. Due to advances in medical diagnosis and treatment, the worldwide TB incidence in new cases per 100,000 is falling at the rate of about 2% per year [4]. In the setting of impaired cell-mediated immunity, primary TB infection or reactivation of latent TB can result in uncontrolled lymphohematogenous spread of *Mycobacterium tuberculosis*. Immunocompromise such as HIV/AIDS infection, use of immunosuppressive drugs, and organ transplant is a strong risk factor for the development of disseminated TB. Miliary TB accounts for a small percentage of TB infection in otherwise immunocompetent adults. Predisposing factors such as malnutrition, alcohol use, pregnancy, silicosis, and underlying malignancy have been identified [1, 2]. Some studies have revealed a female predominance in clinically unrecognized TB [5, 6].

There is no single pathognomonic sign or symptom for miliary TB; therefore, clinical suspicion must be high to achieve timely diagnosis and treatment. Disseminated *Mycobacterium tuberculosis* spreads to vascular beds of various organs, especially those with relatively high blood flow. Thus, miliary TB's ability to affect any organ system mirrors its variable presentation and elusive diagnosis. Symptoms may be rapidly progressive, episodic, or present with a protracted course. Classic TB symptoms include spiking fevers, chills, night sweats, anorexia, weight loss, and cough. End-organ-specific manifestations of disseminated TB may also offer clues for diagnosis, such as choroidal tubercles in the eye, cutaneous lesions, and TB meningitis. Tuberculous lymphadenitis presents with diffuse, nontender lymphadenopathy [1–3, 7, 8]. These symptoms are also highly suspicious for malignancy which can further obscure the definitive diagnosis. Diagnosis may be masked by more classic pathologies such as chronic obstructive pulmonary disease (COPD) exacerbation and pulmonary thromboembolism [5]. Rarely, miliary TB can become fulminant leading to acute respiratory distress syndrome (ARDS), septic shock, multiorgan failure, and death [8, 9].

The term "miliary tuberculosis" is derived from the disease's classic presentation on chest radiograph, resembling millet seeds. However, typical chest radiographic findings may be subtle or absent until late in the disease course. In many cases, miliary TB and especially its cryptic presentation are only diagnosed upon autopsy [5, 6]. Advances in diagnosis tools such as high-resolution computerized tomography (CT) and magnetic resonance imaging (MRI) have allowed for dramatic increases in antemortem diagnosis and are especially useful for identifying extrapulmonary miliary lesions such as in the mesentery, lymph nodes, liver, and spleen [1, 2]. Despite these advances in clinical imaging, difficulty in differentiation between TB lesions and malignant tumors based on clinical and radiological presentation continues [5]. Miliary TB lesions also take up fluorine-18 fluorodeoxyglucose (F-18 FDG) radiotracer on positron emission tomography (PET) CT scan which can either aid in defining extent of known dissemination or can further mimic malignancy and postpone definitive diagnosis [2, 7].

Affected patients may present with nonspecific normochromic anemia, leukopenia or leukocytosis, and elevated erythrocyte sedimentation rate (ESR). When clinical suspicion arises, additional tests may offer further advances toward definitive diagnosis. Testing for TB with skin testing and interferon-gamma release assay (IGRA) is the first of these. IGRA is preferred in those likely infected due to ease of sample acquisition and since a negative TB skin test is common in disseminated disease [1, 8, 10]. A positive IGRA cannot distinguish between active and latent TB, but a negative result may be helpful in ruling out miliary TB. Definitive diagnosis comes from tissue and fluid sampling. For adults with suspected miliary or extrapulmonary TB, sputum samples, fine needle aspirates, and other collected body fluids should be sent for acid-fast bacillus smear microscopy, mycobacterial culture, nucleic acid amplification testing, and histological examination [2, 10]. Culture isolates from mycobacterial culture-positive samples may also be submitted for genotyping and drug susceptibility on an as-indicated basis.

Active TB infection is typically treated with rifamycin, isoniazid, pyrazinamide, and ethambutol for 2 months followed by rifamycin and isoniazid for 4 months, for a total of 6 months of treatment. Most patients with miliary TB receive this empiric treatment and some have shown further improvement with the use of steroids [3, 9, 11]. However, there is no current consensus regarding the optimum duration of treatment for disseminated TB or the use of steroids in treatment [2].

Often in cases of cryptic miliary TB, the suspicion of TB arises too late or not at all. This may be because miliary TB diagnosis is often being overlooked in countries with low incidence of TB [5, 6]. Despite available diagnostic tools and treatment, mortality of miliary TB is still 25–30% in adults [1, 2]. This is often related to delay in diagnosis and subsequent delays in treatment, further emphasizing the need for high clinical suspicion and clinician education of the presentation and appropriate diagnostic steps. Further studies on definitive early diagnosis of disseminated TB and the most effective treatment regimens are also indicated.

4. Conclusions

(i) Miliary tuberculosis is a dramatically variable disease that requires a high index of suspicion and can present insidiously.

(ii) Routine tuberculosis testing in patients presenting with presumed metastatic malignancy may prove beneficial.

(iii) Further studies are needed to determine the most effective treatment regimen and duration for disseminated tuberculosis.

Acknowledgments

The submission of this article was funded by Michael T. Ulrich.

References

[1] S. K. Sharma, A. Mohan, A. Sharma, and D. K. Mitra, "Miliary tuberculosis: new insights into an old disease," *The Lancet Infectious Diseases*, vol. 5, no. 7, pp. 415–430, 2005.

[2] S. K. Sharma, A. Mohan, A. Sharma, and J. J. Manget, "Challenges in the diagnosis & treatment of miliary tuberculosis," *Indian Journal of Medical Research*, vol. 135, no. 5, pp. 703–730, 2012.

[3] K. Chamberlin, S. Orfanos, A. Mukherjee, E. Moy, M. Koganti, and W. Khan, "A case of disseminated tuberculosis mimicking metastatic cancer," *Respiratory Medicine Case Reports*, vol. 25, pp. 239–241, 2018.

[4] Organisation mondiale de la santé, *Global Tuberculosis Report 2018*, World Health Organization, Geneva, Switzerland, 2018.

[5] I. Savic, V. Trifunovic-Skodric, and D. Mitrovic, "Clinically unrecognized miliary tuberculosis: an autopsy study," *Annals of Saudi Medicine*, vol. 36, no. 1, pp. 42–50, 2016.

[6] T. Vasankari, K. Liippo, and E. Tala, "Overt and cryptic miliary tuberculosis misdiagnosed until autopsy," *Scandinavian Journal of Infectious Diseases*, vol. 35, no. 11-12, pp. 794–796, 2003.

[7] C. J. Das, R. Kumar, V. B. Balakrishnan, M. Chawla, and A. Malhotra, "Disseminated tuberculosis masquerading as metastatic breast carcinoma on PET-CT," *Clinical Nuclear Medicine*, vol. 33, no. 5, pp. 359–361, 2008.

[8] M. P. Golden and H. R. Vikram, "Extrapulmonary tuberculosis: an overview," *American Family Physician*, vol. 72, no. 9, pp. 1761–1768, 2005.

[9] B. Barman, I. Tiewsoh, K. Lynrah, B. Wankhar, T. Beyong, and N. Issar, "Miliary tuberculosis with pulmonary and extrapulmonary component complicated with acute respiratory distress syndrome," *Journal of Family Medicine and Primary Care*, vol. 6, no. 3, p. 688, 2017.

[10] D. M. Lewinsohn, M. K. Leonard, P. A. LoBue et al., "Official American thoracic society/infectious diseases society of America/centers for disease control and prevention clinical practice guidelines: diagnosis of tuberculosis in adults and children," *Clinical Infectious Diseases*, vol. 64, no. 2, pp. 111–115, 2017.

[11] L. Ali Chaudhry and S. Al-Solaiman, "Multifocal tuberculosis: many faces of an old menace," *International Journal of Mycobacteriology*, vol. 2, no. 1, pp. 58–69, 2013.

Streptococcus constellatus Causing Empyema and Sepsis, Necessitating Early Surgical Decortication

D. Chrastek, S. Hickman, D. Sitaranjan, I. Vokshi, O. Kakisi, J. Kadlec, W. Bartosik, F. Van Tornout, and V. Kouritas

Department of Thoracic Surgery, Norwich and Norfolk University Hospital NHS Foundation Trust, Norwich, UK

Correspondence should be addressed to D. Chrastek; david.chrastek@nnuh.nhs.uk

Academic Editor: Oguz R. Sipahi

Streptococcus constellatus is an oropharyngeal commensal Gram-positive coccus, frequently associated with the respiratory tract. *S. constellatus* is part of the *Streptococcus anginosus* or *milleri* group, which has traditionally been considered to have propensity to cause empyema and purulent abscesses, a property that is sometimes overlooked as the severity of infections it causes may have a varying degree. In this case, we present the case of a 54-year-old male with known liver cirrhosis who developed a severe empyema during an acute liver failure episode, requiring extensive decortication and prolonged hospital admission.

1. Introduction

Streptococcus constellatus are small catalase-negative coccus, part of the normal flora of the mouth, gut, and urogenital tract but have been known to cause respiratory tract infections [1–3]. Although they are part of the commensal *Streptococcus milleri* group (SMG, also known as the *Streptococcus anginosus* group, SAG), its pathogenic potential is sometimes overlooked [4]. It has been known to cause parapneumonic effusions and abscesses but can normally be eradicated with intravenous antibiotics and occasionally minor surgical procedures such as chest drainage or washout [5]. We herein present the case of a 54-year-old male who developed acute liver failure and left chest empyema, necessitating early surgical intervention with extensive decortication for its treatment.

2. Case Presentation

A 54-year-old male was referred to our department for a left chest empyema following a week's history of progressively worsening shortness of breath, productive cough of white sputum, and an episode of frank hematuria. On presentation, he was visibly icteric with a tender and ascitic abdomen and reduced air entry on the left lung. His past medical history was significant for hepatitis C and liver cirrhosis, alcohol misuse, and a 35-year pack history of tobacco smoking. His family medical history was unremarkable.

Initial CXR showed a large pleural effusion in the left lung (Figure 1). His chest-abdomen-pelvis CT revealed a large, multiloculated pleural effusion on the left side with almost complete collapse of the underlying lung (Figure 2). In his abdomen, ascites was confirmed, as well as hepatic changes consistent with chronic liver disease and an indeterminate hepatic lesion. Based on these findings, a 28 Fr chest drain was inserted initially, and the patient was started on IV piperacillin/tazobactam and clarithromycin on the respiratory ward. From the initial chest drain fluid sample, *S. constellatus* was grown (identified via Vitek MS, Biomerieux, France) and that was sensitive to all antibiotics tested, i.e., penicillin, clarithromycin, amoxicillin, clindamycin, tetracycline, and vancomycin (Vitek MS 2, Biomerieux, France, the disc diffusion method, interpreted according to EUCAST) [6]. Tissue samples were also sonicated prior to inoculation with 5% BA in order to increase the bacterial yield.

Upon admission, he was additionally found with acute liver failure (ALT 157 (U/L), Alk Phos 256 (U/L), Alb 18 (g/L), and INR 2.01). Three days after his admission and despite

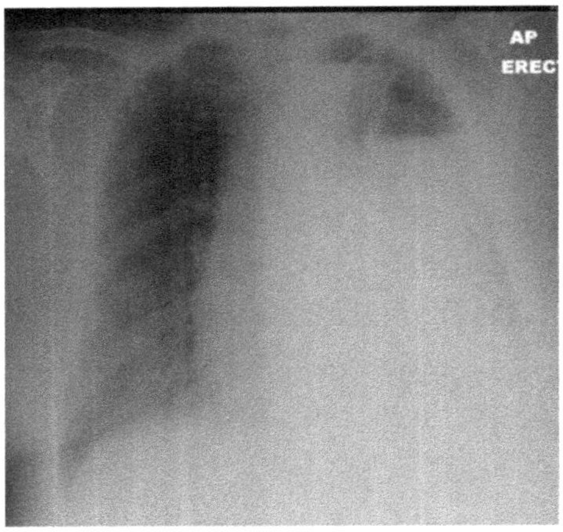

Figure 1: CXR on initial presentation.

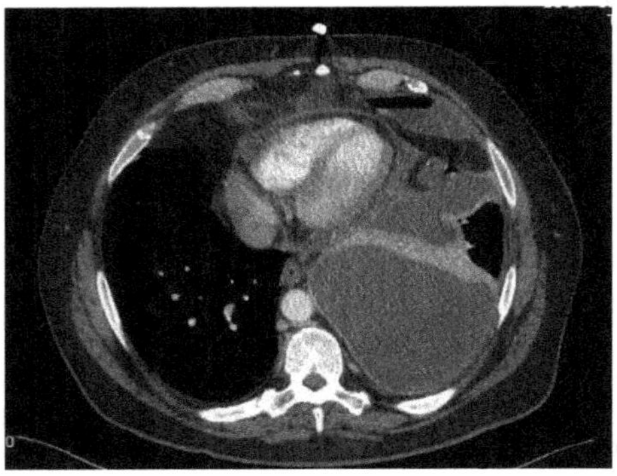

Figure 2: CT on initial presentation.

drainage and piperacillin/tazobactam, he clinically deteriorated becoming septic (according to the Society of Critical Care Medicine criteria—sepsis as having two or more criteria of systemic inflammatory response and with an infection source confirmed or suspected) [7]. For this, he was urgently referred to our department for review during which a surgical intervention was decided. Before surgery, his coagulation imbalances (INR 1.94) were corrected to an extent, with vitamin K initially (10 mg IV 3 doses) and then with fresh frozen plasma (4 units perioperatively).

He underwent VATS exploration with a 3 cm lateral utility incision over the dependent area and 1 camera port anteroinferiorly. Upon entrance into the chest, 1 litre of foul smelling pus was evacuated. A thick mature cortex was noted on the lung, prohibiting it from expansion. A clear plane between the lung and the cortex was created, and therefore, a decortication was performed. Two wide chest drains (28 Fr anterior and tunnelled 32 Fr posterior) were left into the chest, and the lung reexpanded totally after the procedure with minimal air leak (Figure 3). The samples taken during the procedure also grew *S. constellatus*. His postoperative recovery from his chest point of view was uneventful with the anterior drain removed 3 days later. On admission, he was screened for blood-borne viruses and was also found positive for hepatitis C virus (HCV), for which a viral load

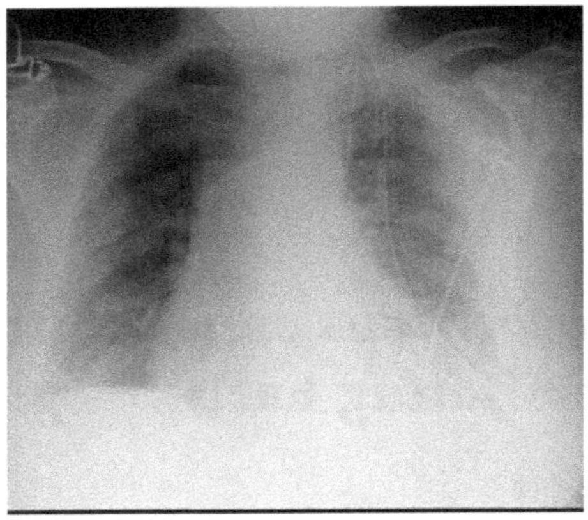

Figure 3: Immediate postoperative CXR.

showed active disease, and he was referred for treatment. He was eventually discharged home without drains, 2 weeks after his operation, remaining in-hospital mainly for investigation of his hepatic lesion.

Two months later, he was readmitted due to raised inflammatory markers and pus leaking from the drain site. Based on the CXR (Figure 4), a surgical 28 Fr drain was reinserted, and he was again started on antibiotics. A CT scan was repeated showing ongoing left-sided consolidation (Figure 5) with small pleural collection. The pus swab taken at this time showed negative for growth of any bacteria, yeast, or fungi. Conservative treatment was decided, and he was finally discharged home with oral antibiotics a couple of days later. Six months after his procedure, he remains well from his chest point of view without any further relapses of his chest infection or pleural collection (Figure 6).

3. Discussion

We herein present a case in which *Streptococcus constellatus* caused a difficulty in treating severe empyema in an immunocompromised patient. The pathogenic potential of commensal bacteria such as *S. constellatus* should not be underestimated especially in patients with immunosuppression, making an aggressive, possibly surgical, treatment necessary. The subspecies *S. constellatus* is known to be a causative organism of respiratory infections, occasionally complicated by easily treatable pleural effusions or abscesses.

A study by Clarridge et al. [5] found that of 41 patients with abscesses caused by *S. constellatus*, the majority (26/41) had infections of the soft tissues, while only 7 cases had pleuropulmonary disease. To add to this, Noguchi et al. [8] studied a cohort of 30 patients with SMG infection, while Kobo et al. [9] studied a cohort of 236; both studies concluded that the *S. constellatus* subspecies was less associated with empyema and less severe infection than other SMG subspecies, such as *S. intermedius*. The patient in our case report, however, suffered from an aggressive *S. constellatus* infection, likely due to immunosuppression secondary to severe hepatic disease caused by hepatitis C, alcoholic cirrhosis, and what was later found to be hepatocellular carcinoma. Literature suggests that while *S. constellatus* is

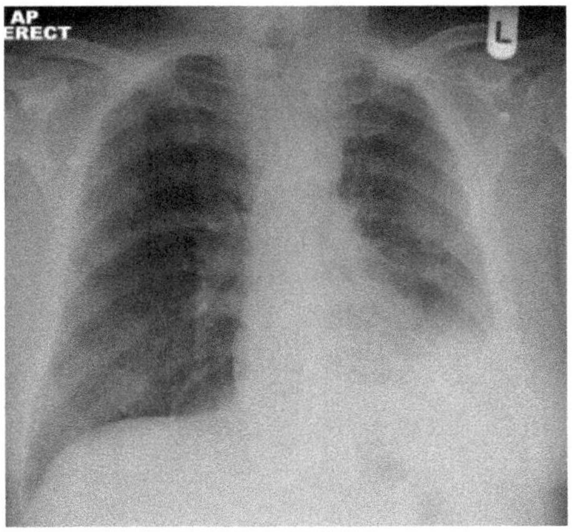

FIGURE 4: CXR on readmission.

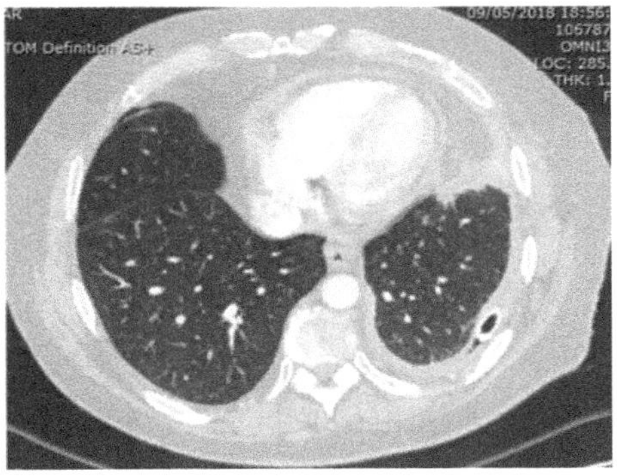

FIGURE 5: CT after readmission and redrainage.

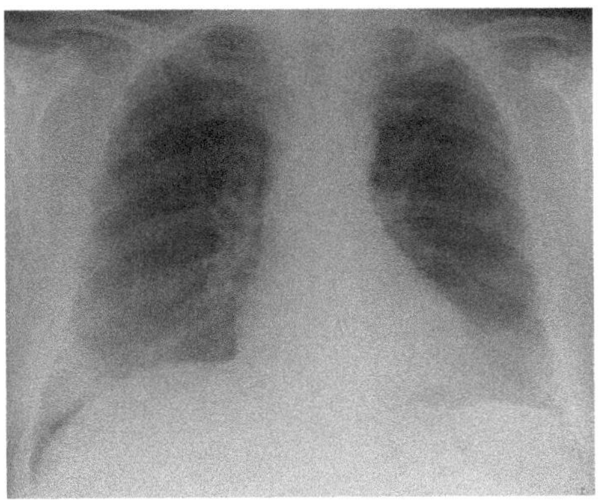

FIGURE 6: Repeat CXR from last outpatient assessment.

a known causative organism in respiratory and pleural infections, its pathogenicity is relatively less severe in comparison to its other SMG siblings. Kobo et al. [9] found interestingly that *S. constellatus* was associated more with bacteremia than with abscess or empyema formation. Clarridge et al. [5] reported that *S. constellatus* infections were sufficiently treated with simple drainage and intravenous antibiotics. Junckerstorff et al. [10] reported that patients growing *S. constellatus* had a shorter hospital stay and a lower 30-day mortality rate than other SMG organisms. There is one other case report by Che Rahim et al. [11] that describes a case of empyema caused by *S. constellatus*, for which decortication was required following a 6-week course of IV antibiotics, with improvement afterwards and no recurrence or sequelae.

In contrast, a surgical intervention was necessitated in our case early on the onset of events because of clinical deterioration in a short period of time because of the liver failure. Also, in the case of our patient, even after treatment with IV antibiotics and an extensive decortication operation, he was readmitted for further issues with his chest. We believe that the likely cause of the severe clinical manifestation of a usually mild organism was due to the patient's other comorbidities, namely, decompensated liver failure and later discovered, hepatocellular carcinoma, as contributing to an overall state of immunosuppression.

Initially, the plan had been to postpone the surgery until the sepsis had settled, and he was haemodynamically stable. Unfortunately, due to his deterioration, he was taken to theatre, and since the cortex was easily removable, a decision was made intraoperatively to complete an extensive decortication in favour of a simple washout and a possible return to theatre. A VATS procedure was more appropriate than open, especially due to the existing coagulation abnormalities and to the overall deteriorated condition of the patient.

In conclusion, *Streptococcus constellatus* normally has relatively low pathogenic potential; however, in this case of an immunocompromised patient, it resulted in sepsis and required extensive decortication. Sepsis is defined as infective source confirmed or expected with 2 or more of the following criteria: temperature >38°C or <36°C, heart rate >90 beats per minute, respiratory rate >20 respirations per minute or $PaCO_2$ <32 mmHg, and WBC >12,000/mm^3, <4,000/mm^3, or >10% bands (7). Regardless of the organism grown, it is always important to consider the potential for simultaneous comorbidities to create an immunocompromised state in patients, which may make early surgical intervention necessary.

Abbreviations

IV: Intravenous
CXR: Chest X-ray
Fr: French
CT: Computed tomography
ALT: Alanine transferase
Alk Phos: Alkaline phosphatase
Alb: Albumin
INR: International normalized ratio
VATS: Video-assisted thoracic surgery.

References

[1] R. A. Whiley, D. Beighton, T. G. Winstanley, H. Y. Fraser, and J. M. Hardie, "*Streptococcus intermedius*, *Streptococcus constellatus*, and *Streptococcus anginosus* (the *Streptococcus milleri* group): association with different body sites and clinical infections," *Journal of Clinical Microbiology*, vol. 30, no. 1, pp. 243-244, 1992.

[2] C. A. Wong, F. Donald, and J. T. Macfarlane, "*Streptococcus milleri* pulmonary disease: a review and clinical description of 25 patients," *Thorax*, vol. 50, no. 10, pp. 1093–1096, 1995.

[3] J.-S. Jerng, P.-R. Hsueh, L.-J. Teng, L.-N. Lee, P.-C. Yang, and K.-T. Luh, "Empyema thoracis and lung abscess caused by viridans streptococci," *American Journal of Respiratory and Critical Care Medicine*, vol. 156, no. 5, pp. 1508–1514, 1997.

[4] N. Akuzawa, T. Hatori, Y. Kitahara, and M. Kurabayashi, "Multiple liver abscesses and bacteremia caused by *Streptococcus constellatus* infection: a case report," *Clinical Case Reports*, vol. 5, no. 1, pp. 69–74, 2017.

[5] J. E. Clarridge, S. Attorri, D. M. Musher, J. Hebert, and S. Dunbar, "*Streptococcus intermedius*, *Streptococcus constellatus*, and *Streptococcus anginosus* ("*Streptococcus milleri* group") are of different clinical importance and are not equally associated with abscess," *Clinical Infectious Diseases*, vol. 32, no. 10, pp. 1511–1515, 2001.

[6] The European Committee on Antimicrobial Susceptibility Testing, *Breakpoint Tables for Interpretation of MICs and Zone Diameters*, The European Committee on Antimicrobial Susceptibility Testing, Växjö, Sweden, 2020, http://www.eucast.org/fileadmin/src/media/PDFs/EUCAST_files/Disk_test_documents/2020_manuals/Manual_v_8.0_EUCAST_Disk_Test_2020.pdf.

[7] M. M. Levy, M. P. Fink, J. C Marshall et al., "2001.CCM/ESICM/ACCP/ATS/SIS International Sepsis Definitions Conference," *Critical Care Medicine*, vol. 31, no. 4, pp. 1250–1256, 2003.

[8] S. Noguchi, K. Yatera, T. Kawanami et al., "The clinical features of respiratory infections caused by the *Streptococcus anginosus* group," *BMC Pulmonary Medicine*, vol. 15, no. 1, p. 133, 2015.

[9] O. Kobo, S. Nikola, Y. Geffen, and M. Paul, "The pyogenic potential of the different *Streptococcus anginosus* group bacterial species: retrospective cohort study," *Epidemiology and Infection*, vol. 145, no. 14, pp. 3065–3069, 2017.

[10] R. K. Junckerstorff, J. O. Robinson, and R. J. Murray, "Invasive *Streptococcus anginosus* group infection: does the species predict the outcome?" *International Journal of Infectious Diseases*, vol. 18, pp. 38–40, 2014.

[11] M. J. Che Rahim, N. Mohammad, and W. S. Wan Ghazali, "Pyopneumothorax secondary to *Streptococcus milleri* infection," *BMJ Case Reports*, vol. 2016, Article ID 2016217537, 2016.

26

A 14-Year-Old Male Patient with Kawasaki Disease Presented with Stroke after COVID-19

Nexhmedin Shala,[1,2] Fisnik Jashari,[1,2] Dren Boshnjaku,[1,2] Argjend Shala,[1,2] Pranvera Ibrahimi,[3,4] Vera Kukaj ,[1,2] and Shemsedin Dreshaj[5,6]

[1]*Clinic of Neurology, University Clinical Center of Kosovo, Pristina 10000, Kosovo*
[2]*Department of Neurology, Faculty of Medicine, University of Pristina "Hasan Prishtina", Pristina 10000, Kosovo*
[3]*Clinic of Cardiology, University Clinical Center of Kosovo, Pristina 10000, Kosovo*
[4]*UBT College, Institute of Medical Sciences and Innovation, Pristina 10000, Kosovo*
[5]*Clinic of Infectious Disease, University Clinical Center of Kosovo, Pristina 10000, Kosovo*
[6]*Department of Infectious Disease, Faculty of Medicine, University of Pristina "Hasan Prishtina", Pristina 10000, Kosovo*

Correspondence should be addressed to Vera Kukaj; vera.kukaj@uni-pr.edu

Academic Editor: Dawei Cui

According to several studies, children represent only about 2% of the patients affected by the current SARS-CoV-2, and most often, they are asymptomatic. However, there is a concern about a vascular inflammatory disease which is similar to Kawasaki disease observed in children and adolescents weeks after infection. We report a case of Kawasaki disease presented with ischemic stroke in a 14-year-old male patient following SARS-Cov-2 infection.

1. Introduction

The COVID-19 pandemic has resulted in over hundred million confirmed cases and millions of deaths. Studies have shown that pediatric patients represent a small percentage of confirmed cases and they display only mild symptoms, making the diagnosis challenging [1, 2]. However, several reports from European countries and North America have described a secondary Multisystem Inflammatory Syndrome in Children (MIS-C) and also patients in their late teens and early twenties who have presented with features of Kawasaki disease (KD) after prior COVID-19 [3]. This alarming complication of COVID-19 in children usually occurs between two and four weeks after infection. Majority of children and adolescents affected by this complication were previously healthy, about 80% of them required intensive care, 2% have died, and many of them developed cardiovascular and clotting complications [4, 5]. Here, we report a clinical case showing an association between SARS-CoV-2 infection and typical KD presented with ischemic stroke. KD affects medium- and small-sized arteries, mainly coronary arteries, and cases complicated with stroke are rarely identified and reported in the literature [6]. To the best of our knowledge, this is the first report of a patient with KD presented with ischemic stroke after COVID-19.

2. Case Description

A 14-year-old male with no chronic medical conditions presented in the Emergency Department with a five-day history of fever, fatigue, bilateral conjunctivitis, cervical lymphadenopathy, hand swelling, and a skin rash on his lateral parts of the body, groin, and both hands (Figures 1 and 2). Because the skin rashes were very prominent, the patient was at first admitted in the clinic of dermatology, and for seven days, he was treated with empirical antibiotics and corticosteroid therapy. He did not develop any significant lower respiratory symptoms. On the third day of being in hospital, his fever resolved and skin rashes began to resolute. On the seventh day of being in hospital, he developed right-

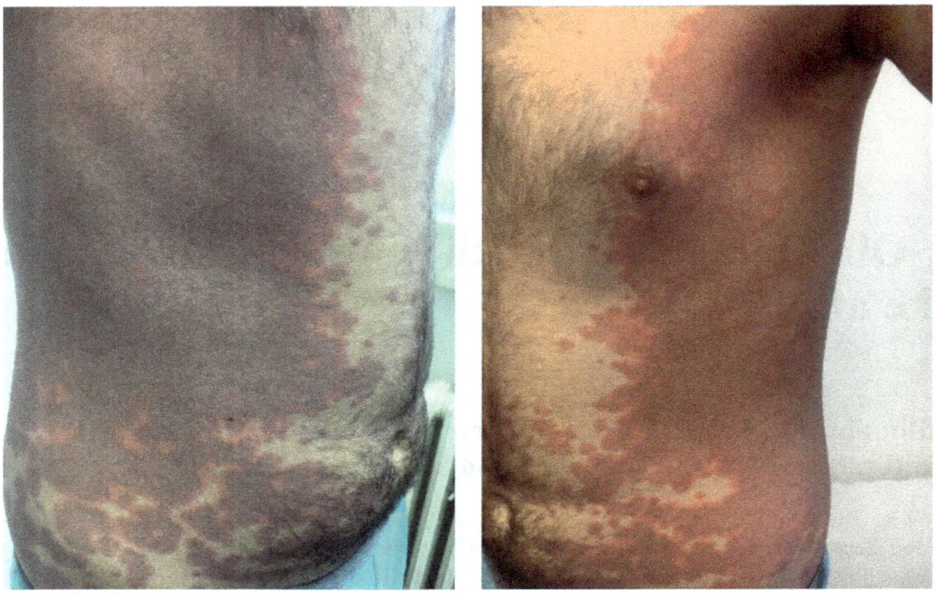

(a) (b)

FIGURE 1: Very prominent skin rashes affecting the lateral parts of the body in both sides.

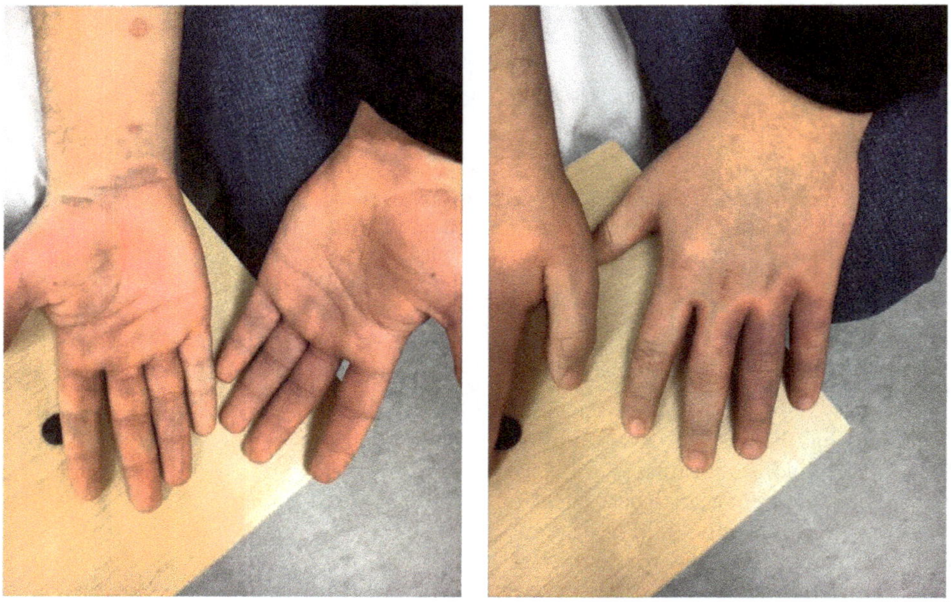

(a) (b)

FIGURE 2: Skin rashes in the distal parts of the upper extremities and palmar edema.

side hemiplegia and aphasia. Brain MRI (Magnetic Resonance Imaging) and MRA (Magnetic Resonance Angiography) were conducted, showing brain ischemia on the terminal branches of the left medial cerebral artery (Figure 3). As a result, the patient was admitted in our Clinic of Neurology for further evaluation and treatment.

His laboratory testing showed increased white blood cell count (WBC) 13 100/mm^3 with increased granulocytes, normal hemoglobin and thrombocyte levels, elevated inflammatory markers (ESR 65 mm/min, CRP 85.1 mg/L), increased d-dimer (4.8 mcg FEU/ml), low albumin level (31.8 g/L), and normal transaminases, bilirubin, blood urea nitrogen, and creatinine level. The patient had mild pyuria (5–10 WBC/hpf), but there was no pathogen isolated in the urine culture. The lumbar puncture was performed showing slight increase of proteins (0.92 g/L) and no blood elements. A plain view chest radiograph showed no significant abnormalities. Electrocardiography showed normal sinus rhythm. Transthoracic

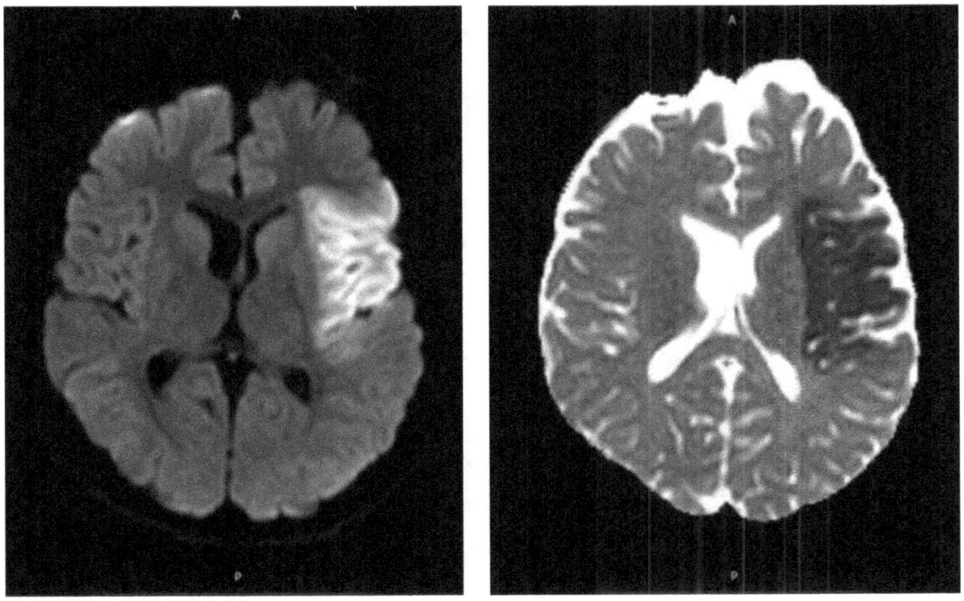

(a) (b)

Figure 3: Axial MRI images (a) diffusion weighted and (b) apparent diffusion coefficient (ADC), showing acute brain ischemia in the territory of the medial cerebral artery.

echocardiography showed normal ejection fraction without coronary artery dilatation. Brain and neck Computed Tomography Angiography (CTA) was normal. However, on transcranial duplex ultrasound, a slight increase of the pulsatility index (PI = 1.18) was observed, suggesting distal resistance due to occlusion of the terminal arterial branches of the left medial cerebral artery (MCA). An autoimmunity panel screening was performed, and the results were negative.

Three weeks before symptom onset, the patients' mother had been confirmed with COVID-19 and displayed mild upper respiratory infection, but our patient was not tested at that time as he had not exhibited fever or any other symptoms of illness. After admission in our hospital, the nasopharyngeal SARS-CoV-2 PCR was negative but serological testing for COVID-19 showed increased IgG levels. Serological (IgM) screening for cytomegalovirus, toxoplasmosis, rubella, HIV, and herpes virus was negative.

KD was diagnosed when our patient met four out of five clinical criteria (generalized rash, peripheral extremity swelling, bilateral nonexudative conjunctivitis, and cervical lymphadenopathy) associated with more than five days of fever. Intravenous immunoglobulin (IVIG) (2 g/Kg) was administrated together with a low dose of aspirin therapy and methylprednisolone 40 mg twice daily. Within 48 hours, the patient improved significantly with near complete resolution of neurological symptoms, and he was able to speak and move, showing only discrete right-side hemiparesis (4/5 muscle strength). Prior to hospital discharge, two weeks later, complete blood count, coagulation profile, d-dimer, albumin level, and CRP were normalized. Also, ischemic changes on brain imaging were decreased (Figure 4). On the follow-up visit, two weeks after hospital discharge, the patient continued to do well without recurring symptoms.

3. Discussion

On 27 April 2020, the United Kingdom National Health Service issued an alert highlighting a multisystem inflammatory syndrome increasingly observed across the United Kingdom, citing a possible association with the SARS-CoV-2. Authors from London, England, [3] and authors from Philadelphia, USA, [7] reported clinical and laboratory features of several patients aged 2–15 years who had been hospitalized with hyperinflammatory shock, all of whom tested positive for SARS-CoV-2 antibodies. Clinical characteristics of these cases shared features with KD and KD shock syndrome, including fever, shock, and variably rash, conjunctivitis, extremity edema, and gastrointestinal symptoms. Centers for Disease Control and Prevention issued a public health advisory and case definition for this hyperinflammatory syndrome, termed MIS-C [8]. They recommended that early diagnosis and treatment of patients meeting full or partial criteria for KD is critical to prevent complications. Patients meeting criteria for KD should be treated with intravenous immunoglobulin (IVIG) and aspirin [9].

Here, we have reported a 14-year-old patient with classical signs of KD presented with ischemic stroke. The diagnosis was challenging because the prior COVID-19 was silent and the skin rashes were very prominent on admission. Therefore, the patient was admitted and empirically treated in the clinic of dermatology at first days, and only after complicated with neurological symptoms, he was transferred to the Neurology Clinic. Prior infection with SARS-CoV-2 was confirmed based on serological testing and prior contact with the infected family member. Brain ischemia was confirmed with MRI. Even though there was not

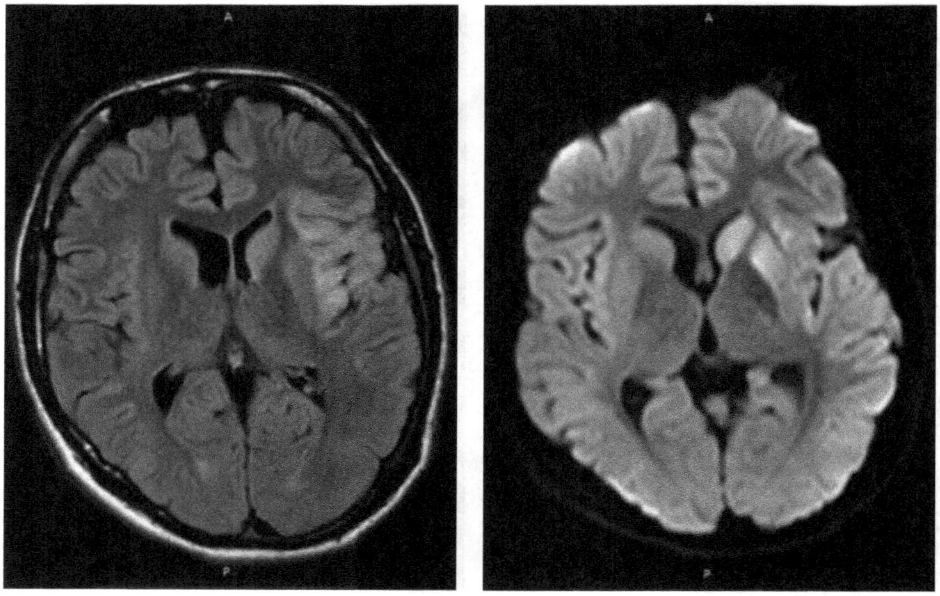

(a) (b)

FIGURE 4: Brian MRI images of the patient, two weeks after neurological symptom onset. Axial (a) fluid-attenuated inversion recovery (FLAIR) MRI scans and (b) diffusion-weighted images (DWI) showing a hyperintense signal and edema of the caudate nucleus head, putamen, and parts of the external capsule and insula on the left side.

any large artery or venous occlusion apparent on CTA, increased pulsatility index was found on the left MCA suggesting distal small diameter arterial segments occlusion. After treatment with IVIG, corticosteroids, and low-dose aspirin, the neurological deficit was resolved.

The exact pathomechanism of the MIS-C is not clear. Given the lag between SARS-CoV-2 infection and MIS-C and the finding that many patients are positive for antibodies and negative for the viral antigen, it has been suggested that abnormal immune response might be the key factor. A potential role of the antibodies in the pathogenesis of KD has been accepted, and the prevalence of such antibodies to target different tissues in the body could explain the multisystem presentation in MIS-C [10].

4. Conclusions

There is a myriad of COVID-19 symptoms and sequelae making the diagnosis challenging. Early diagnosis and prompt treatment of the secondary inflammatory syndromes, including Kawasaki disease, is very important for preventing end-organ damage and long-term complications.

Consent

No written consent has been obtained from the patients as there is no patient identifiable data included in this case report.

References

[1] Y. Dong, X. Mo, Y. Hu et al., "Epidemiology of COVID-19 among children in China," *Pediatrics*, vol. 145, no. 6, Article ID e20200702, 2020.

[2] CDC COVID-19 Response Team, S. Bialek, R. Gierke et al., "Coronavirus disease 2019 in children - United States, february 12-april 2, 2020," *MMWR. Morbidity and Mortality Weekly Report*, vol. 69, no. 14, pp. 422–426, 2020.

[3] S. Riphagen, X. Gomez, C. Gonzalez-Martinez, N. Wilkinson, and P. Theocharis, "Hyperinflammatory shock in children during COVID-19 pandemic," *The Lancet*, vol. 395, no. 10237, pp. 1607-1608, 2020.

[4] E. Whittaker, A. Bamford, J. Kenny et al., "Clinical characteristics of 58 children with a pediatric inflammatory multisystem syndrome temporally associated with SARS-CoV-2," *JAMA*, vol. 324, no. 3, pp. 259–269, 2020.

[5] N. Parri, M. Lenge, and D. Buonsenso, "Coronavirus infection in pediatric emergency departments (CONFIDENCE) research group," *New England Journal of Medicine*, vol. 383, no. 2, pp. 187–190, 2020.

[6] A. Gkoutzourelas, D. P. Bogdanos, and L. I. Sakkas, "Kawasaki disease and COVID-19," *Mediterranean Journal of Rheumatology*, vol. 31, pp. 268–274, 2020.

[7] K. Chiotos, H. Bassiri, E. M. Behrens et al., "Multisystem inflammatory syndrome in children during the coronavirus 2019 pandemic: a case series," *Journal of the Pediatric Infectious Diseases Society*, vol. 9, no. 3, pp. 393–398, 2020.

[8] Centers for Disease Control and Prevention, "Multisystem inflammatory syndrome in children (MIS-C) associated with coronavirus disease 2019 (COVID-19)," 2020, https://emergency.cdc.gov/han/2020/han00432.asp.

[9] R. M. Oates-Whitehead, J. H. Baumer, L. Haines et al., "Intravenous immunoglobulin for the treatment of Kawasaki disease in children," *Cochrane Database of Systematic Reviews*, vol. 2003, no. 4, Article ID CD004000, 2003.

[10] C. R. Consiglio, N. Cotugno, F. Sardh et al., "The immunology of multisystem inflammatory syndrome in children with COVID-19," *Cell*, vol. 183, no. 4, pp. 968–981, 2020.

27

Encephalopathy Associated with Severe Cytomegalovirus Infection in an Immunocompetent Young Woman

Syuichi Tetsuka, Tomohiro Suzuki, Tomoko Ogawa, Ritsuo Hashimoto, and Hiroyuki Kato

Department of Neurology, International University of Health and Welfare Hospital, 537-3 Iguchi, Nasushiobara, Tochigi 329-2763, Japan

Correspondence should be addressed to Syuichi Tetsuka; syuichi@jichi.ac.jp

Academic Editor: Mohamed Dkhil

Primary cytomegalovirus (CMV) infection in healthy young adults is usually an asymptomatic or mononucleosis-like syndrome, whereas in immunocompromised patients, CMV can cause significant disease. In this study, we report an unusual case of primary CMV infection wherein the patient, an immunocompetent 21-year-old woman, presented severe encephalopathy, acute hepatitis, retinitis, and reactivation of latent Epstein–Barr virus. She developed confusion, high fever, headache, and tonic-clonic seizures. Brain magnetic resonance imaging showed high-intensity lesions in the medial temporal lobe and basal ganglia. Liver dysfunction was observed, and abdominal computed tomography revealed splenohepatomegaly. After fundus findings, the patient was diagnosed with CMV retinitis. Upon admission, she was treated with intravenous acyclovir and steroid pulse therapy. Considering both her serious clinical condition and elevated serum levels of interleukin-6, we speculated that her condition was similar to cytokine-storm-induced encephalopathy. On day 2 after admission, she showed prompt recovery from these clinical manifestations. Since blood CMV pp65 antigenemia was found to be positive, we administered ganciclovir for 2 weeks. On the basis of her clinical manifestations and the presence of blood CMV DNA and CMV pp65 antigenemia along with IgM kinetics, we finally diagnosed this patient with severe primary CMV infection. She left our hospital without sequelae 20 days after admission. The incidence of severe CMV disease in immunocompetent young adults might be higher than previously recognized. Noninvasive testing for CMV (such as CMV pp65 antigenemia and CMV DNAemia) is widely available and can help early diagnosis. Short-term glucocorticoid therapy might be beneficial in the treatment of encephalopathy in the early stages of primary CMV infection. Considering such a background, clinicians should keep severe primary CMV infection in mind as a differential diagnosis in the clinical setting.

1. Introduction

Cytomegalovirus (CMV), which establishes a lifelong latency period after primary infection, is a herpes virus that is present everywhere with a worldwide seroprevalence ranging from 45% to 100% [1]. In the past, most people were first infected in the early childhood, but the age of first infection has been rising as the sanitary environment improves in Japan. CMV causes serious diseases in immunocompromised patients and results in significant morbidity and mortality through reactivation of the latent virus or primary infection [2]. Advances in diagnostic technology have revealed that CMV is a common opportunistic infection in fetuses, allograft recipients, bone marrow transplant patients, solid organ transplants, hematopoietic stem cell transplants, and acquired immunodeficiency syndrome (AIDS) patients [3]. Primary CMV infection in healthy young adults is usually asymptomatic in 80% of immunocompetent individuals, and only approximately 20% of patients have mild influenza- or mononucleosis-like symptoms, which include fever, rhinitis and pharyngitis, headache, arthralgia and myalgia, and physical exhaustion [4]. Therefore, the onset of CMV encephalopathy or encephalitis in immunocompetent patients is thought to be extremely rare. However, recently, it seems that the incidence of severe manifestations of CMV infection in immunocompromised individuals has been recognized to be much more common than before. Thus, severe CMV infections, such as encephalopathy, hepatitis, retinitis, gastrointestinal disorders, cardiovascular diseases, pneumonia, and hematological abnormalities in immunocompetent adults, might become a condition that should be considered as one of the differential diagnoses in many future clinical settings [5]. We present a case of an immunocompetent young adult who recovered promptly from severe encephalopathy, acute hepatitis, and retinitis caused by primary CMV infection.

2. Case Presentation

A 21-year-old woman presented to the emergency room at our hospital with a history of confusion, high fever, and headache. Six days before emergency consultation, she had fever in the 38°C range and had a loss of appetite. She had a history of mumps at the age of seven. Other than that, there was nothing remarkable about her medical or medication history. After admission on the same day, her level of consciousness worsened, and she could barely open her eyes when called, but she did not speak, did not get the instructions, and did not move her limbs (Glasgow Coma Scale; E3V1M1). In addition, tonic-clonic seizures that lasted for a few minutes began to occur. Her initial vital signs were as follows: heart rate, 128 beats/min; respiratory rate, 24 breaths/min; blood pressure, 130/81 mmHg; body temperature, 39.9°C; and oxygen saturation, 94% with room air. Neurological examination revealed no neck stiffness and no other gross focal neurological deficits. Results of laboratory investigations are shown in Table 1. Her white blood cell count and C-reactive protein concentration were 11530/μl (neutrophils, 47.0%; lymphocytes, 27.0%; monocytes, 3.0%; and atypical lymphocytes, 23.0%) and 3.34 mg/L, respectively. Also, many atypical lymphocytes were observed in the peripheral blood smear. Ferritin levels were mildly elevated in the serum (68 ng/ml). Liver dysfunction was observed with an elevated aspartate aminotransferase (AST) level (116 IU/L) and an elevated alanine aminotransferase (ALT) level (183 IU/L). Serum creatinine and electrolyte concentrations were normal. Serum levels of interleukin-6 (IL-6) were elevated to 10.3 pg/ml (normal range, <4.0 pg/ml). Both nasopharyngeal swab tests for SARS-CoV-2 RNA and influenza antigen (A and B) were negative results. Based on the presence of liver dysfunction by laboratory investigations at admission, abdominal computed tomography (CT) was performed. An abdominal contrast-enhanced CT revealed a splenohepatomegaly but no sign of neoplasia (Figures 1(a) and 1(b)). Cerebrospinal fluid (CSF) analysis showed lymphocyte-dominant pleocytosis with 186 nuclear cells/mm^3 (180 mononuclear cells/mm^3 and 6 polymorphonuclear cells/mm^3) and protein concentration (41 mg/dL) and glucose concentration (96 mg/dL, with a serum glucose concentration of 140 mg/dL). Fluid-attenuated inversion recovery (FLAIR) images of brain magnetic resonance imaging (MRI) showed high-intensity lesions at the left medial temporal lobe, bilateral caudate nucleus, and left lentiform nucleus (Figures 2(a) and 2(b)). Based on the patient's clinical findings and the results of various laboratory and imaging tests, we diagnosed her with possible meningoencephalitis, including herpes simplex virus encephalitis. On the day of admission, the patient was started on meningoencephalitis treatment with acyclovir (10 mg/kg/IV q8h), ceftriaxone sodium (2 g IV q12h), and fosphenytoin sodium (IV q24h) as antiepileptic drugs and steroid pulse therapy with high doses of intravenous methylprednisolone (1,000 mg) for 3 days.

On the second day of admission, she became afebrile, was able to speak, and was shown to improve her disturbance of consciousness. Serial FLAIR images of brain MRI showed no abnormality and the improvement of previous MRI findings (Figures 2(c) and 2(d)). In the results of laboratory investigations on admission, blood CMV pp65 antigenemia assay was found to be positive (17 pp65-positive cells per 5×10^5 cells) and herpes simplex virus (HSV) DNA was negative in the CSF. Thus, we suspected that encephalopathy was caused by CMV and started to administer ganciclovir (5 mg/kg/IV q12h) instead of acyclovir. As the possibility of CMV infection increased, she consulted an ophthalmologist. As fundus findings, white punctate exudate and petechiae were observed in the retina of the left eye, and a diagnosis of CMV retinitis and uveitis was made (Figures 3(a) and 3(b)). However, symptoms such as decreased visual acuity and visual field impairment had not yet been developed. After that, her general condition recovered rapidly, and after two weeks, she was able to walk and talk normally. In other results of laboratory investigations on admission, blood CMV DNA was detected by polymerase chain reaction (PCR) (1.6×10^3 copies/ml), but CSF CMV DNA was negative (Table 1). The test for Epstein–Barr virus (EBV) DNA in blood was also positive. Anti-CMV IgM antibody levels were elevated (8.54 titers), as were anti-CMV IgG antibodies (15.5 titers) (enzyme-linked immunosorbent assay; positive titer >2.0), in the serum. The human immunodeficiency virus (HIV) antibody testing using rapid tests was negative, and HIV RNA was undetectable in the serum. The number of CD4+ cells was normal. Antinuclear antibody, anti-double-stranded DNA antibody, and hepatitis screening results were negative, and serum immunoglobulin levels (IgG, IgM, IgA, and IgE) were within normal limits. No other potential immunosuppressant factors were recognized in the patient in terms of clinical manifestation or laboratory findings. In addition, the IgM antibody levels of various viruses, including EBV, varicella-zoster virus, and mumps virus, were also elevated in serum. After two weeks of administration of ganciclovir, blood CMV pp65 antigenemia assay became negative and the administration of this drug was terminated. In addition, blood CMV DNA was also negative (Table 1). Two weeks after admission, a retest of CMV antibodies showed that IgM was still positive (7.49 titers), but IgG antibody titer was significantly higher (71.0 titers) than before (15.5 titers) (Table 1). Lower serum levels of IL-6 were observed (2.4 pg/ml). Considering the presence of CMV DNA and pp65 antigenemia along with IgM kinetics, CMV infection in the patient was suggestive of a primary infection. During the subsequent course, her liver function improved, and retinitis did not worsen. She recovered 20 days after admission and was able to leave our

Table 1: Laboratory investigations

Investigations	Result on admission	Results two weeks after the admission	Results four months after the admission
WBC (/μl), (3500–9700)	11530	7600	6800
Differential count (%)	N 47.0, L 27.0, M 3.0, A 23.0	N 68.0, L 25.4, M 6.6, A 0	N 60.5, L 34.9, M 4.6, A 0
Hemoglobin (g/dl), (11.2–15.2)	12.4	12.2	12.5
Platelet count ($\times 10^9$/L), (14.9–37.9)	22.2	30.3	23.1
CRP (mg/dl), (<0.3)	3.34	0.04	0.04
HBV, HCV serology	Negative		
Serum HIV antibody	Negative		Negative
Blood HIV RNA	Negative		
AST (U/l), (8–38)	116	20	21
ALT (U/l), (4–44)	183	22	16
Glucose (mg/dl), (70–109)	140	158	93
CSF counts (cells/mm^3)	WBC 186 (N 6, L 180)	WBC 21 (N 0, L 21)	
CSF glucose (mg/dl), (50–75)	96	58	
CSF protein (mg/dl), (15–45)	41	37	
CSF gram stain and culture	Negative		
CSF TB-PCR	Negative		
CSF fungal culture	Negative		
Nasopharynx influenza antigen (A and B)	Negative		
Nasopharynx COVID-19 RNA	Negative		
Blood CMV pp65 antigenemia (0 pp65-positive cells per 5×10^5 cells)	Positive (17)	Negative (0)	Negative (0)
Blood CMV DNA	Positive (1.6×10^3 copies/ml)	Negative	
CSF CMV DNA	Negative		
Serum anti-CMV IgM (<0.8 titers)	Positive (8.54)	Positive (7.49)	Positive (2.99)
Serum anti-CMV IgG (<2.0 titers)	Positive (15.5)	Positive (71.0)	Positive (42.5)
CSF HSV DNA	Negative		
Serum anti-HSV IgM (<0.8 titers)	Negative (0.28)		
Serum anti-HSV IgG (<2.0 titers)	Negative (<2.0)		
Blood EBV DNA	Positive (2.93 log IU/ml)	Negative	
CSF EBV DNA	Negative		
Serum anti-EBNA IgG (<0.5 titers)	Positive (4.0)	Positive (3.1)	Positive (4.3)
Serum anti-VCA-IgM (<0.5 titers)	Positive (12.7)	Positive (8.9)	Positive (1.4)
Serum anti-VCA-IgG (<0.5 titers)	Positive (8.2)	Positive (8.3)	Positive (8.4)
Serum anti-VZV IgM (<0.8 titers)	Positive (1.32)	Positive (1.48)	Negative (0.62)
Serum anti-VZV IgG (<2.0 titers)	Positive (89.0)	Positive (74.0)	Positive (55.6)
Serum antimumps IgM (<0.8 titers)	Positive (2.9)	Positive (2.58)	Borderline (0.82)
Serum antimumps IgG (<2.0 titers)	Positive (47.0)	Positive (39.0)	Positive (23.5)
Serum interleukin-6 (pg/ml), (<4)	10.3	2.4	

Normal ranges are given in parentheses. WBC, white blood cell; N, neutrophils; L, lymphocytes; M, monocytes; A, atypical lymphocytes; CRP, C-reactive protein; AST, aspartate aminotransferase; ALT, alanine aminotransferase; HBV, hepatitis B virus; HCV, hepatitis C virus; HIV, human immunodeficiency virus; CSF, cerebrospinal fluid; TB, tuberculosis; PCR, polymerase chain reaction; CMV, cytomegalovirus; HSV, herpes simplex virus; EBV, Epstein–Barr virus; EBNA, Epstein–Barr virus nuclear antigen; VCA, virus capsid antigen; VZV, varicella-zoster virus; IgM, immunoglobulin M; IgG, immunoglobulin G.

hospital without sequelae. After 4 months, follow-up laboratory investigations were performed, and blood CMV pp65 antigenemia was confirmed to be negative. The IgM antibody levels of all viruses, including CMV, EBV, varicella-zoster virus, and mumps virus, changed to negative or showed a significant decrease (Table 1). She is on outpatient follow-up and is doing well.

Regarding the relative changes in the patient's IgM and IgG levels over time, CMV IgM four months after admission was observed to decrease to 2.99 titers. Conversely, CMV IgG levels four months after admission were 42.5 titers, which were not significantly different from the values (71.0 titers) two weeks after admission.

3. Discussion and Conclusions

We finally diagnosed this patient with severe primary CMV infection, including encephalopathy, acute hepatitis, and retinitis. With regard to encephalopathy, although this patient exhibited central nervous system involvement, CSF CMV DNA was not detected. Therefore, it is unknown whether the CMV invaded the central nervous system directly. It has been reported that the sensitivity and specificity of CSF CMV DNA by the PCR method in the identification of active CMV infection of the central nervous system were 93.3% and 93.7%, respectively, and the sensitivity and specificity of CSF CMV pp65 antigenemia assay were 84.6%

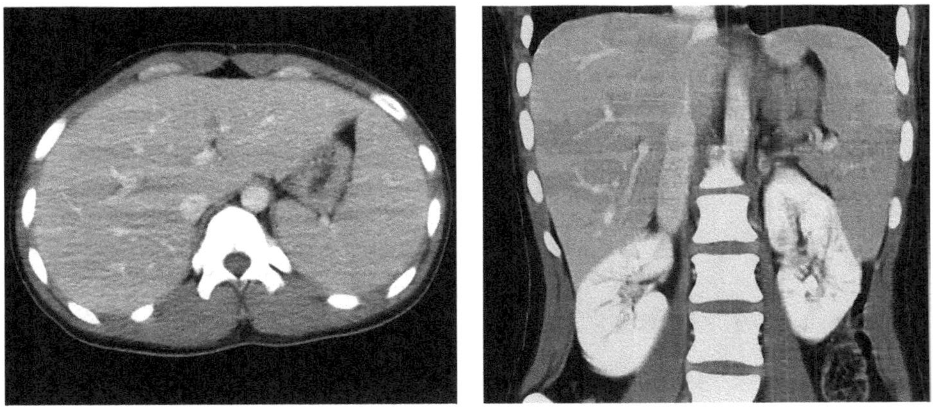

(a) (b)

Figure 1: Abdominal contrast-enhanced CT upon admission. (a) Axial view; (b) Coronal view. There is splenohepatomegaly.

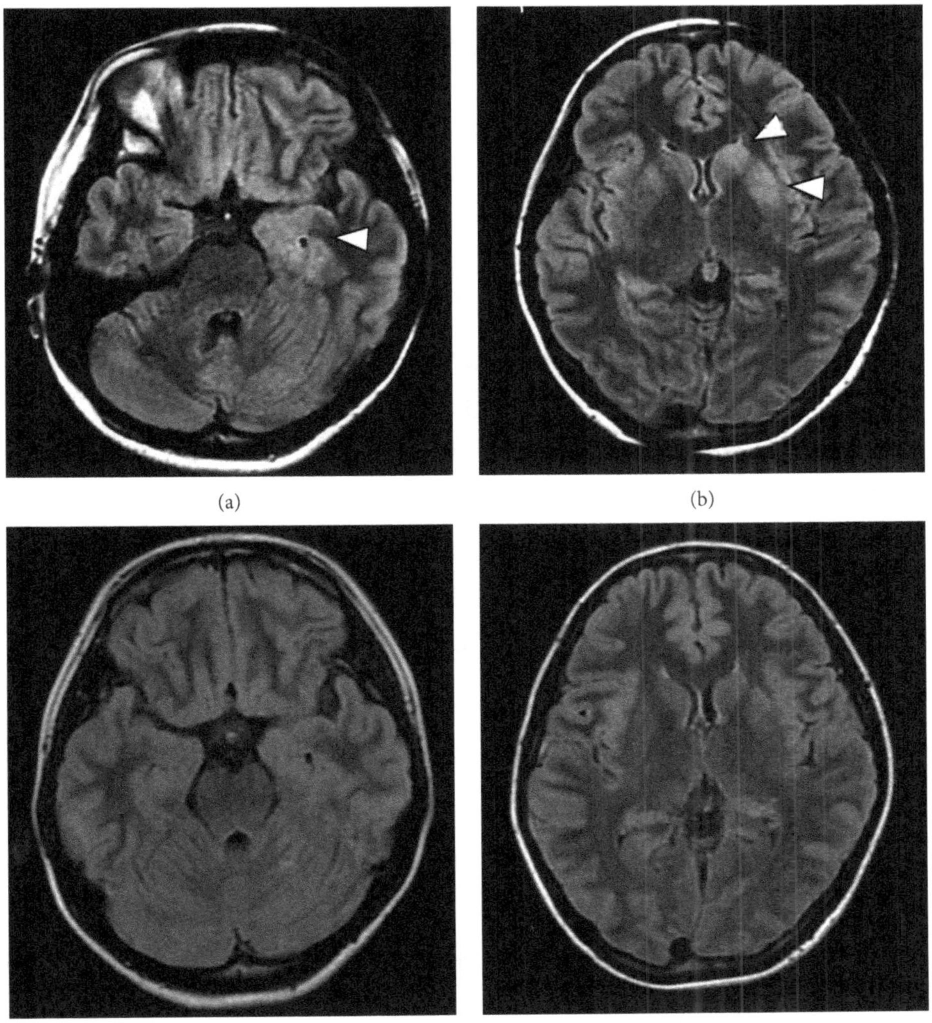

(a) (b) (c) (d)

Figure 2: Brain MRI studies at the onset. Axial view of fluid-attenuated inversion recovery (FLAIR) images showing high-intensity lesions in the left medial temporal lobe (a), bilateral caudate nucleus, and left lentiform nucleus (b). (c), (d) MRI studies on the second day of follow-up. FLAIR images show a normal signal in the medial temporal lobe and basal ganglia and no abnormal lesion. Arrowheads indicate high-intensity lesions.

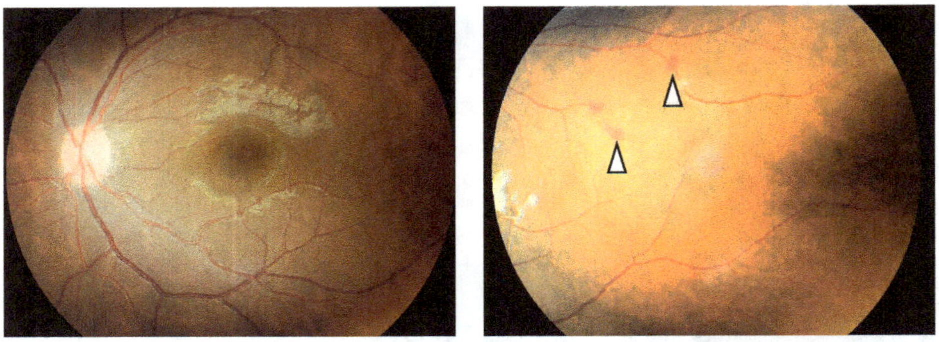

(a) (b)

Figure 3: Fundus appearance on admission. There is white punctate exudate around the macula (a) and petechiae were observed (b) in the retina of the left eye. Arrowheads indicate petechiae.

and 100%, respectively [6]. In the case of latent CMV infection, CMV DNA is not found in the CSF; thus, the detection of CMV DNA in the CSF is a marker of active infections such as CMV encephalitis. Considering such data with laboratory findings, MRI findings, and clinical presentation, we diagnosed encephalopathy, which indirectly causes central nervous system symptoms, instead of encephalitis. On the other hand, blood CMV DNA and CMV pp65 antigenemia were positive. The liver and retina of this patient were considered to be directly invaded by CMV itself, and she developed acute hepatitis and retinopathy. In CMV infections, if healthy adults in whom serum CMV IgG antibody remains negative are first infected, the patients often present with infectious mononucleosis-like symptoms. Fever, liver dysfunction, cervical lymphadenopathy, hepatosplenomegaly, etc. are the main symptoms, and it is difficult to distinguish them from those of the initial infection with the EBV. Moreover, since blood EBV DNA and serum EBV IgM were positive in this case, it is not possible to determine whether CMV or EBV contributed more to acute encephalopathy and acute hepatitis. But, her retinitis was considered to be most likely due to CMV, which is an involvement specific to CMV infection typically. In any case, she had a very rare condition as an immunocompetent young woman.

Several mechanisms have been proposed as the cause of simultaneous positive IgM for EBV and CMV. Given that blood CMV DNA and EBV DNA were detected in this case they include, it is considered that there is the possibility of the two mechanisms: (1) EBV and CMV superinfection and (2) reactivation of latent EBV caused by transient suppression of cell-mediated immunity or settings of acute systemic stress such as cytokine storm caused by CMV infection [7–9]. Furthermore, anti-Epstein–Barr virus nuclear antigen (EBNA) IgG was persistently positive from the beginning; thus, we could rule out the possibility of primary infection of EBV (Table 1). Serum anti-EBNA IgG is detected months after primary infection, which is the recovery period and is an indicator of the history of the infection. The detections of other viral IgM, including varicella-zoster virus and the mumps virus, are insufficient to diagnose viral reactivation; however, such elevated IgM antibodies are frequently observed as nonspecific heterologous IgM during an acute infection. Thus, we diagnosed the patient with only latent EBV reactivation because the other viruses were only indirectly detected. On the other hand, regarding CMV infection, fluctuation in the CMV IgG titers was observed with CMV IgG titers rising from 15.5 titers on admission to 71.0 titers two weeks after the admission. Furthermore, because the presence of CMV DNA and pp65 antigenemia along with IgM kinetics, which were also observed in this case (Table 1), are indicators of a primary infection, we finally diagnosed this patient with severe primary CMV infection, taking into account her clinical findings. If viral replication is out of control by those immune systems, it can lead to severe organ disease and, in some cases, death, particularly in conditions such as AIDS and organ transplantation. In this case, we could make an early diagnosis by using a CMV pp65 antigenemia test and start treating her with ganciclovir on day 2 after admission, which would have led to a good prognosis for her. Diagnosing CMV diseases, just like a lot of other diseases, is difficult in immunocompetent individuals. Although we initially have suspected her suffering from acute HIV infection, considering her manifestations and results of laboratory tests, the differential diagnosis was ruled out based on the negative blood HIV RNA (Table 1). Severe primary CMV infection has a significant diagnostic challenge, especially in immunocompetent young adults, which might lead to delayed diagnosis and adverse health outcomes.

With regard to her experiencing a rapid improvement in clinical symptoms in a short period after the start of treatment, it is supposed that steroid pulse therapy with high doses of glucocorticoid was remarkably effective and she may have had a condition like the so-called cytokine storm. However, steroid administration also has a reverse impact on CMV infection, taking into account her clinical findings. Steroids aggravate the disease, increase the CMV infection rate, and increase the duration of antiviral therapy in patients at high risk of CMV infection [10]. For example, in transplant recipients, steroid bolus for rejection often leads to CMV reactivation [11]. Therefore, as in this case, we consider that high-dose steroid administration should be maintained for a short period in the early stages of the disease and not for a long period, while ruling out potential immunosuppressive conditions [12, 13]. Acute encephalopathy due to cytokine storm is characterized by high levels of serum IL-6, an inflammatory cytokine that plays an important role in cytokine release syndrome [14]. CMV infection induces IL-6, which might contribute to the pathology of the infection [15]. Also, in this case, high levels of IL-6 were observed before steroid pulse therapy, but after treatment, IL-6 also normalized with improvement in clinical symptoms (Table 1). Following the EBV, CMV is the most frequently reported as an infectious trigger for cytokine storm. CMV-related cytokine storm has a poor prognosis as with most other cytokine storm, and there are no randomized controlled trials for the treatment of virus-induced cytokine storm. The treatment is not limited to antiviral drugs, and the combined use of immunomodulatory therapy as in this case is extremely important for improving the prognosis of such patients.

In conclusion, this case report shows a rapid recovery process and good prognosis from severe CMV encephalopathy due to cytokine storm, acute hepatitis, retinitis, and latent EBV reactivation in an immunocompetent young woman. The incidence of severe CMV disease in immunocompetent young adults may be more than previously recognized. The presence of CMV DNA and pp65 antigenemia along with IgM kinetics can be indicators of a primary infection. The experience suggests that early short-term glucocorticoid therapy might be beneficial in severe cases of primary CMV infection with encephalopathy. Also, noninvasive testing for CMV such as the CMV DNAemia and pp65 antigenemia test is widely available and comes with the possibility of promptly obtaining results; thus, it can help early diagnosis if used appropriately. Considering such a background, clinicians should keep severe primary CMV infection in mind as the differential diagnosis in clinical settings.

Consent

The patient provided consent for reporting his case.

Authors' Contributions

All authors contributed equally to this work.

Acknowledgments

The authors would like to thank Enago (https://www.enago.jp) for the English language review.

References

[1] M. J. Cannon, D. S. Schmid, and T. B. Hyde, "Review of cytomegalovirus seroprevalence and demographic characteristics associated with infection," *Reviews in Medical Virology*, vol. 20, no. 4, pp. 202–213, 2010.

[2] M. V. Dioverti and R. R. Razonable, "Cytomegalovirus," *Microbiology Spectrum*, vol. 4, no. 4, 2016.

[3] P. D. Griffiths, "Burden of disease associated with human cytomegalovirus and prospects for elimination by universal immunisation," *The Lancet Infectious Diseases*, vol. 12, no. 10, pp. 790–798, 2012.

[4] O. Picone, C. Vauloup-Fellous, A. G. Cordier et al., "A series of 238 cytomegalovirus primary infections during pregnancy: description and outcome," *Prenatal Diagnosis*, vol. 33, no. 8, pp. 751–758, 2013.

[5] P. I. Rafailidis, E. G. Mourtzoukou, I. C. Varbobitis, and M. E. Falagas, "Severe cytomegalovirus infection in apparently immunocompetent patients: a systematic review," *Virology Journal*, vol. 5, no. 1, p. 47, 2008.

[6] M. Maschke, O. Kastrup, and H.-C. Diener, "CNS manifestations of cytomegalovirus infections," *CNS Drugs*, vol. 16, no. 5, pp. 303–315, 2002.

[7] G. Borges, D. Neves, I. F. Maury, A. Pereira, and M. d. J. Silva, "An unusual case of CMV/EBV ventriculoencephalitis with evolution to primary central nervous system lymphoma in HIV-positive patient," *Case Reports in Infectious Diseases*, vol. 2018, Article ID 7683797, 3 pages, 2018.

[8] A. Heininger, G. Jahn, C. Engel, T. Notheisen, K. Unertl, and K. Hamprecht, "Human cytomegalovirus infections in nonimmunosuppressed critically ill patients," *Critical Care Medicine*, vol. 29, no. 3, pp. 541–547, 2001.

[9] M. Hummel and M. M. Abecassis, "A model for reactivation of CMV from latency," *Journal of Clinical Virology*, vol. 25, pp. 123–136, 2002.

[10] M. Suárez-Lledó, N. Martínez-Cibrián, G. Gutiérrez-García et al., "Deleterious effect of steroids on cytomegalovirus infection rate after allogeneic stem cell transplantation depends on pretransplant cytomegalovirus serostatus of donors and recipients," *Biology of Blood and Marrow Transplantation*, vol. 24, no. 10, pp. 2088–2093, 2018.

[11] S. K. Yadav, S. Saigal, N. S. Choudhary, S. Saha, N. Kumar, and A. S. Soin, "Cytomegalovirus infection in liver transplant recipients: current approach to diagnosis and management," *Journal of Clinical and Experimental Hepatology*, vol. 7, no. 2, pp. 144–151, 2017.

[12] A. Pilotto, S. Odolini, S. Masciocchi et al., "Steroid-responsive encephalitis in coronavirus disease 2019," *Annals of Neurology*, vol. 88, no. 2, pp. 423–427, 2020.

[13] R. C. Da Silva, G. B. Aguiar, C. Kamer, L. Farias, and J. Matsuda, "Acute disseminated encephalomyelitis related to a cytomegalovirus infection in an immunocompetent patient," *Cureus*, vol. 13, p. e12795, 2021.

[14] T. Ichiyama, "Biomarkers for the diagnosis and evaluation in acute encephalopathy," *Acute Encephalopathy and Encephalitis in Infancy and Its Related Disorders*, Elsevier, Amsterdam, Netherlands, pp. 77–79, 2018.

[15] J. F. Carlquist, L. Edelman, D. W. Bennion, and J. L. Anderson, "Cytomegalovirus induction of interleukin-6 in lung fibroblasts occurs independently of active infection and involves a G protein and the transcription factor, NF-κB," *The Journal of Infectious Diseases*, vol. 179, no. 5, pp. 1094–1100, 1999.

Atypical Manifestation of VZV Infection in a Vaccinated Immunocompetent Adult

Deesha Bhojwani, Mohamed Zakarya, and Suha Abu Khalaf

University of Missouri, One Hospital Dr DC043.00, Columbia, MO 65212, USA

Correspondence should be addressed to Deesha Bhojwani; drb17196@gmail.com

Academic Editor: Mohd Adnan

Introduction. Aseptic meningitis can occur from different types of infections of which viral etiologies are the most common. Varicella zoster virus (VZV) nowadays is considered a familiar entity of aseptic meningitis. However, it is usually reported in immunocompromised patients. For cases of VZV meningitis that are observed, a rash has been noted before the onset of meningitis or sometimes after it. *Clinical Case.* We present an uncommon case of VZV meningitis in an 18-year-old immunocompetent male who did not have a rash on presentation and did not develop one during his course either. Cerebrospinal fluid showed lymphocyte-predominant leukocytosis and elevated protein with normal glucose suggestive of aseptic meningitis. Cerebrospinal fluid polymerase chain reaction (CSF PCR) was positive for VZV; cerebrospinal fluid cultures and blood cultures were negative. The patient had complete resolution of symptoms with no complications on intravenous acyclovir therapy and was discharged home on oral valacyclovir therapy. *Conclusion.* It is important to consider varicella zoster virus as an etiology of aseptic meningitis as clinical presentation can be without a vesicular rash and in immunocompetent patients.

1. Introduction

VZV is a human alpha herpes virus that can lead to primary infection which most commonly manifests as varicella/chickenpox. Following primary infection, it becomes latent in ganglionic neurons and adrenal glands. In the setting of immune deficiency, it reactivates to cause herpes zoster (shingles) [1, 2]. Primary varicella infections as well as reactivated infections can lead to central nervous system (CNS) manifestations such as meningitis, encephalitis, or meningoencephalitis in immunocompetent as well as immunocompromised hosts. CNS manifestations are more severe in immunocompromised individuals [3]. Most cases of meningitis/encephalitis due to varicella zoster virus are associated with a rash that develops either at the onset of symptoms or later in the disease course [3]. We present an uncommon case of an 18-year-old immunocompetent male patient who presented with severe headache and fever. CSF studies were suggestive of aseptic meningitis, and the diagnosis of varicella zoster virus (VZV) meningitis was confirmed on CSF PCR. The patient, however, did not develop a rash during the disease course. It is an uncommon presentation of VZV meningitis in an immunocompetent adult without the development of a rash during the clinical course of the disease.

2. Case Presentation

2.1. Patient Information. An 18-year-old man with no significant medical history presented to our hospital with progressively worsening headache and persistent fever of one-day duration. The patient described the headache as the worst headache of his life and was squeezing, band-like in nature. It was associated with photophobia and neck stiffness. The patient also had associated body aches, fatigue, nausea, and multiple episodes of vomiting. His only sick contact was four days prior to his presentation with his friend who had influenza.

2.2. Relevant Past Interventions/History. The patient was vaccinated against varicella at the age of five. He denied any history of febrile exanthems or cold sores in childhood.

Table 1: Physical examination findings.

General	The patient was lying in a dark room with the eyes closed and was distressed due to pain
Head	Atraumatic and normocephalic
Eyes	Anicteric sclera, no conjunctival pallor, or injection
Neck	Nuchal rigidity noted
Respiratory	Unlabored, symmetric chest rise, on room air, no wheezing noted, and chest clear to auscultation bilaterally
Cardiovascular	Tachycardic, patient in sinus rhythm, and no murmurs appreciated on auscultation
Abdomen	Soft, nontender, nondistended, and no hepatosplenomegaly
Neurological	Alert, attentive, and oriented to time; place person, and situation; cranial nerves two to twelve grossly intact; no loss of muscle bulk or tone; sensations to light touch symmetrical and intact in all extremities; strength 5/5 in all extremities, reflexes 2+ at biceps, triceps, knees, and ankles; normal gait; coordination tested by rapid alternating movements intact in all extremities
Skin	Warm, dry, and no mucocutaneous rash noted

Table 2: Vital signs.

Temperature (degree Celsius)	38.4 (location temporal)
Heart rate (beats per minute)	119
Blood pressure (mmHg)	117/59
Respiratory rate (per minute)	20
Oxygen saturation (%)	96% on room air

Table 3: Laboratory findings.

Leukocyte count (per liter)	10.92 × 10 (9)
Hemoglobin (g/dl)	15.2
Platelet count (per liter)	331 × 10 (9)
CSF white blood cell count (per high power field)	109 (critical high >30)
CSF lymphocyte (%)	55%
CSF macrophages/monocytes (%)	4%
CSF neutrophils (%)	41%
CSF protein (mg/dl)	89 (normal 15–45 mg/dl)
CSF glucose (mg/dl)	56 (normal 40–70 mg/dl)
Serum glucose (mg/dl)	118

Table 4: Timeline of clinical events.

Day 0	Fatigue, headache, nausea, vomiting, and neck stiffness
Day 1	The patient was started on IV vancomycin and ceftriaxone. CT head was unremarkable. A lumbar puncture was performed in the emergency room which was suggestive of aseptic meningitis. IV acyclovir started.
Day 2	Patient's headache, nuchal rigidity, nausea, and vomiting significantly improved. Afebrile. CSF PCR positive for VZV. IV vancomycin and ceftriaxone discontinued. The patient continued to be on IV acyclovir
Day 3	Near complete resolution of symptoms. Afebrile. IV acyclovir continued
Day 4	Asymptomatic, afebrile. On IV acyclovir
Day 5	Completed five days of IV acyclovir and discharged home on oral valacyclovir
Day 16	Completed nine days of oral valacyclovir; followed up with primary care provider

2.3. Clinical Findings. The patient was noted to be febrile and tachycardic (Table 1). Nuchal rigidity was present on examination. No mucosal or cutaneous rash was noted on physical examination (Table 2).

2.4. Diagnostic Assessment. The patient had granulocyte-predominant leukocytosis on presentation (Table 3). CT head was performed outside the hospital which was negative for any intracranial abnormalities. Cerebrospinal fluid

Table 5

Author	Patient's age	Rash	Year
Kerr C.	39	Present	2022
Maruki T.	71	Present	2022
Landa E.	69	Present	2022
Yun S.	18	Absent	2022
Lagrine M.	14	Absent	2021
Jia S.	30	Absent	2021
Khalil S.	Not available	Present	2021
Raghunathan	32	Absent	2021
Platanki	56	Information not available	2021
Bateman	36	Present	2021
Bhandari	60	Present	2021
Bhandari	29	Present	2021
Bhandari	22	Present	2021
Sahra S.	31	Present	2021
Imani	32	Present	2020
Ashour A.	39	Absent	2020
Alataby	40	Present	2020
Faluk	45	Present	2020
Sohal	40	Present	2020
Davidson N.	28	Present	2019
Chan	15	Present	2019
Fadhel	44	Absent	2019
Khaliq	28	Present	2018
Ryu	11	Present	2019
Spernovasilis	36	Absent	2018
Suri	24	Absent	2018
Gnoni	29	Present	2018
Kim	16	Present	2017
Kim	8	Present	2017
Itoh	12	Present	2017
Itoh	12	Present	2017
Ganesan	70	Present	2016
Ibrahim	15	Absent	2015
Abe	57	Absent	2015
Sanguankeo	51	Present	2015
Pasedag	18	Absent	2014
El-Safadi	39	Absent	2014
Esposito	14	Present	2013
Goyal	27	Present	2013
Mantero	17	Absent	2013
Kangath	30	Present	2013
Han	7	Present	2011
Klein	53	Absent	2010
Spiegel	14	Absent	2010
Pena	11	Present	2009
Iyer	9	Present	2009
Habib	26	Absent	2009
Leahy	14	Absent	2008
Mpaka	66	Absent	2008
Frantzidou	72	Information not available	2008
Frantzidou	15	Information not available	2008
Haargaard	64	Present	2008
Pirounaki	27	Present	2007
Hartzell	21	Present	2006
Moriuchi	37	Present	1997

studies showed lymphocyte-predominant leukocytosis, elevated protein, and normal CSF glucose (Table 3). Hence, CSF studies were suggestive of aseptic meningitis. CSF meningitis polymerase chain reaction was reactive for varicella zoster virus which confirmed the diagnosis of varicella zoster virus meningitis. Cerebrospinal fluid culture, blood culture, and urine culture remained negative. Human immunodeficiency virus antigen-antibody testing was nonreactive. Herpes simplex virus 1 and 2 polymerase chain reactions were negative.

2.5. Therapeutic Interventions. The patient was started empirically on intravenous (IV) vancomycin (1.5 grams three times daily as per weight-based dosing of ~12 mg/kg/dose with goal vancomycin trough of 15–20 mcg/ml) and ceftriaxone (two grams every twelve hours) prior to lumbar puncture. IV acyclovir (800 mg three times daily) was added to empirical antimicrobial therapy when CSF studies suggested aseptic meningitis. After CSF PCR tested positive for VZV, vancomycin and ceftriaxone were discontinued. The patient was continued on IV acyclovir (10 mg/kg of ideal body weight) for a total of five days. The patient was discharged on oral valacyclovir (2 g every six hours) for nine days to complete a total of fourteen days of antiviral therapy. A timeline of the patient's clinical course is given in Table 4.

2.6. Follow-Up and Outcomes. The patient's clinical condition started to improve after 24 hours of empiric intravenous vancomycin, ceftriaxone, and acyclovir initiation. His clinical condition improved remarkably with the resolution of his symptoms within forty-eight hours of IV acyclovir therapy. The patient was advised to have a close follow-up with a primary care provider after the completion of his antiviral therapy. No rash was noted on examination during his five days of hospitalization. Per patient's mother and primary care provider, no rash developed within one-month postdischarge.

3. Discussion

VZV is associated with numerous manifestations ranging from chickenpox, herpes zoster to CNS manifestations such as meningitis, encephalitis, meningoencephalitis, myelopathy, and cerebellitis [2]. The proposed mechanism of spread of VZV in primary CNS disease is hematogenous spread which involves vesicular trafficking from trigeminal ganglion to cerebral arteries via the ophthalmic branch [3]. Although enterovirus is the most common cause of aseptic meningitis, especially in childhood, VZV is the second most common cause, with 4.4–11% of suspected meningitis cases testing positive for VZV DNA by PCR [3]. Earlier, VZV was not as routinely tested on CSF as enterovirus and HSV 1, 2. However, given better diagnostic studies and wide availability of multiplex PCR testing, the incidence of VZV meningitis has been rising [4].

Primary varicella infections as well as reactivated infections can lead to CNS manifestations in immunocompromised patients and uncommonly in immunocompetent patients. Meningitis and encephalitis are the most common CNS manifestations in adults. VZV infections are usually associated with a rash; however, it is essential to note that cases without a rash have been reported in literature. In primary varicella as well as herpes zoster, CNS manifestations can precede the onset of rash, and hence, even if the rash is absent initially during clinical presentation, it can develop later in the disease course [3]. Additionally, there have been atypical presentations without a rash during the entire clinical course. Even severe manifestation of VZV infection, visceral VZV has been reported in an immunocompromised patient without a rash [5].

There are a total of fifty-five cases of VZV meningitis reported in immunocompetent patients from 1997 to 2022 (Table 5). Of the fifty-five reported cases, eighteen presented without a rash which suggests that our case presentation is uncommon and atypical [6]. Two case reports were reviewed which describe varicella zoster virus meningitis in immunocompetent healthy children at age eight and fourteen who have presented without a rash. The patients had a history of prior varicella infection in both case reports [7, 8]. Ibrahim et al. also reported herpes zoster meningitis in immunocompetent patients without an eruption of a shingles rash [9]. An interesting case has been reported by Spernovasilis et al. of a 36-year-old immunocompetent male with VZV meningitis who presented without a rash [10].

A reduction in neurological morbidity has been observed with antiviral therapy due to which it is essential to diagnose VZV meningitis promptly [4]. Several antiviral agents are effective against VZV; however, acyclovir is the drug of choice given its higher efficacy with lower adverse events. Given the poor bioavailability of oral acyclovir, intravenous (IV) acyclovir is the preferred route [3, 11]. IV acyclovir offers rapid clinical improvement in addition to reduction in long-term complications [12]. Gnoni et al. reported a 29-year-old immunocompetent patient with VZV meningitis that was successfully treated with IV acyclovir for 2 days followed by oral valacyclovir [13]. Valacyclovir is the prodrug of acyclovir that offers three to four times higher oral bioavailability. A dose of two grams every six hours of oral valacyclovir has been found to be equivalent to 10 mg/kg of IV acyclovir every eight hours based on plasma concentration [3, 11].

4. Conclusion

This case provides salient evidence that VZV meningitis can present atypically in young immunocompetent adults. A high index of suspicion is necessary to be able to promptly diagnose and treat this condition before neurological complications ensue. When a CSF infection such as meningitis or encephalitis is suspected, CSF should be routinely tested for VZV along with HSV 1 and 2 [14].

Acknowledgments

The authors wish to extend their appreciation to the staff of the Department of Internal Medicine and the Department of Infectious disease at University of Missouri for extending their support and encouragement towards this report.

References

[1] D. Gilden, "Varicella zoster virus and central nervous system syndromes," *Herpesviridae*, vol. 11, 2004.

[2] M. A. Nagel, C. S. Niemeyer, and A. N. Bubak, "Central nervous system infections produced by varicella zoster virus," *Current Opinion in Infectious Diseases*, vol. 33, no. 3, pp. 273–278, 2020.

[3] A. Grahn and M. Studahl, "Varicella-zoster virus infections of the central nervous system—prognosis, diagnostics and treatment," *Journal of Infection*, vol. 71, no. 3, pp. 281–293, 2015.

[4] J. C. Alvarez, J. Alvarez, J. Tinoco et al., "Varicella-zoster virus meningitis and encephalitis: an understated cause of central nervous system infections," *Cureus*, vol. 12, no. 11, Article ID e11583, 2020.

[5] N. Spernovasilis, M. Raissaki, I. Papakitsou et al., "Visceral varicella-zoster virus infection presenting with severe abdominal pain without a rash in a patient with psoriatic arthritis treated with infliximab biosimilar and steroids: a case report," *Mediterranean Journal of Rheumatology*, vol. 32, no. 3, pp. 280–284, 2021.

[6] S. Bhandari, C. Alme, A. Siller, and P. Jha, "Varicella zoster meningitis in immunocompetent hosts: a case series and review of the literature," *Wisconsin Medical Journal*, vol. 120, no. 1, pp. 74–77, 2021.

[7] M. Lagrine, K. El Fakiri, N. Rada, G. Draiss, N. Soraa, and M. Bouskraoui, "Varicella zoster virus meningitis with absence of rash in an immunocompetent child," *Journal of Medical Case Reports*, vol. 2021, Article ID 2081270, 2 pages, 2021.

[8] G. Szinnai, F. Farron, G. Bär, and U. Heininger, "Herpes zoster and aseptic meningitis in a previously healthy child," *European Journal of Pediatrics*, vol. 162, no. 6, pp. 434-435, 2003.

[9] W. Ibrahim, A. N. Elzouki, A. Husain, and L. Osman, "Varicella zoster aseptic meningitis: report of an atypical case and literature review," *American Journal of Case Reports*, vol. 16, pp. 594–597, 2015.

[10] N. Spernovasilis, A. Milioni, I. Gialamas, E. Kokorakis, and G. Fanti, "Varicella-zoster virus meningitis with hypoglycorrhachia in a young immunocompetent adult without rash: a case report and literature review," *IDCases*, vol. 12, pp. 104–106, 2018.

[11] A. Sauerbrei, "Diagnosis, antiviral therapy, and prophylaxis of varicella-zoster virus infections," *European Journal of Clinical Microbiology & Infectious Diseases*, vol. 35, no. 5, pp. 723–734, 2016.

[12] S. Ciancia, A. Crisafi, I. Fontana, A. De Fanti, S. Amarri, and L. Iughetti, "Encephalitis due to herpes zoster without rash in an immunocompetent 12-year-old girl: case report and review of the literature," *BMC Pediatrics*, vol. 20, no. 1, p. 348, 2020.

[13] M. Gnoni, K. Zaheer, M. M. Vasser et al., "Varicella zoster aseptic meningitis: report of an atypical case in an immunocompetent patient treated with oral valacyclovir," *IDCases*, vol. 13, Article ID e00446, 2018.

[14] J. Parkes-Smith and A. Chaudhuri, "Varicella zoster virus: an under-recognised cause of central nervous system infections?" *Internal Medicine Journal*, vol. 52, no. 1, pp. 100–104, 2022.

Parainfluenza 3 Respiratory Infection Associated with Pericardial Effusion in a Very Low Birthweight Infant

Cristina Aranda Cazón,[1] Luis Arruza Gómez,[2] Gloria Herranz Carrillo,[2] Cristina González Menchén,[1] Zarife Daoud Pérez,[1] José Antonio Martínez-Orgado,[2] and José Tomás Ramos Amador[1]

[1]*Department of Pediatrics, Hospital Clínico San Carlos, Instituto de Investigación Sanitaria del Hospital Clínico San Carlos (IdISSC), Madrid, Spain*
[2]*Division of Neonatology, Hospital Clínico San Carlos, Instituto de Investigación Sanitaria del Hospital Clínico San Carlos (IdISSC), Madrid, Spain*

Correspondence should be addressed to Cristina Aranda Cazón; aranda.cristina@hotmail.com

Academic Editor: Alexandre R. Marra

Parainfluenza 3 virus is a frequent cause of respiratory infections in the pediatric population although it is uncommonly diagnosed in neonates, being usually reported as neonatal intensive care unit microepidemics. We report a case of parainfluenza 3 respiratory infection associated with pericardial effusion in a very low birthweight infant.

1. Case Report

We present the case of a male neonate born at week 25 of gestational age and weighed 720 grams. During pregnancy follow-up, the mother received labetalol because of gestational hypertension. Ultrasound controls during pregnancy were normal, and routine serologies were negative.

At week 25 of gestation, severe preeclampsia was diagnosed. Fetal ultrasound showed intrauterine growth retardation type 1 and redistribution in Doppler flow. Caesarean delivery was indicated due to severe preeclampsia after sulfate magnesium administration for neuronal protection and complete pulmonary maturation. The newborn needed intubation in the delivery room with 100% fraction of inspired oxygen (FiO_2) and intratracheal instillation of surfactant. Then, he was extubated and connected to nasal continuous positive airway pressure (CPAPn). When FiO_2 was decreased to 30%, the patient was transferred to the neonatal intensive care unit (NICU).

At 29 week postconceptional age, the infant was stable with noninvasive ventilation (mean airway pressure (MAP) 6 cmH_2O, FiO_2 0.40). Suddenly, clinical deterioration occurred, involving respiratory distress, increased needs of oxygen therapy, tachypnea, bradycardia, desaturations, and frequent apnea episodes, that required intubation and mechanical ventilation (MAP 12 cmH_2O, FIO_2 0.50). Laboratory tests evidenced lymphocytosis and hypertransaminasemia. Blood culture, urine culture, and cerebrospinal fluid culture were negative (Table 1). Chest X-ray showed bilateral pulmonary infiltrates and significant cardiomegaly (Figure 1(a)). Echocardiography revealed diffuse pericardial effusion involving predominantly right chambers (Figure 2). Contractility and right and left cardiac outputs were preserved as shown in Table 1.

Polymerase chain reaction (PCR) in nasopharyngeal swab was requested the day after the clinical deterioration and was positive for parainfluenza 3 virus (PIV3). The multiplex PCR used was CLART-PneumoVir. It detects 17 respiratory viruses: respiratory syncytial viruses (RSV); RSV group-A; RSV group-B; PIV1; PIV2; PIV3; PIV4; coronaviruses; human metapneumovirus; adenoviruses; enteroviruses; influenza A (including H3N2 and both seasonal and pandemic H1N1), B, and C viruses; rhinoviruses; and bocavirus. Because newborn family members and neonatal intensive care unit staff were asymptomatic before, during or after the episode, nasopharyngeal swabs could not be

Table 1: Diagnostic tests performed.

Test	Results
Blood test before the diagnosis of the pericardial effusion, during sudden clinical deterioration	Leukocytosis 15.08 cells/mm^3 (5–14.5 cells/mm^3; 75% lymphocytes, 12% neutrophils); hemoglobin 12.5 g/dl (10–13 g/dl) and platelet count 280/mm^3 (250–450/mm^3). ALT 203 U/L (6–50 U/L), AST 180 U/L (35–140 U/L), C-reactive protein (CRP) 3, 4 mg/dl (<2 mg/dl); procalcitonine 0.3 ng/ml (<0.5 ng/ml)
Blood culture	Negative
Urine culture	Negative
Cerebrospinal fluid culture	Negative
Chest X-ray	Bilateral pulmonary infiltrates and significant cardiomegaly
Echocardiography	Diffuse pericardial effusion affecting predominantly right chambers. Ejection fraction: 76%; shortening fraction: 41%; LVO: 355 ml/kg/min; RVO: 395 ml/kg/min
PCR in nasopharyngeal swab	Positive for parainfluenza 3 virus
Blood tests after the resolution of the pericardial effusion	Leukocytes 9.8 cells/mm^3(74.4% lymphocytes, 15% neutrophils); hemoglobin 13.1 g/dl and platelet count 255/mm^3. ALT 89 U/L/AST 73 U/L, C-reactive protein (CRP) 1.7 mg/dl; procalcitonine 0.07 ng/ml

obtained from the contacts. Other infectious causes of pericardial effusion were incompatible with the clinical picture: the patient was not treated with drugs that may had caused pericardial effusion, there was no possible traumatic cause (central venous catheter perforation and penetrating trauma), and there were not clinical, analytical, or radiological signs of other causes (tuberculosis, fungal infections, collagen diseases, etc.). Blood culture for other microorganisms, including bacteria and fungi, was negative. Because of this, PIV3 may have been the trigger for the pericardial pathology.

Due to the hemodynamic stability of the patient, a conservative approach was adopted. The patient did not require anti-inflammatory or diuretic therapy to reduce pericardial effusion. Serial echocardiograms and chest X-ray confirmed its reduction until its complete resolution within 5 days (Figure 1(b)). Figure 1 shows the cardiomegaly at the clinical deterioration, with near complete resolution. At 36 weeks postconceptional age, the patient developed severe bronchopulmonary dysplasia (BPD), requiring high-flow nasal cannulae and 40% oxygen supplementation.

2. Discussion

To our knowledge, there are only two cases reported of pericardial effusion associated with parainfluenza viruses in children and none of them in the neonatal period. The first one describes an 8-month-old boy diagnosed with pneumonia and severe combined immunodeficiency. Parainfluenza 3 was isolated in respiratory secretions and pericardial and cerebrospinal fluids. Postmortem evaluation confirmed the presence of the pathogen in the lung, brain, and pericardial samples [1]. The second case is a 9-year-old immunocompetent patient with pericardial effusion in whom parainfluenza 4 was isolated in nasopharyngeal aspirate. The patient was successfully treated with ibuprofen [2]. There are two other cases reported in adults. In the first one, parainfluenza 3 viral infection was considered to be the cause of a fulminant myocarditis with pericardial effusion in a 35-year-old woman with diabetic ketoacidosis and type 1 diabetes [3]. The second one described a 62-year-old woman with pneumonia and pericardial effusion as a result of infection with parainfluenza virus type 4 and thrombotic thrombocytopenic purpura [4].

Parainfluenza virus is an RNA virus belonging to the Paramyxoviridae family, with four types described. It is a prevailing cause of viral respiratory infection in the pediatric population after respiratory syncytial virus, enteroviruses, or human metapneumovirus. Although respiratory viral infections are usual among hospitalized newborns, they are not clinically suspected because the signs and symptoms of infection are nonspecific or too subtle. For this reason, they are seldom diagnosed in the neonatal intensive care unit. There are scarce reports presenting isolated cases like this one as most of the published data refer to neonatal intensive care unit microepidemics in which parainfluenza 3 was just one of the different viruses detected [5]. Those outbreaks are thought to be related to longer stay in the neonatal intensive care unit. As the main route of transmission of this pathogen is through infected secretions, respiratory and contact isolation is essential to prevent disease outbreaks.

Premature infant population may develop parainfluenza virus infection with atypical or even clinically unapparent signs and symptoms [6] as in our patient. Clinical signs are nonspecific (mainly respiratory with increased secretions,

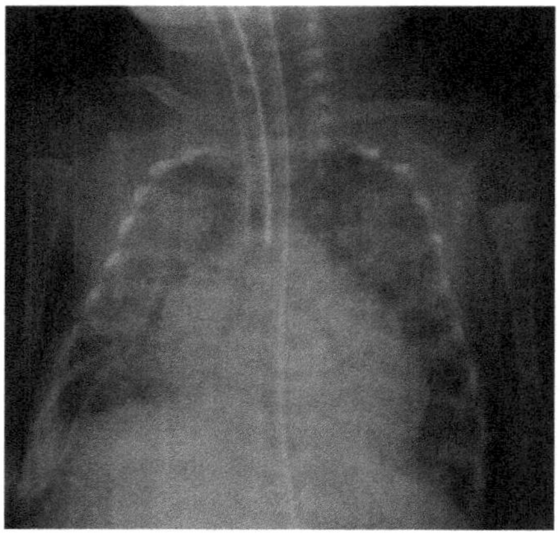

(a)

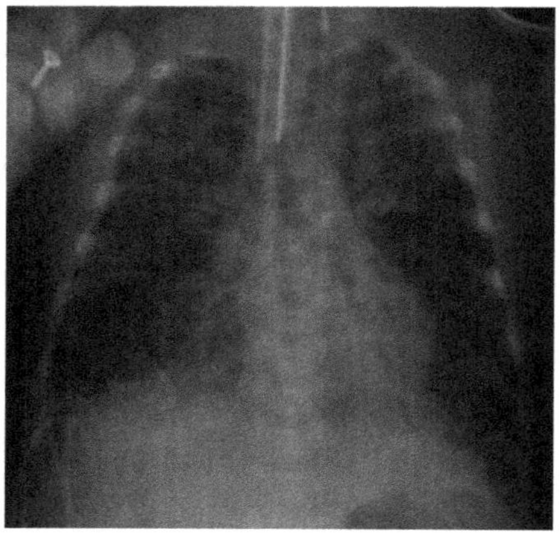

(b)

Figure 1: Acute (a) and convalescent (b) chest radiographs demonstrating cardiomegaly at the time of the clinical deterioration, with near complete resolution five days later.

respiratory distress, coughing, tachypnea, pneumonia, or apnea episodes). Diagnosis requires a high index of suspicion in the presence of suggestive symptoms, since other infecting viruses such as respiratory syncytial viruses, enteroviruses, rhinoviruses, or coronaviruses may induce similar clinical pictures confirmation. Diagnosis is based on the detection of virus-specific RNA using nucleic acid amplification techniques from a respiratory sample such as a nasopharyngeal swab. This technique has been a breakthrough in the diagnosis as it could decrease unnecessary use of empirical antibiotic therapy. Other diagnostic methods are viral culture, usually less available and with longer turnaround time results, and direct viral detection in respiratory secretions by immunofluorescence or enzyme immunoassay, which shows lower sensitivity and specificity than PCR. Currently, there is no specific treatment against parainfluenza virus infections. Management of the infected patient is based on supportive therapy according to the clinical condition.

The main limitation of our case report is the unconfirmed etiological presence of parainfluenza virus

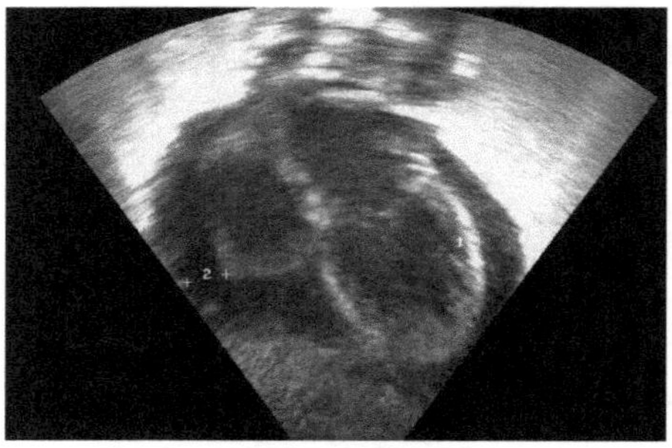

Figure 2: Echocardiography showing pericardial effusion. Dimensions: 1 = 0.43 cm; 2 = 0.41 cm.

in pericardial effusion. Detection of parainfluenza 3-specific RNA from pericardial fluid or blood would offer direct evidence that PIV3 caused the effusion. Pericardial fluid was not obtained due to the invasiveness of the technique in the context of clinical and hemodynamic stability of our patient and spontaneous resolution in 5 days.

In conclusion, parainfluenza 3 infection should be considered during the diagnostic evaluation of neonatal pericarditis. This may prevent possible severe complications and reduce unnecessary use of antibiotics. High index of suspicion is required for rapid diagnosis and appropriate management.

Abbreviations

BPD: Bronchopulmonary dysplasia
FIO_2: Fraction of inspired oxygen
LVO: Left ventricular output
NICU: Neonatal intensive care unit
PCR: Polymerase chain reaction
MAP: Mean airway pressure
RVO: Right ventricular output.

Consent

Informed consent was obtained from the patient's parents.

Authors' Contributions

All authors have participated and worked actively: Drs. Cristina Aranda Cazón, Zarife Daoud Pérez, and José Tomás Ramos Amador have contributed especially from the infectious diseases point of view; Drs. Cristina Aranda Cazón, Luis Arruza Gómez, Gloria Herranz Carrillo, and José Antonio Martínez-Orgado from the neonatology approach; and Dr. Cristina González Menchén contributed mainly as a pediatric cardiologist.

References

[1] J. A. Frank, R. W. Warren, J. A. Tucker, J. Zeller, and C. M. Wilfert, "Disseminated parainfluenza infection in a child with severe combined immunodeficiency," *American Journal of Diseases of Children*, vol. 137, no. 12, pp. 1172–1174, 1983.

[2] A. Ozkaya Parlakay, I. I. Cetin, H. Tezer, B. Gulhan, and T. Revide Sayli, "Parainfluenza virus 4 presenting with pericardial effusion in an immunocompetent child," *Journal of Infection in Developing Countries*, vol. 8, no. 8, pp. 1079–1080, 2014.

[3] N. Ohara, M. Kaneko, H. Kuwano et al., "Fulminant type 1 diabetes mellitus and fulminant viral myocarditis. A case report and literature review," *International Heart Journal*, vol. 56, no. 2, pp. 239–244, 2015.

[4] D. A. Rodríguez-Serrano, M. Nieto-Cabrera, J. Conesa, and E. Culebras-López, "Neumonía como resultado de la infección con parainfluenza tipo virus 4 y púrpura trombocitopénica trombótica," *Medicina Intensiva*, vol. 36, no. 3, p. 235, 2012.

[5] P. M. Smit, S. M. Pronk, J. C. Kaandorp et al., "RT-PCR detection of respiratory pathogens in newborn children admitted to a neonatal medium care unit," *Pediatric Research*, vol. 73, no. 3, pp. 355–361, 2013.

[6] N. J. Bennett, C. M. Tabarani, N. M. Bartholoma et al., "Unrecognized viral respiratory tract infections in premature infants during their birth hospitalization: a prospective surveillance study in two neonatal intensive care units," *Journal of Pediatrics*, vol. 161, no. 5, pp. 814–818, 2012.

30

Successful Treatment of High-Level Aminoglycoside-Resistant *Enterococcus faecalis* Bacteremia in a Preterm Infant with Ampicillin and Cefotaxime

Jennifer Tam,[1,2] **Santina J. Lee**,[3] **Vibhuti Shah**,[4,5] **and Shaun K. Morris**[1,2]

[1]*Division of Infectious Diseases, The Hospital for Sick Children, 555 University Ave., Toronto, ON, Canada*
[2]*Department of Pediatrics, Faculty of Medicine, University of Toronto, 1 King's College Circle, Room 2109, Toronto, ON, Canada*
[3]*Department of Pediatrics and Child Health, University of Manitoba, 840 Sherbrook St., Winnipeg, MB, Canada*
[4]*Department of Paediatrics, Mount Sinai Hospital, 600 University Ave., Toronto, ON, Canada*
[5]*Institute of Health Policy, Management and Evaluation, University of Toronto, 155 College Street, Suite 425, Toronto, ON, Canada*

Correspondence should be addressed to Jennifer Tam; jennifer.marie.tam@gmail.com

Academic Editor: Paola Di Carlo

Enterococcal bloodstream infections are usually treated with single-agent antibiotics. In persistent infections, synergistic combination therapy is often required with a beta-lactam and an aminoglycoside antibiotic. High-level aminoglycoside-resistant (HLAR) enterococci are increasingly prevalent and preclude the use of this combination. The use of ampicillin with a third-generation cephalosporin to treat endovascular HLAR *Enterococcus* infections is becoming more established in the adult population; however, the literature on treatment of such infections in children remains scarce. We report a preterm neonate with persistent HLAR *Enterococcus faecalis* bacteremia from day of life 9 to 17 despite treatment with ampicillin and vancomycin. On day of life 17, antibiotic treatment was switched to ampicillin and cefotaxime, with subsequent clearance of blood cultures on day of life 20. To our knowledge, this is the first report illustrating the use of ampicillin and cefotaxime for an HLAR *E. faecalis* infection in a neonate.

1. Introduction

Uncomplicated enterococcal bloodstream infections are usually treated with single-agent antibiotics. Persistent infections, however, often warrant treatment with a synergistic combination of a beta-lactam and an aminoglycoside antibiotic. High-level aminoglycoside-resistant (HLAR) enterococci are increasingly prevalent and preclude the use of this combination, posing a therapeutic challenge in persistent infections [1].

High-level aminoglycoside resistance is defined as a minimum inhibitory concentration (MIC) of $>500\ \mu$g/mL for gentamicin and an MIC of $>1000\ \mu$g/mL for streptomycin by broth diffusion [1]. The main mechanism of resistance involves the production of aminoglycoside-modifying enzymes, and additionally, mutations in a ribosomal protein for streptomycin [2].

The American Heart Association adult infective endocarditis guidelines currently recommend a combination of ampicillin plus ceftriaxone for HLAR *Enterococcus* infections, as evidence of synergy with this combination continues to grow [1]. The pediatric data for this combination, however, are scarce. Furthermore, ceftriaxone is not typically used in newborns due to risk of biliary sludging and precipitation with calcium-containing intravenous fluids such as total parenteral nutrition. At many institutions including ours, ceftriaxone is not recommended for prolonged use in infants less than 90 days corrected age. Thus, the optimal treatment of a newborn with HLAR *Enterococcus* endovascular infection is not clear.

We report a case of a neonate with persistent positive blood cultures for HLAR *Enterococcus faecalis* treated successfully with a combination of ampicillin and cefotaxime. Informed consent was obtained from the patient's family for this case report.

2. Case

A male infant was born at 26 4/7 weeks of gestation to a 30-year-old G3P2 mother who was blood group A+, HIV-negative, hepatitis B surface antigen-negative, rubella immune, and group B *Streptococcus*-negative. The mother's medical history was significant for cardiomyopathy that resulted in severe congestive heart failure during the pregnancy. This, in combination with fetal intrauterine growth restriction, necessitated induction of labor. The patient was born via vaginal delivery shortly after rupture of membranes. He required resuscitation with positive pressure ventilation and was intubated with subsequent stabilization. Apgar scores were 5 and 7 at 1 and 5 minutes of life, respectively. Birth weight was 490 g (<3rd percentile). He received ampicillin and tobramycin at birth, which were discontinued at 48 hours of life with a negative blood culture.

His postnatal course was complicated by respiratory distress syndrome requiring high-frequency oscillatory ventilation, pulmonary hemorrhage, anemia, thrombocytopenia, patent ductus arteriosus with bidirectional shunt, and grade II intraventricular hemorrhage. He was relatively stable until day of life (DOL) 9 when he developed abdominal distension and lethargy. His only intravenous (IV) access at this time was an umbilical venous catheter inserted shortly after birth. A full sepsis evaluation was performed, and treatment with IV vancomycin and tobramycin was commenced. White blood cell (WBC) counts increased from 19.5 to 30.3×10^9/L, and C-reactive protein (CRP) increased from 18 to 69.7 mg/L over the course of one day. Peripheral blood, cerebrospinal fluid (CSF), and urine catheter cultures were all positive for *Enterococcus faecalis*. The organism was susceptible to ampicillin and vancomycin but was high-level aminoglycoside-resistant. Therefore, on DOL 11 when the blood culture sensitivities were known, vancomycin and tobramycin were discontinued, and ampicillin was started.

Peripheral blood cultures drawn on DOL 12 remained positive for *E. faecalis*, so vancomycin was added again on DOL 13 with the expectation of bloodstream clearance with two agents in a critically ill child. Despite treatment on ampicillin and vancomycin (with an acceptable vancomycin trough level of 8.8 mg/L), peripheral blood cultures continued to be positive on DOL 15 and 17. An umbilical arterial catheter had been removed on DOL 3, and the umbilical venous catheter was removed on DOL 11. No additional central access was placed while blood cultures remained positive. The patient received medications through a peripheral IV line. Investigations to identify a source of persistent infection, including an echocardiogram, abdominal ultrasound, and ultrasound of large vessels, were all unremarkable. Given the persistence of positive blood cultures from DOL 9 to 17, cefotaxime was added to ampicillin on DOL 17 for synergistic effect, and vancomycin was discontinued. A peripheral blood culture drawn on DOL 20 was finally negative.

As no endovascular source was confirmed, it was decided that the patient would complete a 2-week course with ampicillin and cefotaxime from the date of first negative culture. He did not experience any adverse effects to this antibiotic combination. He did not have any recurrence of *E. faecalis* infection but ultimately succumbed to multiorgan failure from his complicated postnatal course and died on DOL 70.

3. Discussion

While enterococci are intrinsically resistant to cephalosporins, there is increasing evidence that the combination of an aminopenicillin and third-generation cephalosporin (primarily cefotaxime or ceftriaxone) has synergistic activity against these organisms. Mainardi et al. demonstrated that amoxicillin and cefotaxime given together against *E. faecalis in vitro* lowered the MIC of each antibiotic significantly, regardless of the *E. faecalis* strain's susceptibility to aminoglycosides [3]. The proposed mechanism was a differential saturation of the penicillin binding proteins (PBPs), with cefotaxime saturating PBPs 2 and 3 and amoxicillin saturating PBPs 4 and 5 [3].

In vivo studies have since supported the effectiveness of the combination of ampicillin and ceftriaxone. For example, in 2007, Gavalda et al. compared 21 patients with HLAR *E. faecalis* endocarditis (age range 6 months to 82 years; median 65 years) with 22 patients with non-HLAR *E. faecalis* (age range 24 to 86 years; median 58 years) who were all treated with ampicillin and ceftriaxone. Clinical cure rates were similar in the two groups, with a 100% clinical and microbiological cure rate in the HLAR *E. faecalis* group who adhered to the study intervention [4].

Pediatric data regarding HLAR enterococci are currently limited to epidemiological studies assessing resistance patterns of blood and urine cultures. To our knowledge, there is only one published report of a pediatric patient in the literature who received the combination of ampicillin and third-generation cephalosporin for a HLAR *E. faecalis* endovascular infection. This patient was a 6-month-old infant who was part of the study by Gavalda et al. assessing ampicillin and ceftriaxone for HLAR *E. faecalis* infective endocarditis; this child demonstrated clinical and microbiologic cure [4]. In general, ceftriaxone is not used in the neonatal population and, instead, cefotaxime is used when a third-generation cephalosporin is warranted. Therefore, our case provides support for the use of the less-studied combination of ampicillin and cefotaxime in treating persistent infection with HLAR *E. faecalis*.

While we cannot be certain that the addition of cefotaxime to ampicillin in our patient was responsible for clearing his HLAR *E. faecalis* infection, we anticipate that the synergistic effect observed in the adult population may also be applied to the pediatric population. Another possible explanation for the persistent bacteremia in our patient may be a theoretical antagonistic effect between ampicillin and vancomycin; this phenomenon is inconsistent in the literature, however, with uncertain clinical significance [5].

To our knowledge, this is the first case illustrating the use of ampicillin and cefotaxime for a HLAR *E. faecalis* infection in a neonate. Further research is required in the pediatric population to assess the efficacy and safety of ampicillin and cefotaxime/ceftriaxone in the treatment of persistent infections with increasingly prevalent HLAR *Enterococcus*.

References

[1] L. M. Baddour, W. R. Wilson, A. S. Bayer et al., "Infective endocarditis in adults: diagnosis, antimicrobial therapy, and management of complications: a scientific statement for healthcare professionals from the American Heart Association," *Circulation*, vol. 132, no. 15, pp. 1435–1486, 2015.

[2] J. W. Chow, "Aminoglycoside resistance in enterococci," *Clinical Infectious Diseases*, vol. 31, no. 2, pp. 586–589, 2000.

[3] J. L. Mainardi, L. Gutmann, J. F. Acar, and F. W. Goldstein, "Synergistic effect of amoxicillin and cefotaxime against *Enterococcus faecalis*," *Antimicrobial Agents and Chemotherapy*, vol. 39, no. 9, pp. 1984–1987, 1995.

[4] J. Gavalda, O. Len, J. M. Miro et al., "Brief communication: treatment of *Enterococcus faecalis* endocarditis with ampicillin plus ceftriaxone," *Annals of Internal Medicine*, vol. 146, no. 8, pp. 574–579, 2007.

[5] E. Cercenado, G. M. Eliopoulos, C. B. Wennersten, and R. C. Moellering, "Absence of synergistic activity between ampicillin and vancomycin against highly vancomycin-resistant enterococci," *Antimicrobial Agents and Chemotherapy*, vol. 36, no. 10, pp. 2201–2203, 1992.

Coronavirus Disease 2019 and Acute Hemorrhagic Edema of Infancy

Mohsen Jari

Department of Pediatric Rheumatology, Imam HosseinChildren,s Hospital, Isfahan University of Medical Sciences, Isfahan, Iran

Correspondence should be addressed to Mohsen Jari; mjari14@yahoo.com

Academic Editor: Mohamed A. Dkhil

Background. Acute hemorrhagic edema of infancy (AHEI) is a small-vessel leukocytoclastic vasculitis, presented with low-grade fever and edema in the face and upper and lower limbs, as well as purpuric/ecchymotic lesions in these regions. AHEI was also reported after viral infections, including herpes simplex virus, rotavirus, and adenovirus. *Case Presentation.* Herein, we reported a case of a 20-month-old boy presented with low-grade fever. Additionally, mild cough and progressive purpuric/ecchymotic lesions were observed in some independent regions and extremity swelling. Laboratory testing showed leukopenia, lymphopenia, and the elevation of both C-reactive protein (CRP) and erythrocyte sedimentation rate (ESR). Thereafter, the result of the reverse-transcriptase polymerase chain reaction (RT-PCR) test on the obtained specimen samples, including nasopharyngeal swab for COVID-19, was positive. The patient was treated with supportive care, and two weeks later, the serology test for COVID-19 resulted positive. *Conclusion.* We should think about children infected with COVID-19, particularly those with skin manifestations.

1. Introduction

Acute hemorrhagic edema of infancy (AHEI) is an immune complex-mediated leukocytoclastic vasculitis, known as a rare disease in children [1]. Age at the time of the onset of this disease is usually between 4 and 24 months. Clinical findings such as low-grade fever, edema of the face and upper and lower limbs, generalized purpura, or ecchymosis rapidly develop over 24–48 hours. Upper respiratory tract infection, gastroenteritis, or vaccination has also been reported to cause this disease [2, 3]. To the best of our knowledge, this is the first report on the association between coronavirus disease 2019 (COVID-19) and AHEI.

2. Case Presentation

A 20-month-old boy was admitted to the pediatric rheumatology clinic of Imam Hossein Children's Hospital, Isfahan University of Medical Sciences, due to fever, mild cough, progressive purpuric/ecchymotic lesions, and extreme swelling in the past 2 days.

The rash initially began on his legs and then rapidly diffused to his forearms, face, and ears.

In physical examination, he was a happy and healthy baby. Besides rash, swelling of his hands and feet and nonexudative bilateral conjunctivitis were visible as well (Figure 1).

He had mild cough for a 5-day duration. Of note, his father was hospitalized due to COVID-19 10 days ago. Review of systems was negative regarding any other problem.

Vital signs were notable for a fever of 38.2°C along with normal respiratory rates and blood pressure.

Laboratory testing demonstrated leukopenia (white blood cell count: 3800/mm^3) and lymphopenia (lymphocyte: 16%). Moreover, the elevation was observed in C-reactive protein (CRP: 47 mg/L) and erythrocyte sedimentation rates (ESR: 19 mm/hr). In addition, serum electrolytes, renal function tests, urinalysis, prothrombin time, and the activated partial thromboplastin time were normal. A reverse-transcriptase polymerase chain reaction (RT-PCR) test was performed on the obtained specimen samples, including

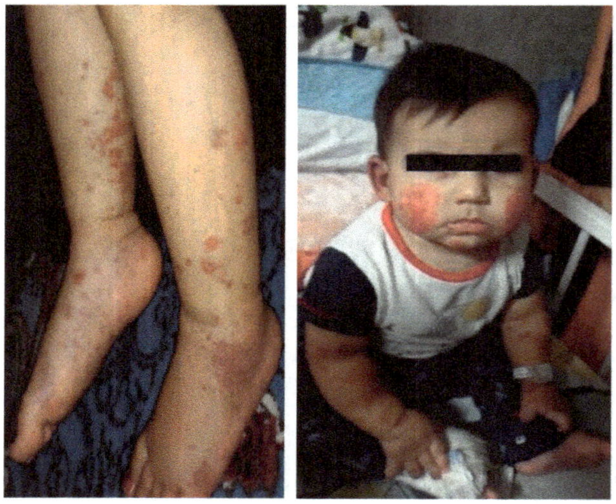

Figure 1: Extremity swelling and purpuric/ecchymotic lesions on the limbs and face.

nasopharyngeal swab for COVID-19, which resulted positive, while the result of the serology test (Ig M and Ig G) for COVID-19 was negative. Additionally, the chest X-ray graph was normal.

The patient was recognized as a case of AHEI triggered by COVID-19. Thereafter, the patient was isolated at home and treated only with supportive care (good nutrition and observation). He had resolution of all symptoms within 5 days. Subsequently, the isolation at home was continued. Two weeks later, a RT-PCR test was performed on the specimen samples, including a nasopharyngeal swab test for COVID-19, which was negative, while the serology test (Ig M) for COVID-19 was positive.

3. Discussion

AHEI was reported after upper respiratory tract infection and viral infections, including herpes simplex virus, rotavirus, and adenovirus. In this regard, vaccinations and antibiotics have been recognized as triggers. AHEI is a leukocytoclastic vasculitis in infants and toddlers aged less than 2 years. This disease is characterized by a purpuric/ecchymotic rash and edema over the limbs, ears, and face. IgA deposits are seen in 10% to 35% of biopsy specimens, so this is a disagreement that it is a mild form of HSP or it is a distinct disease [3, 4]. Usually, AHEI is a self-limited disease, and more than 90% of infected patients completely recover from the disease only with a supportive care within 1–3 weeks after the symptoms' presentation. Of note, systemic involvement, including abdominal pain, intussusception, arthralgia, testicular torsion, and glomerulonephritis, occurred in fewer than 10% of patients diagnosed with AHEI [4, 5].

Diagnosis of AHEI is clinical. Leukocytosis and thrombocytosis and the elevation of C-reactive protein (CRP) and erythrocyte sedimentation rate (ESR) may occur as well. The treatment of AHEI is known as a supportive care, while in the systemic involvement, using corticosteroids remains controversial yet. Corticosteroids can only be considered in a severe systemic involvement and in complications resulted from AHEI3 [3, 4].

The use of both antihistamines and steroids is controversial. Systemic corticosteroids may be used under sever conditions or systemic involvement such as abdominal pain, intussusception, nephritis, scrotal pain, and testicular torsion. Monitoring patients with a rare systemic involvement such as renal involvement is recommended [4, 6].

Currently, the coronavirus disease 2019 (COVID-19) is a pandemic worldwide. COVID-19 increased mortality and morbidity rates in rheumatologic patients due to the underlying immune dysfunction and the treatment with immunosuppressive agents [7].

There are few reports demonstrating that COVID-19 is associated with maculopapular, purpuric, and acroischemic skin lesions. In this regard, few reports suggested that COVID-19 triggers the secretion of some inflammatory products and induces generalized vasculitis. It may be considered as the etiology of these vasculitis-like lesions due to causing endothelial damage [8, 9].

Although no test is suggested in this regard, especially in healthy outpatients, the Italian Rhinologic Society recommended "against the performance of rhinomanometry, acoustic rhinometry, and olfactometry, the self-rating nasal symptoms grading using the Visual Analog Scale or validated questionnaires is the best way to approach these patients. The skin-prick test could also be performed as an alternative. Post-COVID-19 patients could be rather tested clinically and through functional tests, and the Italian Rhinologic Society recommended the evaluation of these patients after 3 consecutive negative swabs (the last one in the previous 48 h)" [10].

Clinical manifestations of coronavirus disease 2019 (COVID-19) are rare or ambiguous among children and adolescents. There are some reports on COVID-19 infection in these age groups, presenting with some types of skin lesions such as erythematous rashes, urticaria, erythematous violaceous patches, purpuric lesions, blisters and ulceronecrotic lesions, and chicken pox-like vesicles.

During the current COVID-19 pandemic, we should think about this infection in all children and adolescents with some skin manifestations [11–13].

4. Conclusions

Some viruses were reported to be associated with AHEI, and our case demonstrated that COVID-19 can precede AHEI as well.

Abbreviations

AHEI:	Acute hemorrhagic edema of infancy
COVID-19:	Coronavirus disease 2019
CRP:	C-reactive protein
ESR:	Erythrocyte sedimentation rate
RT-PCR:	Reverse-transcriptase polymerase chain reaction.

Consent

In this study, the written informed consent form was obtained from the parents to have the case details published.

References

[1] C. S. Moura Garcia, A. Sokolova, and M. L. Torre, "Acute hemorrhagic edema of infancy," *European Annals ofAllergy and Clinical Immunology*, vol. 48, no. 1, pp. 22–26, 2016.

[2] Y. Binamer, "Acute hemorrhagic edema of infancy after MMR vaccine," *Annals ofSaudi Medicine*, vol. 35, no. 3, pp. 254–256, 2015.

[3] H. Chesser, J. M. Chambliss, and E. Zwemer, "Acute hemorrhagic edema of infancy after coronavirus infection with recurrent rash," *Case Reports in Pediatrics*, vol. 2017, Article ID 5637503, 3 pages, 2017.

[4] E. Fiore, M. Rizzi, M. Ragazzi et al., "Acute hemorrhagic edema of young children (cockade purpura and edema): a case series and systematic review," *Journal of the American Academy of Dermatology*, vol. 59, no. 4, pp. 684–695, 2008.

[5] D. F. S. Cunha, A. L. F. Darcie, G. N. Benevides et al., "Acute Hemorrhagic Edema of Infancy: an unusual diagnosis for the general pediatrician," *Autopsy and Case Reports*, vol. 5, no. 3, pp. 37–41, 2015.

[6] J. L. Homme and J. M. Block, "Acute hemorrhagic edema of infancy and common mimics," *American Journal of Emergency Medicine*, vol. 34, no. 5, pp. 936–6, 2016.

[7] P. C. Robinson and J. Yazdany, "The COVID-19 global rheumatology alliance: collecting data in a pandemic," *Nature Reviews Rheumatology*, vol. 16, no. 6, pp. 293-294, 2020.

[8] N. Landa, M. Mendieta-Eckert, P. Fonda-Pascual, and T. Aguirre, "Chilblain-like lesions on feet and hands during the COVID-19 Pandemic," *International Journal of Dermatology*, vol. 59, no. 6, pp. 739–743, 2020.

[9] F. Mazzotta and T. Troccoli, "Monday's case. Acute acroischemia in the child at the time of COVID-19," *DermatologiaPediatrica Bari*, vol. 30, 2020.

[10] G. Motta, D. Passali, G. C. Passali, and E. Cantone, "The Italian society indication for rhinologists during covid-19: Italy phase 2," *International Archives of Otorhinolaryngology*, vol. 24, no. 03, pp. e388–e390, 2020.

[11] C. Guarneri, E. V. Rullo, P. Pavone et al., "Silent COVID-19: what your skin can reveal," *The Lancet Infectious Diseases*, vol. 21, no. 1, pp. 24-25, 2021 Jan.

[12] A. Maniaci, G. Iannella, C. Vicini et al., "A case of COVID-19 with late-onset rash and transient loss of taste and smell in a 15-year-old boy," *American Journal of Case Reports*, vol. 21, Article ID e925813, 2020.

[13] F. D. Algahtani, M. A. Alzain, K. Angawi et al., "Coping during COVID-19 pandemic in Saudi community: religious attitudes, practices and associated factors," *International Journal of Environmental Research and Public Health*, vol. 18, no. 16, Article ID 8651, 2021.

32

An Unusual Case of CMV/EBV Ventriculoencephalitis with Evolution to Primary Central Nervous System Lymphoma in HIV-Positive Patient

Gisela Borges[1] **Diana Neves**[2] **Inês Pintado Maury**[2] **Aida Pereira**[2] **and Maria de Jesus Silva**[1]

[1]*Internal Medicine Department, Hospital Pulido Valente, Lisbon, Portugal*
[2]*Infectious Diseases Department, Hospital Santa Maria, Lisbon, Portugal*

Correspondence should be addressed to Gisela Borges; giselatavborges@gmail.com

Academic Editor: Peter Olumese

Epstein–Barr virus (EBV) is a well-known cause of different types of malignancies particularly Burkitt's lymphoma, nasopharyngeal carcinoma, Hodgkin's lymphomas, and non-Hodgkin's lymphomas including primary central nervous system lymphoma (PCNSL). A higher tendency of malignant transformation associated with EBV has been noticed in immunocompromised patients, such as human immunodeficiency virus (HIV) infected patients. The rapid and effective immune reconstitution is crucial to prevent PCNSL in HIV-positive patients. We present a clinical case of a young patient diagnosed with HIV infection and medicated with antiretroviral therapy (ART) with poor immunological recovery. After two weeks, he developed ventriculoencephalitis, observed in the cranial magnetic resonance imaging (MRI), caused by cytomegalovirus (CMV) and EBV, both with high serum viral load, rapidly evolving to PCNSL. With this unusual clinical case, the authors want to draw attention to the importance of rapid immunological reconstitution in preventing the progression of EBV infection to PCNSL, as well as encouraging the confirmation of the usefulness of early combination of chemotherapy and antiviral therapy, in order to reach a more effective treatment of this herpesvirus infection and associated malignancies.

1. Introduction

HIV infected patients, especially with low CD4+ T cell count, are more susceptible to severe central nervous system (CNS) infections. Several studies have shown that EBV DNA detection in cerebrospinal fluid (CSF) is a good PCNSL marker in this group of patients [1]. Nonetheless, focal brain lesion stereotactic biopsy is the gold standard procedure to establish the final diagnosis. A prompt HIV infection diagnosis and a highly active antiretroviral therapy (HAART) initiation are essential measures to achieve an immunological recovery and consequently prevent EBV infection and its progression to PCNSL [2]. The association between antiviral therapies with specific viral acting chemotherapy (rituximab) may be a more effective therapy against EBV replication and associated PCNSL. The prognosis of patients with EBV associated PCNSL is poor. The average life expectancy varies between two and twelve months after diagnosis [3].

2. Case Report

We present a clinical case of a 31-year-old man diagnosed with HIV-1 infection, with CD4 T cell count of 35 $cells/mm^3$ (4%) and HIV RNA 305349 copies/mL ($\log^{10}$ 5.48) having initiated ART with abacavir/lamivudine and nevirapine. Around two weeks after starting ART, the patient is admitted due to a sudden cognitive impairment (anhedonia and memory loss) with progression to gait change and imbalance. The cranial computerized tomography (CT) scan showed no lesions but the cranial MRI revealed ventriculoencephalitis (Figure 1).

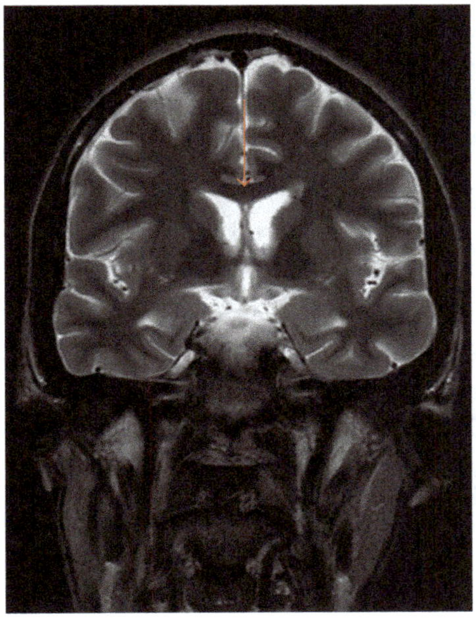

Figure 1: Ventricular hypersignal in cranial MRI (FLAIR), suggestive of ventriculitis.

The cerebrospinal fluid (CSF) had 38 nucleated cells/mm_3, 175 mg/dL proteins and 37 mg/dL glucose (glycaemia 82 mg/dL). The CSF CMV and EBV viral load were 189000 (log^{10} 5.28) and 799 (log^{10} 2.90) copies/mL with negative CSF neurotropic microorganism serologies and molecular identification (HSV 1/2, VZV, *Cryptococcus*, *Brucella*, *Treponema pallidum*, *Borrelia burgdor*feri, JC virus, *Mycobacterium tuberculosis*, and *Toxoplasma gondii*). The final considered diagnostic was mainly CMV-related ventriculoencephalitis and ganciclovir was started.

Nevertheless, the patient started left conjugate horizontal gaze palsy with abducting horizontal saccadic (or jerk-type) nystagmus of the right eye as well as a slight anisocoria with left eye miosis. These changes were enclosed in the one-and-a-half syndrome and left-sided Horner's syndrome. The patient also presented a grade II-III paresis of the right lower limb. The cranial CT scan (performed fifteen days later) revealed a dubious right linear protuberancial hypodensity without signs of intracranial hypertension.

Cranial MRI was repeated one month later revealing improvement of the ventriculitis signs but a larger hippocampus and left mesial temporal region involvement with a discrete increase of the lateral ventricles dimensions.

Due to these clinical and imagiological changes and because we could not exclude tuberculosis infection, classic first-line tuberculostatic therapy was empirically started (stopped after excluding this infection) and foscarnet was added to ganciclovir (until a negative CMV viral load was achieved). At this point, the hypotheses of limbic encephalitis, epileptic activity or paraneoplastic encephalitis could not be excluded. The lumbar puncture was repeated and CSF antineuronal antibodies, HHV-8, and other neurotropic microorganisms were negative.

The electroencephalogram (EEG) showed frontal and frontotemporal bilateral activity with occasional periodic discharges, independent of nonabrupt three-phase bifrontal lesions. Anticonvulsant therapy with levetiracetam and topiramate was started. One month later, the cranial MRI was repeated and a new frontal lesion was detected. The body CT scan was normal. The imagiological reevaluation showed a slight improvement of the frontal lesion with new cerebellum lesions. The suspicion of lymphoproliferative disease was meaningful. Cranial MRI with diffusion and perfusion study with spectroscopy was performed and revealed very suggestive images of CNS lymphoma (Figure 2). For definitive diagnosis, a stereotactic brain biopsy was done. The histological study revealed a polymorphic cellular infiltrate with histiocytes, CD3+ T-lymphocytes, and CD 20+ B-lymphocytes (mixture of numerous small cells and large activated cells with positive hybridization results for EBV-encoded RNA (EBER)). The histology was suggestive of polymorphic lymphoproliferative EBV-positive disease. The molecular studies were not done because the sample was insufficient to perform the clonality analysis (CSF EBV viral load was 12405 copies/mL; CSF HIV and CMV viral load were both undetectable).

At this point, chemotherapy with rituximab was started and radiotherapy was scheduled. Nevertheless, the patient developed a sudden neurological worsening with a generalized tonic-clonic seizure, refractory to the instituted measures, culminating in death.

3. Discussion

The incidence of PCNSL in HIV infected patients is between 2 and 6% (1000 times higher than in general population) and more than 10% in postmortem diagnosis. Risk factors for the development of non-Hodgkin's lymphoma in these patients are low CD4+ T cell count, elevated HIV serum viral load, and chronic hepatitis B and C infection in patients receiving ART [1]. The reported clinical case is about a patient who developed CMV/EBV ventriculoencephalitis that, despite the virological response to antiviral therapy with ganciclovir and foscarnet, evolved to EBV-driven B cell lymphoproliferative disorder that is considered a "grey disorder" (neither benign nor malignant) that usually evolves to PCNSL [4].

Concerning HIV infection, he had a low immunological status on ART with two of the previously mentioned risk factors: CD4+ T cell count 35 cells/mm^3 (4%) and HIV 305349 RNA copies/mL (log^{10} 5.48). It is well known that HAART is able to improve the immune system, being one of the best measures to prevent the EBV infection progression to PCNSL. In HIV infected patients, CMV is usually the most frequent agent associated with CNS infections; nevertheless, the detection of EBV, herpesvirus 6 (HHV-6), and mixed infections may also occur [2]. HIV associated cytomegalovirus (CMV) encephalitis is one of several central and peripheral nervous system infections seen in late-stage disease. Neurologic manifestations of CMV infection include encephalitis, ventriculitis, myelitis, retinitis, radiculoganglionitis, and peripheral neuropathies. These infections usually occur in patients with severe immunodeficiency: CD4+ T cell count typically is lower than 50 cells/mm^3, but even in these patients, viral ventriculoencephalitis cases are rare,

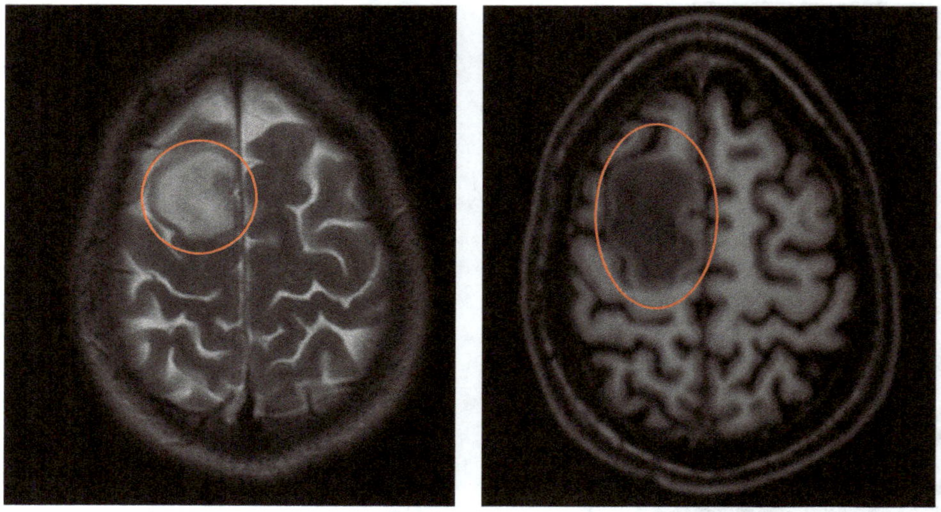

(a) (b)

Figure 2: Cranial MRI in T2 and T1, respectively—frontal lesion corresponding to PCNSL.

which makes this case more interesting. Prior to the development of HAART, 2% of HIV infected patients with CD4+ T cell count less than 50 cells/mm^3 developed CMV neurologic disease [5]. If left untreated, HIV associated CMV encephalitis typically progresses to death in days to weeks. Many studies have shown that EBV DNA detection in CSF is a good lymphoid proliferation and PCNSL diagnostic marker in HIV-positive patients [1].

EBV expresses several genes (latent genes) that participate in the pathogenesis of specific neoplasms, including PCNSL. It has been documented that EBV can be detected in more than 50–60% of lymphoma cases in HIV infected patients [6]. PCNSL accounts for up to 15% of non-Hodgkin's lymphomas in HIV infected patients compared to only 1% in general population. Approximately 20 to 30% of the central nervous system lesions in patients with acquired immunodeficiency syndrome eventually show as PCNSL (approximately half present multiple lesions), with toxoplasmosis and progressive multifocal leukoencephalopathy being the remaining cases. A high level of clinical suspicion is crucial for prompt diagnose and therapeutic management of these patients. Nowadays, there are several suggested therapies for EBV associated PCNSL; however, guidelines have not yet been established. According to the reviewed literature, antiviral therapy efficacy is higher when the virus is in its lithic phase; therefore, one of the new approaches includes induction of this phase by chemotherapy, followed by treatment with antiviral. However, its efficacy has not yet been well studied. On the other hand, monoclonal antibodies, such as anti-CD20 (rituximab), have shown promising results [7]. Although our patient initiated rituximab immediately after the final diagnosis, he had a neurological deterioration culminating in death. This final denouement most likely happened due to the difficult process of reaching the final diagnosis of a disease that itself has a poor prognosis.

References

[1] S. Bossolasco, P. Cinque, M. Ponzoni et al., "Epstein-Barr virus DNA load in cerebrospinal fluid and plasma of patients with AIDS-related lymphoma," *Journal of Neurovirology*, vol. 8, no. 5, pp. 432–438, 2002.

[2] P. A. Martinez, R. Diaz, D. Gonzalez et al., "The effect of highly active antiretroviral therapy on outcome of central nervous system herpesviruses infection in Cuban human immunodeficiency virus-infected individuals," *Journal of Neurovirology*, vol. 13, no. 5, pp. 446–451, 2007.

[3] S. E. Jamal, S. Li, R. Bajaj et al., "Primary central nervous system Epstein-Barr virus-positive diffuse large B-cell lymphoma of the elderly: a clinicopathologic study of five cases," *Brain Tumor Pathology*, vol. 31, no. 4, pp. 265–273, 2014.

[4] C. Y. Ok, L. Li, and K. H. Young, "EBV-driven B-cell lymphoproliferative disorders: from biology, classification and differential diagnosis to clinical management," *Experimental & Molecular Medicine*, vol. 47, no. 1, article e132, 2015.

[5] P. Griffiths, "Cytomegalovirus infection of the central nervous system," *Herpes*, vol. 11, no. S2, pp. 95A–104A, 2004.

[6] L. Geng and X. Wang, "Epstein-Barr virus-associated lymphoproliferative disorders: experimental and clinical developments," *International Journal of Clinical and Experimental Medicine*, vol. 8, no. 9, pp. 14656–14671, 2015.

[7] H. E. Heslop, "Biology and treatment of Epstein-Barr virus-associated non-Hodgkin lymphomas," *Hematology*, vol. 2005, no. 1, pp. 260–266, 2005.

Non-ST Elevation Myocardial Infarction and Severe Peripheral Artery Disease in a 20-Year-Old with Perinatally Acquired Human Immunodeficiency Virus Infection

Purva Sharma, Mohamad Kabach, Samineh Sehatbakhsh, Rashida Tharpe, Shaun Isaac, Robert Chait, and Kleper De Almeida

JFK Medical Center, University of Miami-Palm Beach Regional GME Consortium, Atlantis, FL, USA

Correspondence should be addressed to Purva Sharma; purva7sharma@gmail.com

Academic Editor: Alexandre R. Marra

Human immunodeficiency virus (HIV) infection confers an increased risk of cardiovascular disease, including acute coronary syndrome (ACS). Patients with perinatally acquired HIV may be at increased risk due to the viral infection itself and exposure to HAART in utero or as part of treatment. A 20-year-old female with transplacentally acquired HIV infection presented with symptoms of transient aphasia, headache, palpitations, and blurry vision. She was admitted for hypertensive emergency with blood pressure 203/100 mmHg. Within a few hours, she complained of typical chest pain, and ECG showed marked ST depression. Troponin I levels escalated from 0.115 to 10.8. She underwent coronary angiogram showing 95% stenosis of the right coronary artery (RCA) and severe peripheral arterial disease including total occlusion of both common iliacs and 95% infrarenal aortic stenosis with collateral circulation. She underwent successful percutaneous intervention with a drug-eluting stent to the mid-RCA. Patients with HIV are at increased risk for cardiovascular disease. Of these, coronary artery disease is one of the most critical complications of HIV. Perinatally acquired HIV infection can be a high-risk factor for cardiovascular disease. A high degree of suspicion is warranted in such patients, especially if they are noncompliant to their ART.

1. Introduction

Human immunodeficiency virus (HIV) infection is associated with an increased risk of cardiovascular disease through various mechanisms including premature atherosclerosis from endothelial inflammation and platelet dysfunction as well as from cART therapy involving protease inhibitors resulting in dyslipidemia and insulin resistance [1]. One of the most important cardiac presentations is coronary artery disease leading to acute coronary syndrome (ACS). Patients with perinatally acquired HIV infection may be at an increased cardiac risk due to a combination of in utero HIV exposure and long-term exposure to cART [2]. We present a case of a 20-year-old African American female who acquired HIV infection through transplacental transmission and presented to us with ACS.

2. Case Report

A 20-year-old African American female with HIV infection since birth, acquired by transplacental transmission, presented to the emergency department with symptoms of transient aphasia lasting a few seconds. She described associated headache, palpitations, and blurry vision for the past 24 hours. Apart from HIV infection, she had no other significant past medical history and denied any surgeries in the past. She had no history of alcohol or tobacco use or illicit drug use. On presentation, her blood pressure was 203/100 mmHg and pulse was regular with 118 beats/minute. The rest of her exam was pertinent for tachycardia, palpable thrill, and a displaced point of maximal impulse. Remainder of the physical examination was unremarkable.

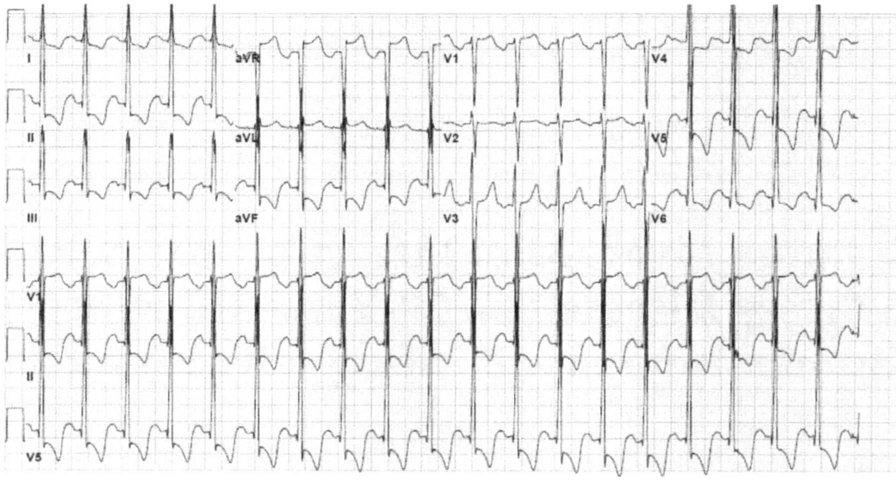

FIGURE 1: EKG showing ST segment depressions in inferolateral leads.

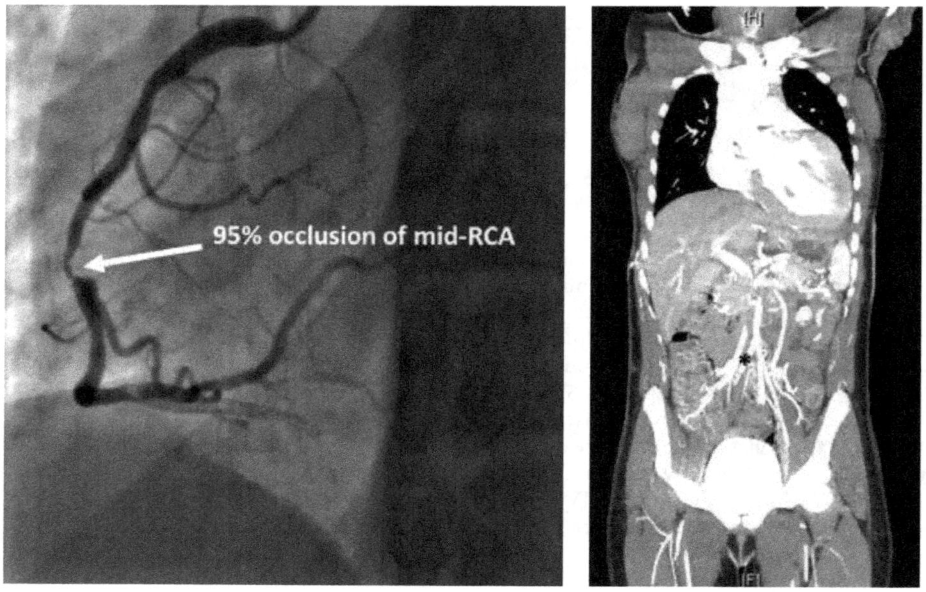

(a) (b)

FIGURE 2: (a) 95% stenosis of the right coronary artery (RCA). (b) 95% infrarenal aortic stenosis with collateral circulation.

Her initial laboratory tests were notable for microcytic anemia (Hb 7.3, MCV 64), hypokalemia (3.4 mEq/L), and elevated creatinine (1.4 mg/dL). She also had an elevated troponin level of 0.115, and her NT-proBNP was 23,245. Her CD4 count was 78 cells/μL, and HIV-1 ribonucleic acid viral load was 9018 copies/ml. Upon presentation, her electrocardiogram (ECG) showed sinus tachycardia with a ventricular rate in the 100 s and some nonspecific ST-T wave changes. Her chest radiograph and CT scan of the brain were normal. Further imaging of the brain such as MRI was not performed. She was admitted to the intensive care unit for hypertensive emergency and was started on an esmolol drip. However, within a few hours of admission, she complained of typical chest pain. A repeat ECG showed marked ST depression in the inferolateral leads, suggestive of ischemia (Figure 1). She was started on ACS protocol with aspirin, clopidogrel, and unfractionated heparin drip. Echocardiogram revealed moderate left ventricular hypertrophy with moderate-to-severe left ventricular dysfunction and ejection fraction (EF) of 30–35%. Her troponin I levels escalated from 0.115 to 10.8. She underwent coronary angiogram which showed 95% stenosis of the right coronary artery (RCA). It also revealed stenosis of the distal aorta. Due to this finding, a peripheral CT angiogram was done for further evaluation of the arterial system which showed severe peripheral arterial disease including total occlusion of both common iliac arteries and 95% infrarenal aortic stenosis with collateral circulation (Figures 2(a) and 2(b)). She underwent successful percutaneous intervention with a drug-eluting stent to the mid-RCA. The patient was discharged on dual antiplatelet therapy, high-intensity statin, a beta blocker and spironolactone, and cART.

3. Discussion

Patients with HIV infection are at increased risk for cardiovascular disease [3].

Of these, ACS is now one of the most critical complications of HIV. Since the advent of efficient antiretroviral therapies and the consequent longer patient life span, an increased risk for myocardial infarction has been observed in HIV-infected patients compared with the general population in Western countries [4]. HIV infection leads to chronic immune activation which plays a role in the pathogenesis of HIV-related atherosclerosis and CAD [5]. Post et al. studied the association between HIV infection and subclinical atherosclerosis through CT angiography. They found that coronary artery plaque, especially noncalcified plaque, is more prevalent and extensive in HIV-infected men, independent of CAD risk factors [6]. In our patient, although none of the imaging studies reported atherosclerosis, subclinical atherosclerosis cannot be ruled out. Also, there was a suspicion for fibromuscular dysplasia in our patient, given the findings of the CT angiogram which could be explained by the vascular endothelial dysfunction due to HIV infection. Endothelial dysfunction is known to be one of the important mechanisms by which HIV affects the blood vessels. In a study by Torriani et al., it was shown that the endothelial function improved after starting ART regimens [7].

HIV infection is associated with increased risk of acute myocardial infarction although the mechanism behind this is not clearly understood [8]. Studies have shown that both HIV infection and the concomitant use of ART play a role in increased AMI risk. However, infection with virus itself could be the main cause as studies have shown that viral load suppression results in lower cardiovascular disease risk [9]. HIV-related cardiomyopathy is a significant manifestation of cardiac disease in HIV-infected patients. Left ventricular diastolic dysfunction appears to be the most common manifestation [10], although systolic dysfunction is also observed with moderate frequency, particularly among untreated HIV-infected patients. In a prospective multicenter study of 196 children infected with HIV through vertical transmission, baseline echocardiogram and follow-up every 4 months for 2 years was obtained. The study showed that subclinical cardiac abnormalities such as dilated cardiomyopathy (depressed contractility and dilatation) and inappropriate LV hypertrophy were commonly seen as part of perinatally acquired HIV [11].

In our patient, the systolic function was reduced with ejection fraction of 30%–35%, and Doppler readings were consistent with grade 1 diastolic dysfunction. The etiology of the patient's cardiomyopathy could be attributed to the long-standing hypertension as well as HIV infection.

Our patient had a known history of noncompliance to her HAART medications, and her CD4 count was low at the time of presentation with a high viral load. We could thus hypothesize that the uncontrolled viral replication in our patient was one of the major risk factors for cardiovascular disease. Many studies have shown that adherence to HAART is the critical behavior underlying many of the long-term outcomes for children and adolescents with HIV [12]. Thus, this would be one of the major challenges as seen in our patient and would require counselling the patient and their family.

Another possibility also considered was HIV-related Takayasu's arteritis (TA) which is described by the American College of Rheumatology as a HIV-associated rheumatic disease and can present with ACS. Features that led to this being considered included her age under 40, hypertension, CT imaging that showed diffuse narrowing in the distal aorta, and a markedly elevated ESR/CRP [13]. Our patient did not have aneurysms which, while well described in the literature, are not pathognomonic of TA [14].

4. Conclusion

We thus conclude that perinatally acquired HIV infection can be a high-risk factor for CVD. In our patient, the fact that she was noncompliant with her medication also put her at risk for accelerated atherosclerosis. A high degree of suspicion is warranted in such patients, especially if they are noncompliant to their ART. Further studies are needed to assess CVD risk and to establish guidelines on CVD risk management.

References

[1] V. A. Triant, "Cardiovascular disease and HIV infection," *Current HIV/AIDS Reports*, vol. 10, no. 3, pp. 199–206, 2013.

[2] S. E. Lipshultz, S. Chanock, S. P. Sanders, S. D. Colan, A. Perez-Atayde, and K. McIntosh, "Cardiovascular manifestations of human immunodeficiency virus infection in infants and children," *American Journal of Cardiology*, vol. 63, no. 20, pp. 1489–1497, 1989.

[3] T. Wang, R. Yi, L. A. Green, S. Chelvanambi, M. Seimetz, and M. Clauss, "Increased cardiovascular disease risk in the HIV-positive population on ART: potential role of HIV-Nef and Tat," *Cardiovascular Pathology*, vol. 24, no. 5, pp. 279–282, 2015.

[4] F. Boccara, S. Lang, C. Meuleman et al., "HIV and coronary heart disease: time for a better understanding," *Journal of the American College of Cardiology*, vol. 61, no. 5, pp. 511–523, 2013.

[5] S. M. Crowe, C. L. V. Westhorpe, N. Mukhamedova, A. Jaworowski, D. Sviridov, and M. Bukrinsky, "The macrophage: the intersection between HIV infection and atherosclerosis," *Journal of Leukocyte Biology*, vol. 87, no. 4, pp. 589–598, 2010.

[6] W. S. Post, M. Budoff, L. Kingsley et al., "Associations between HIV infection and subclinical coronary atherosclerosis," *Annals of Internal Medicine*, vol. 160, no. 7, pp. 458–467, 2014.

[7] F. J. Torriani, L. Komarow, R. A. Parker et al., "Endothelial function in human immunodeficiency virus-infected antiretroviral-naive subjects before and after starting potent

antiretroviral therapy. The ACTG (AIDS clinical trials group) study 5152s," *Journal of the American College of Cardiology*, vol. 52, no. 7, pp. 569–576, 2008.

[8] M. S. Freiberg, C. C. H. Chang, L. H. Kuller et al., "HIV infection and the risk of acute myocardial infarction," *JAMA Internal Medicine*, vol. 173, no. 8, p. 614, 2013.

[9] W. M. El-Sadr, D. Abrams, M. Losso, H.-T. General De Agudos, J. M. Ramos Mejia, and C. Rappoport, "CD4+ count-guided interruption of antiretroviral treatment," *New England Journal of Medicine*, vol. 355, no. 22, pp. 2283–2296, 2006.

[10] J. S. Cardoso, B. Moura, L. Martins, A. Mota-Miranda, F. R. Gonçalves, and H. Lecour, "Left ventricular dysfunction in human immunodeficiency virus (HIV) infected patients," *International Journal of Cardiology*, vol. 63, no. 1, pp. 37–45, 1998.

[11] S. E. Lipshultz, K. A. Easley, E. J. Orav et al., "Left ventricular structure and function in children infected with human immunodeficiency virus: the prospective P2C2 HIV multicenter study," *Circulation*, vol. 97, no. 13, pp. 1246–1256, 1998.

[12] R. C. Vreeman, M. L. Scanlon, M. S. McHenry, and W. M. Nyandiko, "The physical and psychological effects of HIV infection and its treatment on perinatally HIV-infected children," *Journal of the International AIDS Society*, vol. 18, no. 7, 2015.

[13] W. P. Arend, B. A. Michel, D. A. Bloch et al., "The American College of Rheumatology 1990 criteria for the classification of Takayasu arteritis," *Arthritis and Rheumatism*, vol. 33, no. 8, pp. 1129–1134, 2010.

[14] C. Marks and S. Kuskov, "Pattern of arterial aneurysms in acquired immunodeficiency disease," *World Journal of Surgery*, vol. 19, no. 1, pp. 127–132, 1995.

Cerebral Venous Thrombosis as Rare Presentation of Herpes Simplex Virus Encephalitis

José Leite,[1] **Ana Ribeiro**,[2] **Diana Gonçalves**,[1] **João Sargento-Freitas**,[3] **Luís Trindade**,[2] **and Victor Duque**[2]

[1]*Department of Internal Medicine, Coimbra University Hospital Centre, Coimbra, Portugal*
[2]*Department of Infectious Diseases, Coimbra University Hospital Centre, Coimbra, Portugal*
[3]*Department of Neurology, Coimbra University Hospital Centre, Coimbra, Portugal*

Correspondence should be addressed to José Leite; ze.pedro.leite@gmail.com

Academic Editor: George N. Dalekos

Herpes simplex virus 1 is a prevalent neurotropic pathogen that infects and establishes latency in peripheral sensory neurons. It can migrate into the central nervous system and cause encephalitis. The association between herpes simplex virus encephalitis and cerebral venous thrombosis is rare, with a very limited number of case reports described in the literature, despite the recognized thrombogenic effects of the virus. A 44-year-old man was brought to the emergency department with generalized tonic-clonic seizures requiring sedation and ventilation to control it. Initial brain computed tomography revealed cortical and subcortical edema on the left frontal lobe, and a subsequent contrast-enhanced exam showed absence of venous flow over the anterior half of the superior sagittal sinus. Cerebrospinal fluid polymerase chain reaction was positive for herpes simplex virus type 1, and the patient was started on acyclovir and anticoagulation, with clinical improvement. Acyclovir administration was maintained for 14 days and oral anticoagulation for one year, with no recurrence of thrombotic events or other complications. A well-timed treatment has a validated prognostic impact on herpes simplex encephalitis, making early recognition of its clinical aspects of main importance.

1. Introduction

Herpes simplex virus 1 (HSV-1) infection is common, with a seropositivity prevalence greater than 60% worldwide [1, 2]. HSV-1 is a neurotropic pathogen that infects and establishes latency in peripheral sensory neurons, but it can migrate into the central nervous system with potentially devastating results. Herpes simplex virus encephalitis (HSE) is an atypical presentation of the infection, with significant mortality and morbidity if not promptly recognized and adequately managed [2]. Despite the prothrombotic effects of the virus [3], the association between HSE and cerebral venous thrombosis (CVT) is extremely rare, with, to the best of our knowledge, only three cases described in the literature [4–6].

2. Case Presentation

A 44-year-old white man, with a previous history of gouty arthritis and type 2 diabetes diagnosed two years earlier, was admitted to the emergency department for a reported episode of generalized tonic-clonic seizure at home, lasting 2 minutes. The patient had no recent history of fever or flu-like symptoms but reported a moderate occipital headache in the previous four days. On the initial clinical examination, the patient was lucid and oriented, hemodynamically stable, and with fever (auricular temperature of 38°C). A thorough neurological examination revealed neither meningism signs nor any focal neurological deficit. Fundoscopic examination was normal. Apart from evidence of tongue biting, he had no visible oral or genital vesicular lesions or any skin rash. There were no palpable lymph nodes.

During the observation period in the emergency room, several convulsive episodes were observed, with postcritical agitation and disorientation, requiring sedation with propofol and intubation for airway protection.

A brain computed tomography (CT) scan was performed, revealing cortical and subcortical edema of the left anterior frontal region and a local linear hyperdensity suggestive of a discrete subarachnoid haemorrhage. A cerebral CT venography revealed venous thrombosis in the anterior two-thirds of the superior longitudinal sinus (Figure 1).

The patient had no prior personal or family history of epilepsy or thrombotic events. There was no history of cancer. His long-term medication was metformin 700 mg and allopurinol 300 mg once a day. He had good metabolic control of type 2 diabetes with a hemoglobin A1c count of 6.2% and no evidence of end-organ damage. Uric acid was in the normal range.

Complete blood count and renal and hepatic function were normal. He had a normal leukocyte count and a red cell distribution width of 13.9%. Inflammatory markers were slightly elevated, the erythrocyte sedimentation rate was 43 mm/h, and the C-reactive protein was 233.3 nmol/L (normal <4.76 nmol/L).

Two sets of blood cultures were collected but had no bacterial growth after 5 days of incubation. An anteroposterior view of a chest X-ray was obtained and showed no evidence of opacities or consolidations. His electrocardiogram had a normal sinus rhythm.

The cytochemical study of cerebrospinal fluid (CSF) revealed 2 leucocytes/mm^3, a protein level of 230 mg/L, and a glucose level of 10 mmol/L (serum level of 14 mmol/L). The CSF multiplex polymerase chain reaction was positive for HSV-1 and negative for all the other microorganisms tested (HSV-2, enterovirus, varicella zoster virus, human herpes virus 6, cytomegalovirus, *N. meningitidis*, *H. influenzae*, *E. coli* K1, *S. agalactiae*, *L. monocytogenes*, and *C. neoformans*). Serology for HSV was IgG positive and IgM negative and negative for both HIV and syphilis.

The autoimmune study (antinuclear antibodies, anticardiolipin antibodies, and lupus anticoagulant) was negative or normal. Complement C3 and C4 test and homocysteine were normal. Protein C, protein S, and antithrombin III levels were normal. The molecular study of genetic thrombophilias was negative for prothrombin 20210G>A mutation but revealed heterozygosity for factor V Leiden (mutation 1691G>A).

The diagnosis of CVT secondary to HSV-1 infection in a patient with heterozygosity for factor V Leiden was made. The treatment was started with enoxaparin 1 mg/kg twice daily, levetiracetam 1500 mg bid, and acyclovir 800 mg tid for 14 days. The patient had a positive clinical evolution during hospitalization, with no more seizures and no neurological deficits at discharge. The selected oral anticoagulant was rivaroxaban 20 mg id, maintained for 12 months, without any new convulsive or thromboembolic episodes registered.

3. Discussion

HSV-1 is estimated to affect more than 60% of world population and is the main etiological agent of sporadic encephalitis [1, 2]. The diagnosis is suggested by altered mental status, with or without fever, associated with laboratory and imaging evidence of inflammation of the central nervous system. A clinical picture of headache, seizures, and focal neurological deficits should make one think of herpetic encephalitis. CSF may usually present moderate lymphocytic pleocytosis (10–200 lymphocytes/mm^3). Brain CT has low sensitivity and diagnostic specificity, with brain magnetic resonance imaging (MRI) being the examination of choice for the diagnosis of encephalitis, although it is not always available in an emergency room. The definitive diagnosis is made by a positive multiplex PCR for HSV in the CSF. This test has high sensitivity (96%) and specificity (99%) and supplanted virus cultures as the test of choice for definitive diagnosis [2]. HSV serology is of little interest in the acute setting [2].

If clinical suspicion is high, treatment should be initiated as soon as possible. The early introduction of acyclovir is the modifiable factor with the most significant impact on prognosis [2]. Empirical treatment is indicated for suspected cases, given the potential benefit compared to the relative innocuity of the drug. The delay in therapy initiation is one of the factors responsible for poor prognosis, along with age and altered mental status at presentation [2]. A dose of 30 mg/kg/day (10 mg/kg tid) is recommended for 14 to 21 days, depending on the clinical response. Untreated HSV-1 encephalitis typically had a high mortality rate (about 70%) that significantly decreased to 5–15% with the advent of acyclovir [2]. Although it seems to improve the outcome in animal models, the role of corticosteroids in the treatment of HSE is not yet well established, and their use is reserved for situations in which there is significant brain edema and mass effect [2].

Recurrence is uncommon in adults and is generally less severe than the initial episode. It is, however, more related to immune-mediated phenomena than to virus activity itself [2].

The most frequent complications of HSE are seizures and brain edema. HSE may rarely present or evolve with intracranial bleeding [7], most often in the form of scattered petechial haemorrhages. This complication may occur even after the initiation of treatment, and the lack of clinical improvement or sudden clinical worsening should raise suspicion of a vascular complication.

Endothelial cell (EC) injury is a common feature of viral infections and can alter hemostasis.

Herpesviridae infections, particularly, inhibit anticoagulant functions and induce a procoagulant phenotype. However, if on one hand the vasculopathy associated with the varicella zoster virus is well known, having a wide clinical range that goes from transient ischemic attacks and cerebral and subarachnoid haemorrhages to spinal-cord infarction [8], on the other hand the vascular involvement in herpes simplex infections is not so conspicuous.

There are several mechanisms, studied in vitro, that were proposed as contributing factors to increased thrombotic risk in HSV infections [3]. By infecting EC, HSV-1 and HSV-2 reduce heparan sulfate proteoglycan synthesis and expression, therefore preventing antithrombin III binding to its surface. The expression of thrombomodulin is also reduced, affecting protein C activation.

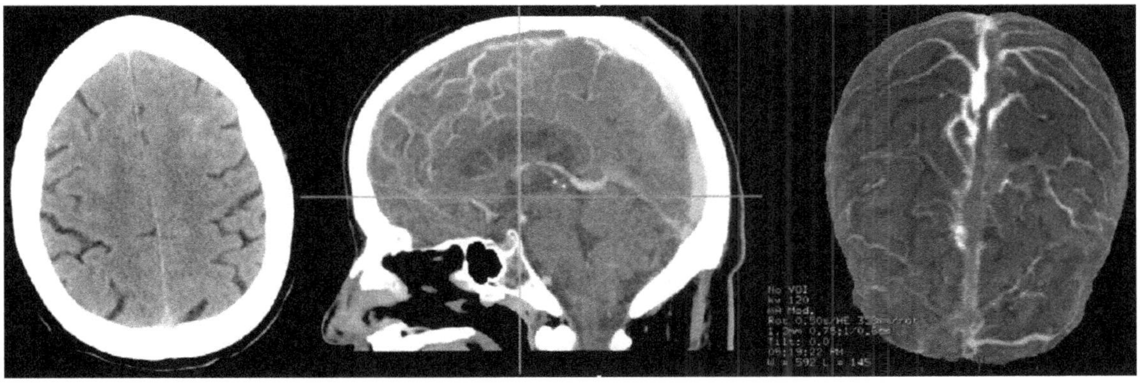

(a) (b) (c)

Figure 1: Brain computed tomography images. (a) Initial CT scan reveals loss of cortical-subcortical discrimination in the left frontal lobe and a local linear hyperdensity indicating subarachnoid haemorrhage. (b) CT venography: sagittal cut showing absence of permeability of the anterior two-thirds of the superior longitudinal sinus consistent with thrombosis. (c) 3D reconstruction of the CT venography.

Changes in the EC membrane lead to enhanced thrombin generation, increasing platelet binding and decreasing prostacyclin synthesis. Another mechanism proposed is that HSV infection increases endothelial binding sites for inflammatory cells and platelets, with subsequent release of inflammatory cytokines and potentiation of a prothrombotic EC surface.

Although the prothrombotic effects of HSV-1 are recognized and debated in the literature, CVT is an extremely rare event in a proven association with herpetic encephalitis [3]. To our knowledge, there are only another three cases reported in the literature (Table 1). All patients were aged between 30 and 50 years and had a similar clinical presentation, with seizures and headaches being the predominant symptoms. In three of the four cases, the diagnosis of HSE and CVT was made simultaneously and in one case [6], there was a clinical worsening during HSE treatment that led to CVT diagnosis. In two of the cases, there was an identifiable risk factor for venous thromboembolism. Our patient is the only one that received a direct anticoagulant as maintenance treatment after the acute phase. There were no neurological deficits at hospital discharge in any case nor were any recurrences of the symptoms reported.

CVT has a prothrombotic risk factor identified in 85% of the cases [9], either genetic or acquired. Its clinical manifestations are vast, from headaches to nausea and vomiting or signs of intracranial hypertension, focal neurological syndromes, and encephalopathy. The diagnosis is usually made by contrast-enhanced CT or MRI. The therapeutic approach should be anticoagulation, even in the presence of intracerebral haemorrhage [9–11]. The initiation of anticoagulation should be done with low-molecular weight heparin or conventional heparin until the patient is stable and then switching to oral anticoagulation with warfarin that should be continued for 3 months (in the presence of transient risk factors) or 6–12 months (in the presence of nonmodifiable risk factors). Indefinite anticoagulation should be considered in the presence of major risk factors, namely, severe thrombophilia (antithrombin deficiency, protein C or S, antiphospholipid syndrome, and homozygosity for factor V Leiden) [11]. Factor V Leiden is the genetic risk factor most often found in patients with venous thrombosis. Heterozygosity has a prevalence of 3–8% in the European population. The risk of cerebral venous thrombosis is 3–5 times normal in heterozygotes [12].

The role of direct anticoagulants in the anticoagulation of cerebral thrombotic events is still not consensual. Although its therapeutic role in pulmonary and lower limb venous thrombosis is already widely supported and recommended, cerebral venous thrombosis relies on a considerably different pathophysiological basis, and its use for this purpose should be considered off-label [10, 13]. The available literature relies essentially on a small series of clinical cases [11, 14], and therefore the quality of evidence is still considered very low. There is no evidence of inferiority in relation to warfarin, either in terms of efficacy or safety [12, 13], but its use requires close counseling and follow-up. In the described clinical case, the authors consider that the association of a genetic risk factor with HSV-1 central nervous system infection caused the thrombotic event. Anticoagulation with rivaroxaban was chosen after a multidisciplinary team discussion on the available therapeutic options.

4. Conclusion

HSV-1 encephalitis in association with CVT is a rare event with very few cases reported.

The management of both events requires early therapeutic measures with great impact on the prognosis.

The role of direct oral anticoagulants as a therapeutic arsenal for thrombotic events is expanding, but its use in the treatment of CVT requires more scientific support and should be adapted to each clinical case individually.

Table 1: Comparison between cases of HSV encephalitis associated with CVT reported in the literature.

Case number	Year of publication	Patient's age	Patient's sex	HSV clinical presentation	Diagnosis of CVT	Risk factors identified for venous thromboembolism	CVT treatment	Outcome
Case 1 [4]	2005	48	Male	Seizures, high fever, history of headaches, and flu-like symptoms	Simultaneous	None	LMWH acute phase followed by warfarin for 6 months	Favourable, no deficits
Case 2 [5]	2012	30	Female	Seizures, high fever, confusion, and headaches	Simultaneous	Pregnancy	LMWH until delivery	Favourable, no deficits
Case 3 [6]	2018	31	Male	Seizures, headache, and photofobia	Day 6 of treatment: worsening headache, upper limb weakness	None	Intravenous heparin acute phase followed by warfarin for 1 year	Favourable, no deficits
Our case	—	44	Male	Seizures, low fever, and history of headaches	Simultaneous	Factor V Leiden heterozygosity	LMWH acute phase followed by rivaroxaban 1 year	Favourable, no deficits

LMWH: low-molecular-weight heparin.

Consent

Written informed consent was obtained from the patient for publication of this case report and the accompanying images.

Authors' Contributions

All authors contributed to the diagnosis and treatment of the male patient and to preparing the final manuscript. This manuscript was drafted together with ABRR and DFSLG. The case report was reviewed by Professors JSF and VMJD, who are specialists on the subject, and recommended corrections were made. All of the authors have read and accepted the final version of this case report.

References

[1] C. M. Menendez and D. J. J. Carr, "Defining nervous system susceptibility during acute and latent herpes simplex virus-1 infection," *Journal of Neuroimmunology*, vol. 308, pp. 43–49, 2017.

[2] M. J. Bradshaw and A. Venkatesan, "Herpes simplex virus-1 encephalitis in adults: pathophysiology, diagnosis, and management," *Neurotherapeutics*, vol. 13, no. 3, pp. 493–508, 2016.

[3] A. C. Nicholson and D. P. Hajjar, "Herpesviruses in atherosclerosis and thrombosis," *Arteriosclerosis, Thrombosis, and Vascular Biology*, vol. 18, no. 3, pp. 339–348, 1998.

[4] K. H. Chan, R. T. F. Cheung, W. M. Liu, W. Mak, and S. L. Ho, "Cerebral venous thrombosis in a gentleman presenting with fever, convulsion and frontotemporal haemorrhages," *Journal of Clinical Neuroscience*, vol. 12, no. 2, pp. 186–188, 2005.

[5] R. Öcal, Ö. Coşkun, C. Bulut, S. Kinikli, G. Kutlu, and L. E. İnan, "Cerebral venous thrombosis in a subject with herpes encephalitis: case report," *Turkiye Klinikleri Journal of Medical Sciences*, vol. 32, no. 4, pp. 1191–1194, 2012.

[6] A. Lal, M. C. Dhamne, A. C. Hui, and A. Ahmad, "Herpes simplex virus (HSV) encephalitis in a young man: an unusual course," *BMJ Case Reports*, vol. 2018, article bcr-2017-222499, 2018.

[7] A. Rodríguez-Sainz, I. Escalza-Cortina, L. Guio-Carrión et al., "Intracerebral hematoma complicating herpes simplex encephalitis," *Clinical Neurology and Neurosurgery*, vol. 115, no. 10, pp. 2041–2045, 2013.

[8] D. Gilden, R. J. Cohrs, R. Mahalingam, and M. A. Nagel, "Varicella zoster virus vasculopathies: diverse clinical manifestations, laboratory features, pathogenesis, and treatment," *Lancet Neurology*, vol. 8, no. 8, pp. 731–740, 2009.

[9] J. Stam, "Thrombosis of the cerebral veins and sinuses," *New England Journal of Medicine*, vol. 352, no. 17, pp. 1791–1798, 2005.

[10] W. Ageno, J. Beyer-Westendorf, D. A. Garcia, A. Lazo-Langner, R. D. McBane, and M. Paciaroni, "Guidance for the management of venous thrombosis in unusual sites," *Journal of Thrombosis and Thrombolysis*, vol. 41, no. 1, pp. 129–143, 2016.

[11] J. M. Ferro, M.-G. Bousser, P. Canhão et al., "European Stroke Organization guideline for the diagnosis and treatment of cerebral venous thrombosis - endorsed by the European Academy of Neurology," *European Journal of Neurology*, vol. 24, no. 10, pp. 1203–1213, 2017.

[12] J. L. Kujovich, "Factor V leiden thrombophilia," *Genetics in Medicine*, vol. 13, no. 1, pp. 1–16, 2010

[13] C. Geisbüsch, D. Richter, C. Herweh, P. A. Ringleb, and S. Nagel, "Novel factor xa inhibitor for the treatment of cerebral venous and sinus thrombosis," *Stroke*, vol. 45, no. 8, pp. 2469–2471, 2014.

[14] S. I. Patel, H. Obeid, L. Matti, H. Ramakrishna, and F. E. Shamoun, "Cerebral venous thrombosis," *Neurologist*, vol. 20, no. 5, pp. 80–88, 2015.

35

Acute Brucellosis Presenting with Bleeding Tendency due to Isolated Severe Thrombocytopenia

M. Aon[1] and T. Al-Enezi[2]

[1]*Department of Medicine, Faculty of Medicine, Cairo University, Giza, Egypt*
[2]*Department of Medicine, Jahra Hospital, Al-Jahra, Kuwait*

Correspondence should be addressed to M. Aon; maon2004@cu.edu.eg

Academic Editor: Tomoyuki Shibata

Mild anemia and leukopenia are the most common hematologic findings in the course of acute brucellosis. Severe form of thrombocytopenia is less frequently reported. We describe a case of acute brucellosis in a 20-year-old man, who presented with fever, purpuric skin lesions, epistaxis, and hematuria. The absolute platelet count was 2×10^9/L. The patient was diagnosed as suffering from brucellosis on the basis of a strongly positive serologic reaction and was treated with antibiotics and a short course of corticosteroids, with a rapid rise in platelet count. *Brucella* infection can cause immune-mediated thrombocytopenia that is reversible after appropriate antimicrobial therapy and steroid treatment.

1. Introduction

Brucellosis is one of the most important and widespread zoonoses in the world. In humans, brucellosis can be caused by *B. melitensis*, *B. abortus*, *B. suis*, and *B. canis* [1]. Mild hematological abnormalities, such as anemia and leukopenia, are common in the course of human brucellosis; however, they generally resolve with treatment of the disease. Thrombocytopenia is less common, and it is rarely severe enough to cause bleeding [2, 3]. Hereby, we describe an acute brucellosis patient who presented with bleeding manifestations (epistaxis, gingival bleeding, and hematuria) and severe thrombocytopenia consistent with immune thrombocytopenic purpura.

2. Case Report

A 20-year-old male patient with no past medical history presented to the emergency room (at Jahra Hospital, Kuwait) with history of fever associated with malaise and arthralgia for 7 days. On arrival in the causality, he was febrile (39°C). Rest of the physical examination was normal. A history of ingesting unpasteurized camel's milk was reported, and a serological test for brucellosis was positive. A complete blood count (CBC) showed hemoglobin 145 g/L, WBCs 7.6×10^9/L with 45.6% lymphocytes and 49.2% neutrophils, and platelets 4×10^9/L. Other laboratory tests showed urea 3.6 mmol/L, creatinine 75.25 μmol/L, total bilirubin 16.1 μmol/L, ALT 48 IU/L, and AST 52 IU/L. There was severe isolated thrombocytopenia (4000), but no evidence of skin or mucous membranes bleeding. He denied use of any over-the-counter drugs, painkillers, or NSAIDs. The ER physician advised for hospital admission but he refused. Therapy with doxycycline and rifampicin was prescribed, but then he left against medical advice. Two days later, he returned to the emergency room with complaints of epistaxis, gingival bleeding, and hematuria. No hematemesis or melena was reported. He was febrile with a body temperature of 38.7°C, an arterial blood pressure of 110/75 mmHg, and a heart rate of 72 beats/min. There was nonitchy flat purpuric rash, particularly on his lower extremities. His physical examinations of the cardiovascular, respiratory, abdominal, and central nervous systems were normal. Repeat CBC showed hemoglobin 128 g/L, WBCs 4.9×10^9/L with 51.8% lymphocytes and 41.1% neutrophils, and platelets 2×10^9/L. A peripheral blood smear examination showed normal RBCs, WBCs morphology, and marked thrombocytopenia with occasional giant platelets and no platelet clumps. When true thrombocytopenia was confirmed and to exclude other causes of thrombocytopenia, malaria blood film, coagulation profile, fibrinogen level, antinuclear antibody (ANA), double-stranded DNA antibody (anti-ds DNA), and serological tests for HbsAg, anti-HCV, HIV, cytomegalovirus, and Ebstein–Barr virus all were unremarkable. *Brucella* agglutination test was positive (titer 1 : 1280). We considered a diagnosis of brucellosis with immune thrombocytopenic purpura. Due to the very low platelet count and the mucous membrane hemorrhage, 12 units of platelets were infused. Treatment with intravenous immunoglobulin (IVIg) was initiated at a dose of 500 mg/kg/day, combined with prednisolone (1 mg/kg/day), doxycycline (100 mg/12 hours), and rifampicin (600 mg/day). Fever resolved on the second day of treatment, platelet count started to rise, and bleeding manifestations improved. On the 6th day, his platelet count was 66000, and he was discharged from hospital on tablet prednisolone of 25 mg daily with gradual tapering, tablet rifampin of 600 mg daily, and capsule doxycycline of 100 mg twice a day for total six weeks. Blood cultures performed on specimens obtained at the time of admission showed no growth. He was planned for follow-up one month after discharge from the hospital, but he did not show up. A follow-up phone call confirmed that all his symptoms resolved and he finished his treatment course.

3. Discussion

Brucellosis is a chronic granulomatous infection caused by Gram-negative coccobacilli of the genus *Brucella* and transmitted to humans through direct contact with infected animals or through consumption of unpasteurized dairy products [4]. Human brucellosis remains the commonest zoonotic disease worldwide with more than 500,000 new cases annually. The annual incidence in Kuwait is 33.9 cases per million. Despite the developing economy and advancing technology, consumption of raw milk products is still common and the region is considered an endemic area [5].

Most of the *Brucella* patients (44.8–60.5%) have a history of raising livestock or occupations carrying a risk for brucellosis. Consumption history of dried raw meat or dairy products is present in 24.6–35.1% of cases [3, 6]. The study case was infected through drinking unpasteurized milk. Studies showed that raw milk consumption is the commonest route of infection in Kuwait [7, 8].

Human brucellosis is a disease of protean manifestations. The most frequent symptoms are fever, malaise, sweating, arthralgia, headache, and back pain. Physical examination may reveal fever, hepatomegaly, or splenomegaly. *Brucella* infection may involve any organ or tissue in the body, e.g., the locomotor, genitourinary, gastrointestinal, hematological, cardiovascular, respiratory, and central nervous systems [6].

Date from the largest case series in the literature showed that the most common laboratory findings were high CRP levels (58.4%), high ESR (51.3%), anemia (40.3%), lymphocytosis (28.2%), and transaminase elevation (24.8%). The standard tube agglutination test was positive in 94.1% of cases [3].

In brucellosis, the blood count is often characterized by mild leukopenia and relative lymphocytosis along with anemia [9]. Although laboratory abnormalities with regard to the hematological system are common in the course of human brucellosis, isolated thrombocytopenia is less common (1–8%), and it is rarely severe enough to cause bleeding [2, 10].

Isolated thrombocytopenia complicating *Brucella* infection results from multiple possible mechanisms. Among the proposed mechanisms are hypersplenism, bone marrow suppression, disseminated intravascular coagulation, and hemophagocytosis [11]. Immune-mediated thrombocytopenia, which has not received major attention, is an important mechanism encountered during the course of brucellosis. An immune response is activated in the course of brucellosis which may cause an autoimmune hemolysis and destruction of platelets. Immune thrombocyte destruction may significantly threaten life due to severe bleeding [12].

The main mechanism of thrombocytopenia in our patient was possibly related to brucellosis-induced antibodies reacting with thrombocytes. Normal coagulation profile, normal fibrinogen level, and absence of schistocytes in the peripheral blood film were against DIC. There was no splenomegaly, so we cannot refer the thrombocytopenia to splenomegaly and hypersplenism. There was no evidence of bone marrow suppression as WBCs, RBCs, and reticulocytes were all within the normal limit. Bone marrow suppression and hypersplenism are usually associated with pancytopenia. In the study case, only isolated thrombocytopenia was observed. To exclude other causes of thrombocytopenia, the virology panel, malaria blood film, ANA, and anti-ds DNA were tested and results came negative.

Evidence for an immune mechanism may include rapid response to corticosteroids, positive Coombs tests, or the presence of antiplatelet antibodies. Antiplatelet antibodies can be difficult to detect by the usual tests and have a little correlation between their titer and the degree of thrombocytopenia. A negative assay for antiplatelet antibodies does not exclude the diagnosis of immune thrombocytopenia [10].

Combining therapies (corticosteroids and IVIg) is appropriate for the emergency treatment of primary immune thrombocytopenia patients with uncontrolled bleeding and severe thrombocytopenia especially when an urgent increase in platelet count is required, e.g., before surgical procedures or with active central nervous system (CNS), gastrointestinal (GI), or genitourinary bleeding [13].

In brucellosis, thrombocyte recovery usually occurs within 1–3 weeks of initiating appropriate antimicrobial therapy. However, in cases of severe thrombocytopenia, an urgent treatment institution of glucocorticoids will result in an increased platelet count and can be used to control bleeding until the antimicrobial therapy takes effect [14]. If a patient has mild-to-moderate thrombocytopenia with no life-threatening bleeding, antibrucellosis treatment should be started only. It is suggested that corticosteroids should be started along with antibrucellosis treatment in cases of which platelet count is <10 000 [11].

Although we initiated treatment with IVIg and steroids, we believe that, in most cases of *Brucella*-associated thrombocytopenia, treatment with corticosteroids along with antibrucellosis treatment will suffice. The rapid response to treatment supports the notion that immune-mediated one is the culprit mechanism.

The percentage of cases with positive cultures ranges from 11.4 to 38. Serology is the preferred method for the diagnosis of brucellosis when bacterial isolation is not possible. Titers ≥1 : 160 are considered diagnostic in conjunction with a compatible clinical presentation. In endemic areas, using a titer ≥1 : 320 may be more specific [3, 15].

In conclusion, brucellosis should always be kept in mind for the differential diagnosis of isolated thrombocytopenia in endemic areas. Patients should be investigated for brucellosis in the presence of fever or a travelling history to countries where the disease is endemic. Although it is rare, if diagnosed properly, dramatic response to the treatment is expected.

References

[1] L. B. Lopes, R. Nicolino, and J. P. A. Haddad, "Brucellosis-risk factors and prevalence: a review," *Open Veterinary Science Journal*, vol. 4, no. 1, pp. 72–84, 2010.

[2] E. Crosby, L. Llosa, M. M. Quesada, C. P. Carrillo, and E. Gotuzzo, "Hematologic changes in brucellosis," *Journal of Infectious Diseases*, vol. 150, no. 3, pp. 419–424, 1984.

[3] T. Buzgan, M. K. Karahocagil, H. Irmak et al., "Clinical manifestations and complications in 1028 cases of brucellosis: a retrospective evaluation and review of the literature," *International Journal of Infectious Diseases*, vol. 14, no. 6, pp. e469–e478, 2010.

[4] T. M. Abdallah, O. M. Abd elbagi, A. OsmanKaroum, and A. A. Abdallah Ali, "Acute brucellosis as unusual cause of immune thrombocytopenia: a case report and review of the literature," *Asian Pacific Journal of Tropical Biomedicine*, vol. 4, no. 9, pp. 751–754, 2014.

[5] G. Pappas, P. Papadimitriou, N. Akritidis, L. Christou, and E. V. Tsianos, "The new global map of human brucellosis," *Lancet Infectious Diseases*, vol. 6, no. 2, pp. 91–99, 2006.

[6] B. Jia, F. Zhang, Y. Lu et al., "The clinical features of 590 patients with brucellosis in Xinjiang, China with the emphasis on the treatment of complications," *PLOS Neglected Tropical Diseases*, vol. 11, no. 5, pp. 1–10, 2017.

[7] A. R. Mousa, K. M. Elhag, M. Khogali, and A. A. Marafie, "The nature of human brucellosis in Kuwait: study of 379 cases," *Clinical Infectious Diseases*, vol. 10, no. 1, pp. 211–217, 1988.

[8] A. R. Lulu, G. F. Araj, M. I. Khateeb, M. Y. Mustafa, A. R. Yusuf, and F. F. Fenech, "Human brucellosis in Kuwait: a prospective study of 400 cases," *QJM: An International Journal of Medicine*, vol. 66, no. 1, pp. 39–54, 1988.

[9] B. Aygen, M. Doganay, B. Sumerkan, O. Yildiz, and U. Kayaba, "Clinical manifestations, complications and treatment of brucellosis: a retrospective evaluation of 480 patients," *Médecine et Maladies Infectieuses*, vol. 32, no. 9, pp. 485–493, 2002.

[10] E. J. Young, A. Tarry, R. M. Genta, N. Ayden, and E. Gotuzzo, "Thrombocytopenic purpura associated with brucellosis: report of 2 cases and literature review," *Clinical Infectious Diseases*, vol. 31, no. 4, pp. 904–909, 2000.

[11] M. Yilmaz, O. Tiryaki, M. Namiduru et al., "Brucellosis-induced immune thrombocytopenia mimicking ITP: a report of seven cases," *International Journal of Laboratory Hematology*, vol. 29, no. 6, pp. 442–445, 2007.

[12] Z. Abbaspour Rad, B. Sajedi, S. Akbarieh, A. H. Heydari, S. B. Ali, and A. M. Mojdehi, "A case report of isolated thrombocytopenia induced by brucellosis," *Asian Pacific Journal of Tropical Disease*, vol. 7, no. 3, pp. 181-182, 2017.

[13] D. Provan, R. Stasi, A. C. Newland et al., "International consensus report on the investigation and management of primary immune thrombocytopenia," *Blood*, vol. 115, no. 2, pp. 168–186, 2010.

[14] E. Gurkan, F. Baslamisli, B. Guvenc, B. Bozkurt, and C. Unsal, "Immune thrombocytopenic purpura associated with *Brucella* and toxoplasma infections," *American Journal of Hematology*, vol. 74, no. 1, pp. 52–54, 2003.

[15] Z. Memish, M. W. Mah, S. Al Mahmoud, M. Al Shaalan, and M. Y. Khan, "*Brucella* bacteraemia: clinical and laboratory observations in 160 patients," *Journal of Infection*, vol. 40, no. 1, pp. 59–63, 2000.

36

Acute Cytomegalovirus Illness in an Immunocompetent Adult Causing Intravascular Hemolysis and Suspected Hemophagocytic Lymphohistiocytosis

Ross P. Elliott,[1] Brian P. Freeman,[2] Jeffery L. Meier,[3,4] and Rima El-Herte[5]

[1]*Internal Medicine Residency Program, MercyOne Medical Center and Clinics, Des Moines, IA 50314, USA*
[2]*Mission Cancer and Blood, Des Moines, IA 50309, USA*
[3]*Iowa City Veterans Affairs Health Care System, Iowa City, IA 52246, USA*
[4]*Division of Infectious Diseases, Department of Internal Medicine, University of Iowa Carver College of Medicine, Iowa City, IA 52242, USA*
[5]*Division of Infectious Diseases, Department of Medicine, Creighton, University School of Medicine and CHI Health, Omaha, NE 68124, USA*

Correspondence should be addressed to Rima El-Herte; rimael-herte@creighton.edu

Academic Editor: Zarrin Basharat

Background. Primary cytomegalovirus (CMV) infection of the immunocompetent host usually produces little-to-no illness. Occasionally, the infection results in mononucleosis syndrome, protracted fever, hepatitis, tissue-invasive disease, or Guillain-Barré syndrome. Hemolytic anemia and hemophagocytic lymphohistiocytosis (HLH) are rare complications that have not been reported to co-occur. Having hemolytic anemia in conjunction with more common findings of fever and hepatitis complicates the diagnosis of HLH. *Case Presentation.* A 34-year-old male with previously good health presented with a prolonged febrile illness, jaundice, and anemia. An extensive work-up during hospitalization revealed intravascular hemolytic anemia, leukopenia, hepatosplenomegaly, and biopsy evidence of extensive lymphohistiocytic infiltration of the liver with microgranulomata and sinusoidal hemophagocytosis. Soluble CD25 level was mildly elevated at 1200.3 pg/mL and the HScore calculation (fever, bicytopenia, hepatosplenomegaly, aspartate aminotransaminase 99 IU/L, ferritin 1570 ng/mL, fibrinogen 488 mg/dL, and triglycerides 173 mg/dL) suggested a moderate probability of reactive HLH. Primary CMV infection was diagnosed based on CMV IgM positivity, low CMV IgG avidity index, and low-grade CMV DNAemia. The CMV antigen was not detected in the liver biopsy, and the bone marrow biopsy was unremarkable. The illness began to improve before he received oral valganciclovir for 5 days, and he was in good health 10 months later. *Conclusion.* Acute CMV illness in an immunocompetent adult can present with hemolytic anemia and clinicopathologic abnormalities consistent with a form fruste of HLH. The illness is likely due to an excessive or unbalanced immune response that may self-correct.

1. Introduction

Human cytomegalovirus (CMV) causes debilitating or fatal diseases in people with immature or profoundly defective cellular immune systems. CMV disease of this severity is rarely encountered in people without these immune system abnormalities. While CMV is the most common cause of the heterophile antibody-negative mono syndrome in adolescents and adults, most CMV infections go unnoticed in immunocompetent people. Occasionally, the first episode of CMV infection in an immunocompetent person causes a self-limited prolonged febrile or atypical monolike illness that is usually accompanied by liver test abnormalities signifying hepatitis [1]. Rarely does the infection progress to a tissue invasive disease that involves the gastrointestinal tract, lung, eye, or other organs [2]. The immunologic response to the acute infection may also at times go awry to produce hemolysis, immune thrombocytopenia, myocarditis, skin eruptions, Guillain-Barré syndrome, meningoencephalitis, and, in rare cases, hemophagocytic lymphohistiocytosis (HLH) [3]. Awareness of the unusual presentations of the acute CMV infection in the immunocompetent host is key to early diagnosis and directing test utilization and disease management.

2. Case Presentation

A 34-year-old Caucasian male was in his usual state of good health until July 2020 when he presented with a 1-week history of fever up to 39.3°C, sore throat, headaches, cough, and malaise. Having developed this during the SARS-CoV-2 pandemic, he presented to a COVID-19 testing site where jaundice was noted. He was triaged to the emergency room and then hospitalized. He tested negative for SARS-CoV-2 infection by polymerase chain reaction (PCR). A review of the system was negative for oral ulcers, change in vision, enlarged lymph nodes, chest or abdominal discomfort, dyspnea, nausea, vomiting, diarrhea, genital lesions, dysuria, hematuria, arthralgia, myalgia, neurological change, memory deficit, or rash. He had a cholecystectomy two years ago. He reported no illicit drug use, recent travel, or exposure to sick contacts, tuberculosis, ticks, animals, vaping, herbs, or supplements. He had two young children, both in daycare, and his wife was pregnant. The family medical history was unremarkable; no immunodeficiency, malignancy, autoimmunity, or severe infections. He had used over-the-counter acetaminophen and ibuprofen at the recommended doses. Laboratory tests revealed white blood cell count (WBC) 4.6 k/mm3 (range, 4.5–11 k/mm^3) with neutrophils 55.6%, lymphocytes 24.2%, and monocytes 13.8%; hemoglobin (Hgb) 13.6 g/dL (range, 13.5–17.5 g/dL); platelets 155 k/mm^3 (range, 150–450 k/mm^3); peripheral smear with reactive lymphocytes; alkaline phosphatase 94 IU/L (range, 20–140 IU/L); alanine transaminase (ALT) 219 IU/L (range, 5–55 IU/L); aspartate aminotransaminase (AST) 99 IU/L (range, 5–45 IU/L); total bilirubin 8 mg/dL (range, 0.2–1.5 mg/dL); indirect bilirubin 7.1 mg/dL (range, 0.1–1.4 mg/dL); and normal serum creatinine. Urine analysis showed clear orange urine at pH 6.0 (range, 4.5–7) with specific gravity 1.205 (range, 1.010–1.030), protein 20 mg/dL (negative), ketones 20 mg/dL (negative), urobilinogen >20 (range, 0.1–1.8 mg/dL) and negative values for bilirubin, blood, glucose, nitrite, and leukocyte esterase. Serological testing was negative for hepatitis A virus IgM, hepatitis B virus surface antigen, hepatitis B virus core IgM, hepatitis C virus antibody (Ab), human immunodeficiency virus (HIV) p24 antigen (Ag), HIV-1 and HIV-2 Abs, antinuclear antigen Ab, liver-kidney microsomal Ab, mitochondrial Ab, and antismooth muscle Ab. Ceruloplasmin was normal. Iron level was 219 mcg/dL (range, 35–160 mcg/dL), normal TIBC, elevated iron saturation at 83% (range, 30–50%), and low transferrin at 161 mg/dL (range 200–430 mg/dL). IgG level was normal at 957 mg/dL (range, 650–1600 mg/dL). Blood cultures were negative. Abdominal ultrasound showed moderate hepatomegaly and changes consistent with fatty liver disease. Abdominal MRI showed similar changes plus splenomegaly (16 cm). The patient was discharged home on hospital day 3.

On the following day, he was readmitted because of worsening symptoms and normocytic anemia. The Hgb of 12.5 g/dL on the day of entry steadily decreased to 8.7 g/dL on day 8 of this hospitalization. Other remarkable blood count results included WBC 4.2 k/mm^3 (range, 4.5–11 k/mm^3), neutrophils 1.9 k/mm^3 (range, 1.8–7.7 k/mm^3), and platelets 155 k/mm^3. Peripheral smear revealed an increase in reactive lymphocytes but a normal lymphocyte count and no schistocytes. Other remarkable laboratory findings included AST 56 IU/L, ALT 120 IU/L, total bilirubin 7.7 mg/dL, indirect bilirubin 6.7 mg/dL, ferritin 1570 ng/mL (range, 24–336 ng/mL), fibrinogen 488 mg/dL (range, 200–450 mg/dL), triglycerides 173 mg/dL (range, <149 mg/dL), LDH 341 IU/L (range, 135–220 IU/L), haptoglobin 1 mg/dL (range, 40–280), absolute reticulocyte count 0.1947 million/mm^3 (range, 0.62–1.88 million/mm^3), plasma free Hgb 60 mg/L (range, 0–9 mg/dL), no urinary hemosiderin, and negative Coomb's test.

Computed tomography of the chest, abdomen, and pelvis showed hepatosplenomegaly without lymphadenopathy. To investigate the cause of the liver abnormalities, a percutaneous liver biopsy was performed on day 2 of hospitalization. This showed portal triad inflammation involving lymphocytes, eosinophils, and granulomatous inflammation (Figure 1), as well as rare lobular microgranulomata (Figure 2). Liver sinusoids had excessive numbers of Kupffer cells (Figure 3) and T-lymphocytes (Figure 4). Occasional benign appearing histiocytes/Kupffer cells had findings of hemophagocytosis of red blood cells and probable leukocytes (Figure 5). Immunohistochemical stains for CMV, HSV-1, and HSV-2 Ags were negative. In situ hybridization for EBV EBER RNA was negative. Special stains for acid-fast bacilli and fungi were negative. Additional testing performed on blood for the HLH possibility included a soluble CD25 (IL-2 receptor) level that was elevated at 1200.3 pg/mL (range, 175.3–858.2). Natural killer cell activity was not assessed.

The infectious disease workup revealed CMV IgM and IgG in serum and CMV DNA in plasma at 41 IU/mL (reference value, undetected; quantification range, 35–10^6 IU/mL). Primary CMV infection was later confirmed by evidence of a low CMV IgG avidity index of 0.18 (cut off >0.7 for past infection). EBV viral capsid antigen (VCA) IgG and IgM were positive, EBV nuclear antigen IgG >8 (EBNA antibody), and plasma EBV DNA was absent. The blood was negative by PCR for HHV8, ehrlichia, anaplasma, and *Coxiella burnetii* DNA. Also negative in the blood were brucella IgG and IgM, ehrlichia and anaplasma Abs, parvovirus B19 IgM, *Rickettsia rickettsii* Abs, and tuberculosis interferon gamma release assay. Histoplasma Ag in blood and urine; blastomyces Ag in urine, CSF, and blood were negative. Flow cytometry applied to the blood was negative for blasts and atypical lymphoid proliferation. Bone marrow biopsy performed on day 6 of the hospitalization (blood count Hgb 9.8 g/dL), showed normocellular marrow for age with 1+ polychromasia, normal trilineage hematopoiesis, increased storage iron, and no hemophagocytosis, malignancy, CMV Ag, EBV EBER RNA, or stainable acid-fast bacilli and fungi.

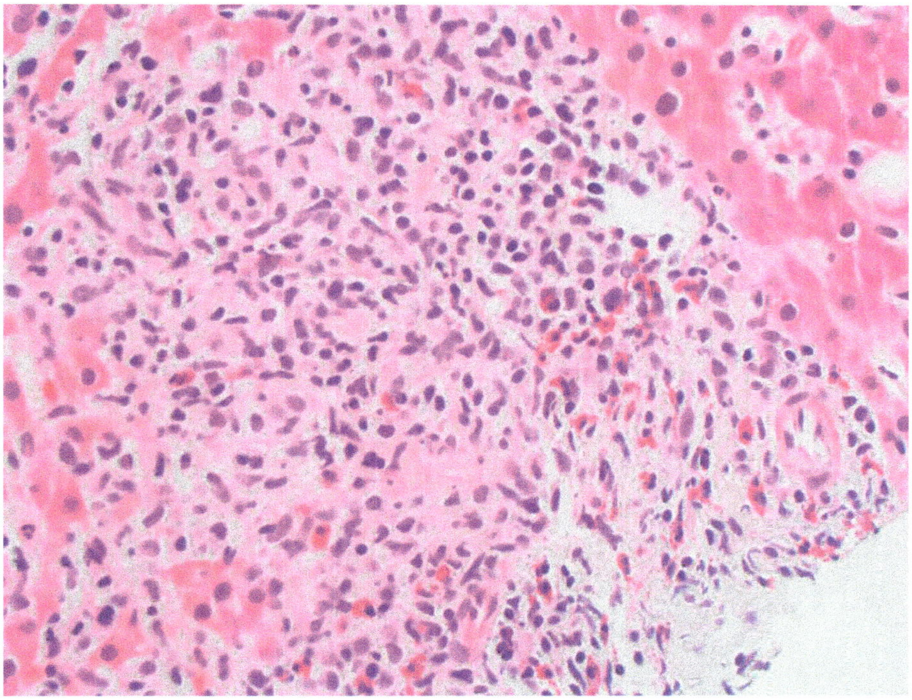

FIGURE 1: Liver portal triad is expanded by lymphocytes, eosinophils, and noncaseating granulomatous inflammation. H&E stain of liver tissue. No interface hepatitis or proliferating bile ductules. Original magnification, 400x.

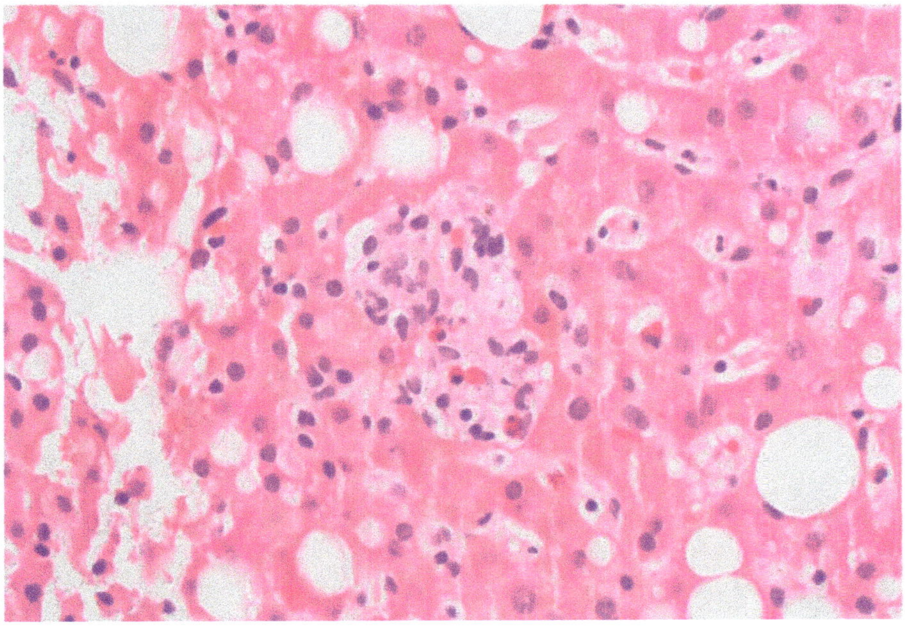

FIGURE 2: Lobular microgranuloma in the liver. H&E stain of liver tissue. Original magnification, 400x.

3. Outcome and Follow-up

The patient's condition was improving before he was given oral valganciclovir for 5 days and discharged home. He received no corticosteroids, immune globulin, or other immunomodulatory therapy. After discharge from the hospital, he had four face-to-face follow-up visits over 10 months. At 5 weeks after the onset of illness, the patient had returned to his usual activity level and had no symptoms of CMV DNAemia. At four months, the cytopenia had resolved (WBC 4.0 k/mm3, Hgb 14.3 g/dL, and platelets 210 k/mm^3), liver transaminases had normalized, and total bilirubin had improved. At 10 months, the labs showed Hgb 14.5 g/dL, total bilirubin 3.7 mg/dL,

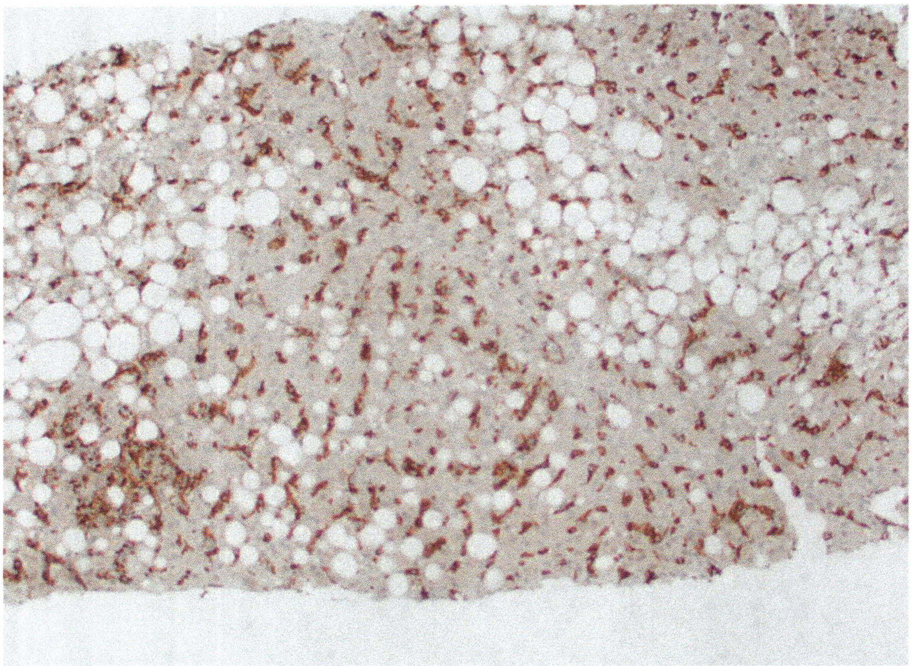

Figure 3: Immunohistochemical staining of CD68-positive macrophages/Kupffer cells (brown stain) in the liver. An excessive number of macrophages are located in sinusoids.

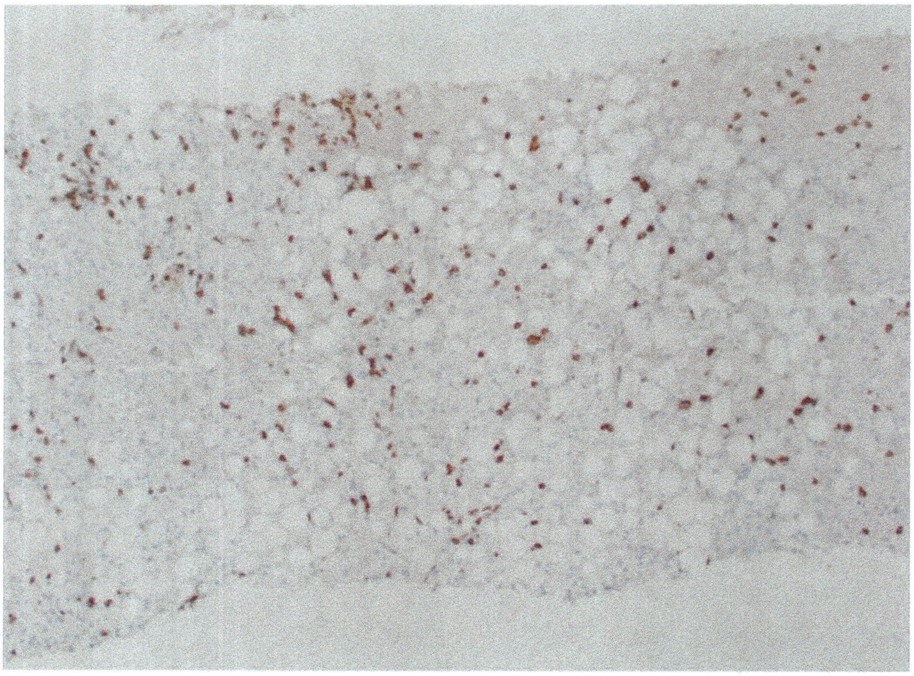

Figure 4: Immunohistochemical staining of CD3-positive T-lymphocytes (brown stain) in the liver. An excessive number of T-lymphocytes are in sinusoids.

direct bilirubin 1 mg/dL, ferritin 280 ng/mL, and haptoglobin 49 mg/dL. The persistent elevation in indirect bilirubin levels could be from residual compensated hemolysis or previously unrecognized Gilbert syndrome. The patient elected to not return for further follow-up.

4. Discussion

The extensive workup that was undertaken for our patient revealed hepatosplenomegaly, hepatitis, hemolytic anemia, and neutropenia. Atypical lymphocytes were not present. Testing for many possible etiologies resulted in the diagnosis

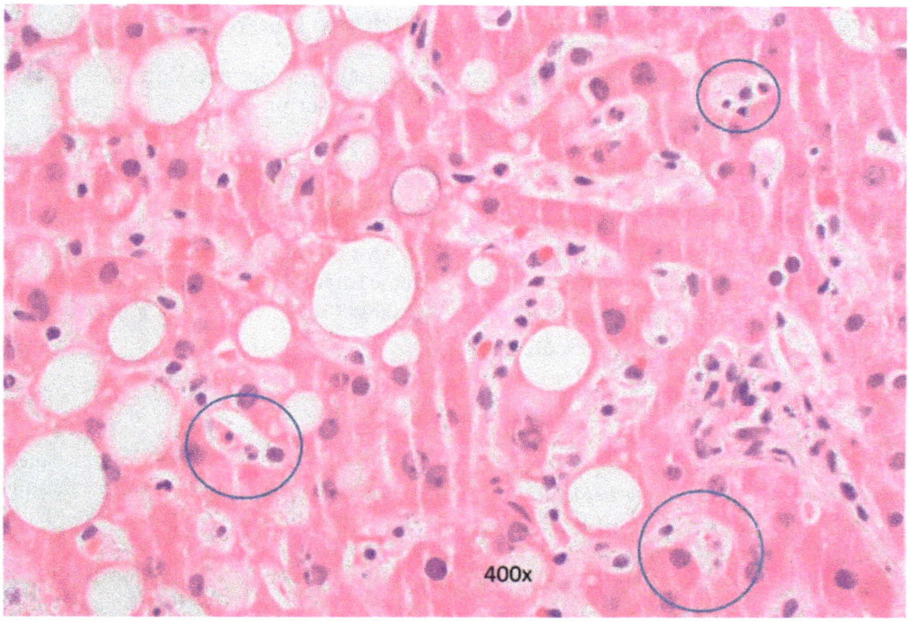

FIGURE 5: Sinusoidal histiocytic hemophagocytosis. H&E stain of liver tissue. Examples of mature red cells within histiocyte cytoplasm as well as probable degenerate neutrophils within histiocytes are circled. Original magnification, 400x.

of primary CMV infection. The diagnosis was based on laboratory findings of low CMV IgG avidity index, CMV IgM positivity, and low-grade CMV DNAemia, in conjunction with a compatible clinical presentation that is discussed below. Serologic evidence of low CMV IgG avidity index or CMV IgG seroconversion confirms a primary CMV infection diagnosis in immunocompetent people, whereas CMV IgM positivity is a product of a primary infection, reactivation/re-infection, or false-positive test [4, 5]. The patient's two young children in daycare may have put him at a higher risk of acquiring CMV, because young children frequently acquire CMV in the daycare setting, shed the virus in high amounts in oral secretions and urine, and transmit CMV to adults via close oral contact with infectious saliva [3, 6]. While acute EBV infection can also produce fever, hepatitis, and hemolytic anemia, our patient's EBV serologies signaled a past EBV infection with immune reactivation (EBV VCA IgM and IgG positivity with highly positive EBNA antibody) or false-positive EBV VCA IgM. Primary CMV infection commonly produces EBV VCA IgM positivity [7, 8]. The lack of EBV DNA in plasma also makes EBV-driven infectious mononucleosis, or HLH, unlikely [9, 10]. Tests for several other possible infectious causes of the patient's illness were negative.

Acute hemolytic anemia is a rare complication of primary CMV infection that was first recognized over 50 years ago [11–13]. Hemolytic anemia arises from intravascular or extravascular hemolysis. CMV may induce antibodies directed against red blood cell surface Ags that may be detected by the direct Coombs test. The majority of case reports of CMV-associated acute hemolysis have indicated the Coombs test was negative and the hemolysis was recognized several days after the onset of any symptoms, as was the situation for our patient. Hepatosplenomegaly is common in these cases and may foster extravascular hemolysis by hepatic and splenic macrophages. Our patient had hepatosplenomegaly with liver biopsy evidence of extensive lymphohistiocytic infiltration and macrophages containing ingested erythrocytes. The self-limited course of acute hemolytic anemia is not unusual [14, 15]. Corticosteroids have been used in severe cases of CMV-induced hemolytic anemia [15, 16], which is in line with the view that corticosteroids may be beneficial in treating the acute hemolytic anemia resulting from EBV-induced infectious mononucleosis [17].

Abnormal liver tests are one of the most common findings in people presenting with symptomatic primary CMV infection [1]. This is usually the consequence of an excessive immunologic response and mononuclear cell infiltration in the liver that may take weeks to resolve. Evidence of active CMV replication is commonly absent in the liver tissue at the time it is examined. The enlarged liver of our patient was marked by a portal and sinusoidal T-lymphocytic and histiocytic infiltration and sinusoidal hemophagocytosis of lymphocytes and RBCs. Microgranulomas were also present. These are features of immune system hyperactivation, including macrophage activation, that are triggered by various types of infections, malignancies, and autoimmune conditions [18]. Histopathologic abnormalities of this type can be associated with or without HLH [18, 19]. HLH is a rare complication of CMV infection in people with acquired or congenital immunodeficiency. Seven cases of CMV-induced HLH have been reported in immunocompetent hosts [20–26], and none of these cases had concomitant hemolytic anemia. These published HLH cases represent the extreme of the illness, and none were reported to be self-limited. The diagnosis of secondary HLH is usually based on criteria provided in the HLH-2004 guideline from the Histocyte Society [27] or in the HScore [28]. The HLH diagnosis per the HLH-2004 guideline requires having 5 of 8 criteria: fever, splenomegaly, cytopenia (2 or 3 lineages), hypertriglyceridemia (triglycerides ≥ 265 mg/dl), hypofibrinogenemia (fibrinogen ≤ 150 mg/dl), hemophagocytosis of bone marrow, spleen, or lymph node, low or absent NK cell activity, elevated ferritin (≥500 ug/L), and elevated soluble CD25 (≥2,400 U/mL) [27]. Our patient met 4 of 8 HLH-2004 guideline criteria for secondary HLH. The HScore differs from the HLH-2004 guideline by including criteria of immunosuppression, hepatomegaly, and elevated AST level and not including NK activity or soluble CD25 level [28]. Our patient did not have immunosuppression or bone marrow hemophagocytosis. His calculated HScore put him at a moderate probability of having reactive HLH. Because EBV-induced infectious mononucleosis and hemolytic anemia elevate ferritin levels [29], an acute CMV monolike illness with hemolytic anemia may do the same. Our patient's CD25 level was not in a range typically observed in HLH cases. Notably, neither the HLH scoring system requires evidence of hemophagocytosis nor lists liver hemophagocytosis as an HLH criterion. However, liver biopsy evidence of lymphohistiocytic infiltration and sinusoidal hemophagocytosis in the setting of an acute systemic inflammatory illness should prompt the consideration of HLH [19, 30].

Our patient's primary CMV infection produced clinical and pathological abnormalities that are consistent with a form fruste of HLH. The illness began to improve before the patient received 5 days of oral valganciclovir and the patient had not received corticosteroid or another hemolysis- or HLH-directed treatment. This suggests that a primary CMV infection presenting in an immunocompetent host as incomplete HLH does not necessarily require HLH-directed therapy. In contrast, the severity of illness and mortality risk from full-blown HLH usually necessitates an HLH-directed intervention, such as corticosteroid, cytotoxic drug, other immunomodulatory agents, and/or hematopoietic stem cell transplantation. Antiviral therapy, such as oral valganciclovir or IV ganciclovir, is often given to inhibit viral replication in the hope of silencing the driver of immune hyperactivation. It was not until HLH was suspected in this patient that CMV infection was considered in the differential diagnosis. Recognizing the varied spectrum of CMV-associated illnesses is key to early diagnosis and directing test utilization and disease management.

5. Learning Points

(i) Acute CMV infection in the immunocompetent host can cause self-limited hemolytic anemia.

(ii) Acute CMV infection can induce lymphohistiocytic infiltration and hemophagocytosis in the liver.

(iii) Intravascular hemolysis complicates the use of current criteria to classify a patient as having HLH.

Consent

This report has no personal identifying information. The local institutional review board has approved this work.

Authors' Contributions

Both Jeffery Meier and Rima El-Herte contributed equally to the manuscript.

Acknowledgments

J.L.M.'s effort and cost of publication were supported by the Department of Veteran Affairs Merit Award (I01 BX004434).

References

[1] T. G. Wreghitt, E. L. Teare, O. Sule, R. Devi, and P. Rice, "Cytomegalovirus infection in immunocompetent patients," *Clinical Infectious Diseases*, vol. 37, no. 12, pp. 1603–1606, 2003.

[2] P. I. Rafailidis, E. G. Mourtzoukou, I. C. Varbobitis, and M. E. Falagas, "Severe cytomegalovirus infection in apparently immunocompetent patients: a systematic review," *Virology Journal*, vol. 5, no. 1, p. 47, 2008.

[3] C. S. Crumpacker and S. Wadhwa, "Cytomegalovirus," *Mandell, Douglas and Bennett's Principles and Practice of Infectious Diseases*, Elsevier, Philadelphia, PA, USA, 2015.

[4] H. E. Prince and M. Lape-Nixon, "Role of cytomegalovirus (CMV) IgG avidity testing in diagnosing primary CMV infection during pregnancy," *Clinical and Vaccine Immunology*, vol. 21, no. 10, pp. 1377–1384, 2014.

[5] C. Perillaud-Dubois, E. Bouthry, A. Jadoui, A. L. Leng, A. M. Roque-Afonso, and C. Vauloup-Fellous, "Positive predictive values of CMV-IgM and importance of CMV-IgG avidity testing in detecting primary infection in three different clinical settings. A French retrospective cohort study," *Journal of Clinical Virology*, vol. 132, Article ID 104641, 2020.

[6] T. B. Hyde, D. S. Schmid, and M. J. Cannon, "Cytomegalovirus seroconversion rates and risk factors: implications for congenital CMV," *Reviews in Medical Virology*, vol. 20, no. 5, pp. 311–326, 2010.

[7] A. Guerrero-Ramos, M. Patel, K. Kadakia, and T. Haque, "Performance of the architect EBV antibody panel for determination of Epstein-Barr virus infection stage in immunocompetent adolescents and young adults with clinical suspicion of infectious mononucleosis," *Clinical and Vaccine Immunology*, vol. 21, no. 6, pp. 817–823, 2014.

[8] F. de Ory, M. E. Guisasola, J. C. Sanz, and I. Garcia-Bermejo, "Evaluation of four commercial systems for the diagnosis of Epstein-Barr virus primary infections," *Clinical and Vaccine Immunology*, vol. 18, no. 3, pp. 444–448, 2011.

[9] S. Y. Jiang, J. W. Yang, J. B. Shao, X. L. Liao, Z. H. Lu, and H. Jiang, "Real-time polymerase chain reaction for diagnosing infectious mononucleosis in pediatric patients: a systematic review and meta-analysis," *Journal of Medical Virology*, vol. 88, no. 5, pp. 871–876, 2016.

[10] S. Yu, Q. Yang, J. Wu et al., "Clinical application of Epstein-Barr virus DNA loads in Epstein-Barr virus-associated diseases: a cohort study," *Journal of Infection*, vol. 82, no. 1, pp. 105–111, 2021.

[11] P. J. Toghill, M. E. Bailey, R. Williams, R. Zeegen, and R. Bown, "Cytomegalovirus hepatitis in the adult," *The Lancet*, vol. 289, no. 7504, pp. 1351–1354, 1967.

[12] R. R. Coombs, "Cytomegalic inclusion-body disease associated with acquired autoimmune haemolytic anaemia," *British Medical Journal*, vol. 2, no. 5607, pp. 743-744, 1968.
[13] Case Records of the Massachusetts General Hospital, "Weekly clinicopathological exercises. Case 52-1968," *New England Journal of Medicine*, vol. 279, no. 26, pp. 1444–1452, 1968.
[14] W. Veldhuis, M. Janssen, W. Kortlandt, A. Houte, and M. Ree, "Coombs-negative severe haemolytic anaemia in an immunocompetent adult following cytomegalovirus infection," *European Journal of Clinical Microbiology & Infectious Diseases*, vol. 23, no. 11, pp. 844–847, 2004.
[15] C. A. Horwitz, K. Skradski, E. Reece et al., "Haemolytic anaemia in previously healthy adult patients with CMV infections: report of two cases and an evaluation of subclinical haemolysis in CMV mononucleosis," *Scandinavian Journal of Haematology*, vol. 33, no. 1, pp. 35–42, 2009.
[16] F. Taglietti, C. M. Drapeau, E. Grilli et al., "Hemolytic anemia due to acute cytomegalovirus infection in an immunocompetent adult: a case report and review of the literature," *Journal of Medical Case Reports*, vol. 4, no. 1, p. 334, 2010.
[17] S. E. Straus, J. I. Cohen, G. Tosato, and J. Meier, "Epstein-Barr virus infections: biology, pathogenesis, and management," *Annals of Internal Medicine*, vol. 118, no. 1, p. 45, 1993.
[18] V. Prendki, J. Stirnemann, M. Lemoine et al., "Prevalence and clinical significance of Kupffer cell hyperplasia with hemophagocytosis in liver biopsies," *The American Journal of Surgical Pathology*, vol. 35, no. 3, pp. 337–345, 2011.
[19] J. De Gottardi, M. Montani, A. Angelillo-Scherrer, A. Rovo, and A. Berzigotti, "Hepatic sinusoidal hemophagocytosis with and without hemophagocytic lymphohistiocytosis," *PLoS One*, vol. 14, no. 12, Article ID e0226899, 2019.
[20] A. Hot, M. H. G. Madoux, J. P. Viard, B. Coppere, and J. Ninet, "Successful treatment of cytomegalovirus-associated hemophagocytic syndrome by intravenous immunoglobulins," *American Journal of Hematology*, vol. 83, no. 2, pp. 159–162, 2008.
[21] A. K. Bonnecaze, W. G. Willeford, P. Lichstein, and J. Ohar, "Acute cytomegalovirus (CMV) infection associated with hemophagocytic lymphohistiocytosis (HLH) in an immunocompetent host meeting all Eight HLH 2004 diagnostic criteria," *Cureus*, vol. 9, no. 3, Article ID e1070, 2017.
[22] S. M. Patil, P. P. Beck, T. P. Patel et al., "Cytomegalovirus pneumonitis-induced secondary hemophagocytic lymphohistiocytosis and SIADH in an immunocompetent elderly male literature review," *IDCases*, vol. 22, Article ID e00972, 2020.
[23] A. Singh, A. Singh, A. Chauhan, V. Padole, D. Chhabra, and R. Upneja, "The great masquerader: hemophagocytic lymphohistiocytosis secondary to cytomegalovirus infection in an immunocompetent young man," *Journal of Family Medicine and Primary Care*, vol. 9, no. 7, 2020.
[24] M. Atim-Oluk, "Cytomegalovirus associated haemophagocytic lymphohistiocytosis in the immunocompetent adult managed according to HLH-2004 diagnostic using clinical and serological means only," *European Journal of Microbiology and Immunology*, vol. 3, no. 1, pp. 81–89, 2013.
[25] H. Tsuda and K. Shirono, "Successful treatment of virus-associated haemophagocytic syndrome in adults by cyclosporin A supported by granulocyte colony-stimulating factor," *British Journal of Haematology*, vol. 93, no. 3, pp. 572–575, 1996.
[26] Y. T. Tseng, W. H. Sheng, B. H. Lin et al., "Causes, clinical symptoms, and outcomes of infectious diseases associated with hemophagocytic lymphohistiocytosis in Taiwanese adults," *Journal of Microbiology, Immunology, and Infection*, vol. 44, no. 3, pp. 191–197, 2011.
[27] J. I. Henter, A. Horne, M. Arico et al., "HLH-2004: diagnostic and therapeutic guidelines for hemophagocytic lymphohistiocytosis," *Pediatric Blood and Cancer*, vol. 48, no. 2, pp. 124–131, 2007.
[28] L. Fardet, L. Galicier, O. Lambotte et al., "Development and validation of the HScore, a score for the diagnosis of reactive hemophagocytic syndrome," *Arthritis & Rheumatology*, vol. 66, no. 9, pp. 2613–2620, 2014.
[29] C. Dematapitiya, C. Perera, W. Chinthaka et al., "Cold type autoimmune hemolytic anemia-a rare manifestation of infectious mononucleosis; serum ferritin as an important biomarker," *BMC Infectious Diseases*, vol. 19, no. 1, p. 68, 2019.
[30] C. de Kerguenec, S. Hillaire, V. Molinie et al., "Hepatic manifestations of hemophagocytic syndrome: a study of 30 cases," *American Journal of Gastroenterology*, vol. 96, no. 3, pp. 852–857, 2001.

37

Streptococcus thoraltensis Bacteremia: First Described Case as a Fever of Unknown Origin in Human

Nikolaos Petridis, Athanasia Apsemidou, Georgios Kalopitas, Georgios Pilianidis, and Iakovos Avramidis

First Department of Internal Medicine, G. Papanikolaou General Hospital, Thessaloniki, Greece

Correspondence should be addressed to Nikolaos Petridis; nikosmed1@gmail.com

Academic Editor: Larry M. Bush

Streptococcus thoraltensis has mainly been reported to cause infections in animals. Its clinical significance as a human pathogen has not yet been fully elucidated and needs further investigation. We describe here a case of bacteremia attributed to *S. thoraltensis* in a 55-year-old female patient admitted to our department due to fever of unknown origin. To the best of our knowledge, this is the first reported case of *S. thoraltensis* bacteremia in a human and the first reported case of *S. thoraltensis* as a cause of fever of unknown origin in human.

1. Introduction

Streptococcus thoraltensis is a recently described species that has been isolated from several animal species [1]. According to the literature, this rare and unusual species of streptococci has recently been isolated from human samples. A recent study revealed *S. thoraltensis* as a predominant colonizing isolate in the nasal cavity and oropharynx in 29 fuel workers [2]. To the best of our knowledge, only one case of *S. thoraltensis* isolation from both the maternal placenta and newborn tracheal aspirate cultures and four cases from the subgingival plaque in patients undergoing tooth extraction have been reported in the literature [3–5].

2. Case Presentation

A 55-year-old female patient with past medical history of osteoporosis and hyperlipidemia was admitted to our department for a 2-month history of high-grade fever, up to 39°C, mainly occurring in the evening, which was responding to acetaminophen. She denied night sweats, anorexia, fatigue, weight loss, chest pain, shortness of breath, other joint pain, abdominal pain, recent travel, or a family history of autoimmune disease, although she reported traumatic dental procedure 6 months prior to admission.

On presentation, her vital signs revealed a temperature of 36.7°C, heart rate of 74 bpm, and blood pressure of 100/70 mmHg. Her physical examination was unremarkable, except for a systolic heart murmur, heard best over the aortic, pulmonic, and mitral area with radiation into the neck. Laboratory studies revealed thrombocytopenia with 123.000 μL platelets, white blood cell count of 4.3×10^9 L with neutrophils as the predominant type, and mild normocytic anemia (Hct: 34.7%; Hb: 11.7 g/d). The C-reactive protein (CRP) was 1.43 mg/dL (nl: <0.5), the erythrocyte sedimentation rate (ESR) was 32 mm/h, and creatine phosphokinase (CPK) was also elevated as 335 U/L (reference range: <180 U/L).

From three blood cultures obtained on the 1st, 2nd, and 3rd day of her hospitalization, when she was febrile, *Streptococcus thoraltensis* was identified, while infection caused by Brucella, *Mycobacterium tuberculosis*, Coxiella, and Leishmania was excluded. The suspicion of an infective endocarditis (IE) was raised, and a transthoracic and transesophageal echo was performed. However, there was no evidence of IE, and only mild aortic stenosis was revealed. A

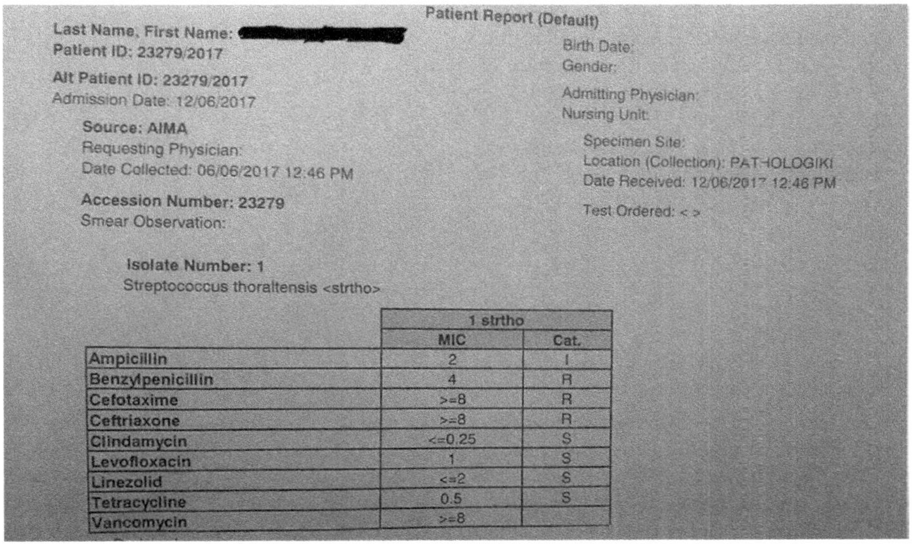

Patient Report (Default)

Last Name, First Name: [redacted]
Patient ID: 23279/2017
Alt Patient ID: 23279/2017
Admission Date: 12/06/2017

Birth Date:
Gender:
Admitting Physician:
Nursing Unit:

Source: AIMA
Requesting Physician:
Date Collected: 06/06/2017 12:46 PM

Specimen Site:
Location (Collection): PATHOLOGIKI
Date Received: 12/06/2017 12:46 PM

Accession Number: 23279
Smear Observation:

Test Ordered: < >

Isolate Number: 1
Streptococcus thoraltensis <strtho>

	1 strtho	
	MIC	Cat.
Ampicillin	2	I
Benzylpenicillin	4	R
Cefotaxime	>=8	R
Ceftriaxone	>=8	R
Clindamycin	<=0.25	S
Levofloxacin	1	S
Linezolid	<=2	S
Tetracycline	0.5	S
Vancomycin	>=8	

FIGURE 1: Susceptibility test of *Streptococcus thoraltensis* isolate.

panoramic X-ray showed no lesions. Additionally, as part of the diagnostic procedure, a chest, abdomen, and pelvis computed tomography (CT) scan was performed and revealed no abscesses and masses.

Due to the fact that the patient continued to have high-grade fevers and the systolic heart murmur, empirical antibiotic treatment with ampicillin/sulbactam and gentamicin was initiated on day 4. Susceptibility testing was performed on the initial isolate and revealed intermediate sensitivity to these agents, as determined by the E-test method (Figure 1). The patient responded 48 hours after the initiation of the treatment. The duration of the antibiotic therapy was fourteen days. The patient had experienced no recurrence of fever, the subsequent blood cultures were negative, and the inflammation markers decreased (CRP: 0.3 mg/dl; ESR: 10 mm/h).

3. Discussion

We searched the literature including PubMed and individual references for publications of review articles, single cases, or case series with the following keywords: "Streptococcus thoraltensis" and "human." There have been documented only five cases of *S. thoraltensis* isolation from human samples. To the best of our knowledge, this is the first reported case of *S. thoraltensis* bacteremia.

A significant limitation to this report is the method used to identify the pathogen due to the fact that the automated VITEK 2 system lacks the specificity of the 16S rRNA gene sequence, although a proper gold standard for the identification of streptococci is not available [6–8]. Nevertheless, identification of *S. thoraltensis* from three individual cultures presents a strong case to implicate this organism.

The characteristic of our patient's infection was high fever mainly occurring in the evening and relatively low levels of inflammation markers which nevertheless were decreased after the treatment initiation. Although our patient had a good clinical outcome, the case was clinically challenging regarding the lack of *S. thoraltensis* cases and the unknown proper duration of treatment in this isolate's bacteremia. Regarding the source of the infection, it remains unknown, considering the long period between the dental procedure and the initiation of her symptoms (>4 months). Hence, her bacteremia can be considered community acquired of unknown origin.

S. thoraltensis has mainly been reported to cause infections in animals. Its clinical significance as a human pathogen has not yet been fully elucidated and needs further investigation. Whether this case represents an isolated and rare bacteremia or an emerging infection will be established by novel possible cases.

References

[1] R. Facklam, "What happened to the streptococci: overview of taxonomic and nomenclature changes," *Clinical Microbiology Reviews*, vol. 15, no. 4, pp. 613–630, 2002.

[2] S. S. AlWakeel, "Microbiological and molecular identification of bacterial species isolated from nasal and oropharyngeal mucosa of fuel workers in Riyadh, Saudi Arabia," *Saudi Journal of Biological Sciences*, vol. 24, no. 6, pp. 1281–1287, 2017.

[3] S. Dhotre, N. Suryawanshi, B. Nagoba, and S. Selkar, "Rare and unusual isolates of viridans streptococci from the human oral cavity," *Indian Journal of Pathology and Microbiology*, vol. 59, no. 1, pp. 47–49, 2016.

[4] S. Dhotre, N. Suryawanshi, and B. Nagoba, "Isolation of Streptococcus thoraltensis from human oral cavity," *Indian Journal of Dentistry*, vol. 5, pp. 140-141, 2014.

[5] M. Vukonich, H. Moline, M. Chaussee, B. Pepito, and M. K. Huntington, "Case report: chorioamnionitis attributed to Streptococcus thoraltensis," *South Dakota Medicine*, vol. 68, no. 7, pp. 298-299, 2015.

[6] J. Barry, A. Brown, V. Ensor et al., "Comparative evaluation of the VITEK 2 advanced expert system (AES) in five UK hospitals," *Journal of Antimicrobial Chemotherapy*, vol. 51, no. 5, pp. 1191–1202, 2003.

[7] F. Wallet, C. Loiez, E. Renaux, N. Lemaitre, and R. J. Courcol, "Performances of VITEK 2 colorimetric cards for identification of gram-positive and gram-negative bacteria," *Journal of Clinical Microbiology*, vol. 43, no. 9, pp. 4402–4406, 2005.
[8] M. Haanpera, J. Jalava, P. Huovinen, O. Meurman, and K. Rantakokko-Jalava, "Identification of alpha-hemolytic streptococci by pyrosequencing the 16S rRNA gene and by use of VITEK 2," *Journal of Clinical Microbiology*, vol. 45, no. 3, pp. 762–770, 2007.

38

Candida krusei Empyema Thoracis: A Community-Acquired Infection Requiring a High Index of Suspicion

Hazim Bukamur, Waseem Ahmed, Yazan Numan, Ibrahim Shahoub, and Fuad Zeid

Department of Pulmonary Medicine, Joan C. Edwards School of Medicine, Marshall University, Huntington, WV, USA

Correspondence should be addressed to Hazim Bukamur; Bukamur@marshall.edu

Academic Editor: Raul Colodner

Empyema thoracis is a serious condition characterized by the accumulation of purulent fluid in the pleural cavity, typically following a pneumonia, subdiaphragmatic abscess, or esophageal rupture. Fungal empyema thoracis is a rare form of this condition with especially high mortality, in which the most frequently isolated fungus is *Candida* spp. This article presents a 74-year-old female with *Candida krusei* pneumonia and a complicated hospital course, initially presenting with nausea, vomiting, and dysphagia. She was initially suspected to have community-acquired pneumonia and was started on azithromycin and ceftriaxone. Worsening respiratory function led to the diagnosis of hydropneumothorax. Pleural fluid and an independent sample of pus and pleural tissue grew *Candida krusei*, giving the diagnosis of fungal empyema. With further respiratory deterioration, the patient was intubated and switched to piperacillin/tazobactam and micafungin. Decortication with extensive pleural peel and removal of foul-smelling pus and food particles within the chest was performed. This further lead to confirmation of esophageal perforation, and she was started on voriconazole and meropenem. After developing septic shock, the patient was managed with phenylephrine and vasopressin. Finally, after improving she was weaned off pressors and extubated, followed by an esophagogastroduodenoscopy (EDG) with pneumatic balloon dilation and WallFlex stent placement. This patient's case demonstrated an example of empyema thoracis, which required a high index of suspicion since the presentation was with a community-acquired infection. *Candida* empyema thoracis may be a complication of operation, gastroesophageal fistula, and spontaneous esophageal rupture. On the other hand, the course of this patient's hospital stay progressed from esophageal perforation to *Candida krusei* pneumonia, empyema, and pneumothorax. Thus, community-acquired fungal empyema should be considered in patients with respiratory symptoms and suspected esophageal perforation; nevertheless, after a diagnosis of fungal empyema, esophageal perforation should also be ruled out in addition to other causes like pneumonia, subphrenic abscess, and hematogenous spread. Improved communication between clinicians and microbiologists can lead to early diagnosis and a reduction in the morbidity and mortality of this condition.

1. Introduction

Empyema thoracis is a serious condition characterized by the accumulation of purulent fluid in the pleural cavity, typically following a pneumonia, subdiaphragmatic abscess, or esophageal rupture. Fungal empyema thoracis is a rare form of this condition with especially high mortality, in which the most frequently isolated fungus is *Candida* spp [1]. A high index of suspicion is required to diagnose this condition, as it may present as a community-acquired infection [2].

2. Case Presentation

A 74-year-old female with a history of schizophrenia, dementia, COPD, and a CVA presented to the Emergency Department with nausea and vomiting for 3 days, as well as dysphagia for 2 weeks, which all began after drinking hot water. Her vital signs on presentation were BP of 122/77 millimeter of mercury (mmHg), HR of 75 beats per minute (bpm), RR of 16 breaths/minute (br/min), oxygen saturation of 95% on room air, and temperature of 97.7°F. The chest examination revealed decreased air entry and diffuse rhonchi bilaterally. The remainder of physical examination was unremarkable. Her labs showed WBCs of 10,300/mm^3, creatinine of 0.77 mg/dl, and a negative urine analysis. The chest X-ray (CXR) revealed left lower lobe consolidation with a left-sided pleural effusion. The abdominal X-ray exhibited dilation of the esophagus. The patient refused a modified barium swallow and a CT of the abdomen. She was started on azithromycin and ceftriaxone for community-acquired pneumonia.

On the third day of admission, she became short of breath, with vitals of HR 130 bpm, BP 86/43 mmHg, RR 38 br/min, temperature 98.6°F, and oxygen saturation 93% on 3 L/min of oxygen. On examination, the patient was cyanotic, using accessory muscles, taking rapid shallow breaths, with decreased air entry and hyper-resonance to percussion on the right side of the chest. The CXR showed a large right-sided hydropneumothorax, and the esophagus was air-filled down to the distal segment (Figure 1). Surgery was consulted, and a chest tube was inserted on the right side, which removed 1.85 liters of pleural fluid. Analysis of the pleural fluid showed WBCs 17424/cmm, RBCs 1728/cmm, neutrophils 95%, lymphocytes 3%, macrocytes 2%, albumin 1.2, amylase 816, glucose < 1, LDH 1559, pH 7.41, and protein 2.7. The pleural fluid grew *Lactobacillus*, and the pleural fluid and sputum culture then grew *Candida krusei*, which was isolated again from a second confirmatory sample of pus, indicating its clinical significance and satisfying the criteria for fungal empyema [2]. Susceptibility testing revealed intermediate sensitivity to 5-flucytosine with minimal inhibitory concentration (MIC) 16.0 mg/L and good sensitivity to itraconazole with MIC of 0.25 mg/L (sensitivity was not done for micafungin). Three sets of blood cultures were negative.

Thereafter, the patient was intubated and transferred to the ICU. The antibiotics were switched to piperacillin/tazobactam and micafungin. CT of the chest without contrast showed bilateral pleural fluid collections, which were larger and more complex appearing on the right (Figure 2). Cardiothoracic surgery was consulted, after which right decortication was performed, with extensive pleural peel and removal of foul-smelling pus and food particles within the chest. Pleural tissue culture grew *C. Krusei*. To further confirm the diagnosis of esophageal rupture, a limited Gastrografin swallow was done through the preexisting NG tube while it was pulled back into the distal esophagus. This revealed a leak in the right distal esophagus, after which a barium swallow exposed esophageal perforation with contrast extravasation into the right pleural cavity (Figure 3), that was confirmed by CT scan.

Infectious diseases was consulted, who then switched the medications to voriconazole and meropenem. Subsequently, the patient developed septic shock during the course of her ICU stay and was started on phenylephrine and vasopressin. After two weeks, the patient improved, was weaned off pressors, and was extubated. An EGD was performed, with pneumatic balloon dilation to 20 mm and WallFlex stent placement. Finally, the patient improved and was discharged from the ICU to the general medical floor.

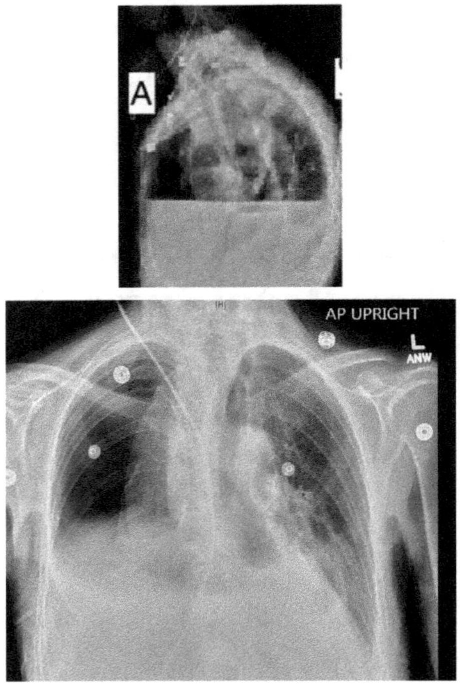

FIGURE 1: CXR showing a large right-sided hydropneumothorax, and the esophagus was air-filled down to the distal segment.

3. Discussion

Empyema is, by definition, pus in the pleural space. Pus is a thick, viscous, yellowish fluid formed in infected tissue, composed of WBCs, tissue debris, necrotic tissue, and pathogens [3]. Fungal empyema thoracis is a rare but severe form of invasive candidiasis with high mortality. The most frequently isolated microorganisms in this condition are *Candida* species, whereas other filamentous fungi are rare, as only sporadic cases have been reported. Interestingly, *Candida* empyema thoracis has been reported as a complication of operation, gastropleural fistula, and spontaneous esophageal rupture [4].

In a retrospective analysis of 128 cases of culture-positive pleural effusion, Ishiguro et al. demonstrated that isolation of *Candida* species could be an important clue for empyema due to gastrointestinal perforation [5]. In this case presentation, the patient presented with dysphagia and was diagnosed with esophageal perforation complicated by *C. krusei* pneumonia, empyema, and pneumothorax.

The diagnosis of fungal bronchopulmonary infection is difficult to confirm because fungi isolated from the sputum may represent either pathogens or saprophytes, and invasive diagnostic procedures such as bronchoscopy or lung biopsy are usually necessary [6]. The diagnosis of fungal empyema thoracis requires that the following criteria be met:

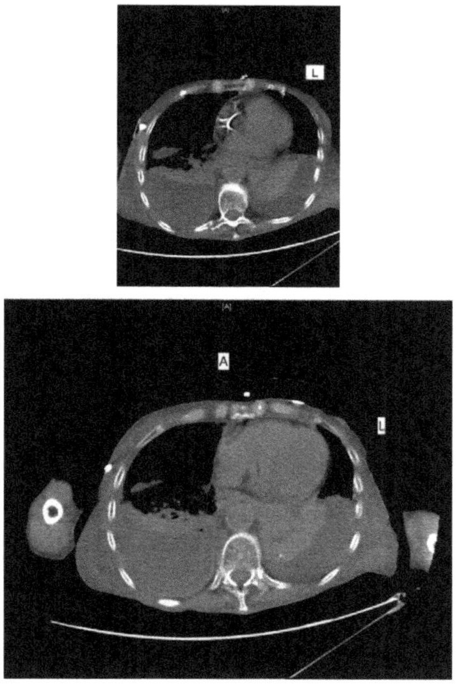

FIGURE 2: CT of the chest without contrast showing bilateral pleural fluid collections, which were larger and more complex appearing on the right.

(1) isolation of fungal species from exudative thoracentesis fluid, (2) significant signs of infection, such as fever (body temperature > 38.3°C) and leukocytosis (WBCs > 10,000/μL), and (3) isolation of the same fungus from pleural fluid and other specimens, including blood, sputum, or surgical wounds, that showed evidence of tissue invasion [2]. The patient in our case presentation was afebrile, with leukocytosis, and *Candida krusei* was isolated from the thoracentesis fluid as well as sputum and tissue cultures from the thoracotomy, thus satisfying two of the criteria mentioned above.

Although the prevalence of *C. krusei* remains low among yeast infections, its intrinsic resistance to fluconazole raises epidemiological and therapeutic concerns. Echinocandins have *in vitro* activity against most *Candida* spp. and are the first-line agents in the treatment of candidemia. Although resistance to echinocandins is still rare, individual cases of *C. krusei* resistance have been reported in recent years, especially with strains that have been under selective pressure [7]. Review of 25,470 isolates of yeasts and 3,216 isolates of filamentous fungi showed voriconazole to have broad-spectrum activity against pathogenic yeasts including intrinsically fluconazole-resistant isolates such as *C. krusei*, dimorphic fungi, opportunistic molds like *Aspergillus* spp., and amphotericin-B-resistant *Aspergillus terreus*, *Fusarium* spp., and *Scedosporium apiospermum*. It displays excellent clinical efficacy in patients with fluconazole-resistant and fluconazole-susceptible *Candida* infections, invasive bone and central nervous system aspergillosis, and various refractory fungal infections [8]. In our case presentation, the patient was first treated empirically with micafungin and then switched to voriconazole after receiving susceptibility testing results.

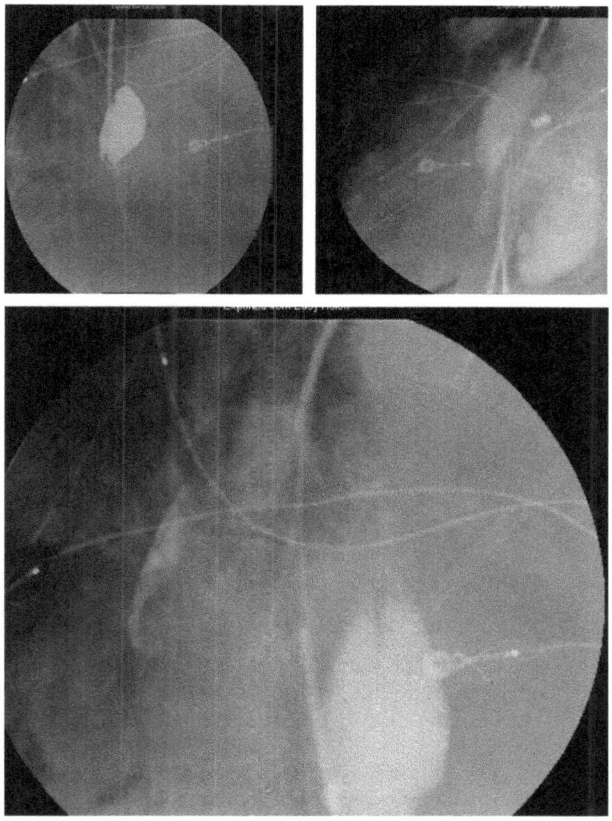

FIGURE 3: A barium swallow showing contrast extravasation into the right pleural cavity confirming esophageal perforation.

There are several surgical options available for management of the pleural fluid in patients with empyema, including tube thoracostomy, intrapleural instillation of fibrinolytics, thoracoscopy with breakdown of adhesions or decortication, thoracotomy with breakdown of adhesions and decortication, and open drainage procedures [3]. Some physicians recommend a formal thoracotomy when the patient's condition allows it, since it may lead to an early discharge without tubes and open draining wounds. Pothula and Krellenstein retrospectively studied 90 patients with this hypothesis, which resulted in low morbidity (10%) and very low mortality (8%). The mortalities in the formal thoracotomy group were mostly related to underlying disease and age [9]. The patient in our case presentation had chest tube insertion and bilateral pleural fluid collections shown on CT of the chest, after which right decortication was performed.

4. Conclusion

Infections of the pleural cavity remain an important cause of morbidity and mortality despite advances in diagnostic modalities and therapy. We are presenting this case and are confident that it will be a valuable addition to medical literature in raising awareness about community-acquired fungal empyema in patients presenting with respiratory symptoms and suspected esophageal perforation. Additionally, in the presence of a fungal empyema, esophageal rupture should also be considered and ruled out in addition to other causes like pneumonia, subphrenic abscess, and hematogenous spread [10]. In our case, we think that the fungal empyema happened secondary to esophageal rupture as other causes had been excluded with negative blood culture, no subphrenic abscess in CT abdomen, and no recent trauma or thoracic surgical intervention. In order to accurately diagnose fungal empyema, a high level of suspicion is required, as it may be due to a community-acquired infection. Furthermore, there is a need for improved communication between clinicians and microbiologists for early decision making, which will reduce the morbidity and mortality [11]. Finally, empirical systemic antimycotic therapy should always be considered in an ideal multidisciplinary approach to the management of patients with esophageal rupture [10].

References

[1] N. Pal, A. De, M. Mondal, and P. K. Maiti, "*Candida albicans* as a rare causative agent of pyopneumothorax," *International Journal of Current Microbiology and Applied Sciences*, vol. 4, no. 7, pp. 716–719, 2015.

[2] V. P. Bardkar, M. Mathur, S. D. Kulkarni, and S. Kumar, "Thoracic empyema due to *Candida albicans*: case report," *Indian Journal of Pathology and Microbiology*, vol. 51, no. 2, pp. 286–288, 2008.

[3] R. W. Light, "Parapneumonic effusions and empyema," *Proceedings of the American Thoracic Society*, vol. 3, no. 1, pp. 78–80, 2006.

[4] T. M. Bauer, V. Dupont, and W. Zimmerli, "Invasive candidiasis complicating spontaneous esophageal perforation (Boerhaave syndrome)," *American Journal of Gastroenterology*, vol. 91, no. 6, pp. 1248–1250, 1996.

[5] T. Ishiguro, N. Takayanagi, T. Ikeva et al., "Isolation of *Candida* species is an important clue for suspecting gastrointestinal tract perforation as a cause of empyema," *Internal Medicine*, vol. 49, no. 18, pp. 1957–1964, 2010.

[6] S. C. Ko, K. Y. Chen, P. R. Hsueh, K. T. Luh, and P. C. Yang, "Fungal empyema thoracis," *Chest*, vol. 117, no. 6, pp. 1672–1678, 2000.

[7] A. Forastiero, V. G. Gil, O. R. Menendez et al., "Rapid development of *Candida krusei* echinocandin resistance during caspofungin therapy," *Antimicrobial Agents and Chemotherapy*, vol. 59, no. 11, pp. 6975–6982, 2015.

[8] J. Pemán, M. Salavert, E. Cantón et al., "Voriconazole in the management of nosocomial invasive fungal infections," *Therapeutics and Clinical Risk Management*, vol. 2, no. 2, pp. 129–158, 2006.

[9] V. Pothula and D. J. Krellenstein, "Early aggressive surgical management of parapneumonic empeymas," *Chest*, vol. 105, no. 3, pp. 832–836, 1994.

[10] A. Cascio, M. Barone, V. Micali et al., "On a fatal case of *Candida krusei* pleural empiema in a pregnant woman with spontaneous esophageal perforation," *Mycopatholgia*, vol. 169, no. 6, pp. 451–455, 2010.

[11] V. K. Srinivasnakshatri, P. Subramani, K. N. Venkateshwaraprasad, and P. Varma, "A fatal case of fungal empeyma due to *Candida krusei* and *Candida tropicalis*: a rare occurrence with an atypical presentation," *Journal of Clinical and Diagnostic Research*, vol. 8, no. 11, pp. DD01–DD02, 2014.

Add-On Therapy with Ertapenem in Infections with Multidrug Resistant Gram-Negative Bacteria: Pediatric Experience

Sevgen Tanır Basaranoglu, Yasemin Ozsurekci, Kubra Aykac, Kamile Oktay Arıkan, Ayse Buyukcam, Ali Bulent Cengiz, Mehmet Ceyhan, and Ates Kara

Pediatric Infectious Disease Department, İhsan Doğramacı Children's Hospital, Hacettepe University, Ankara, Turkey

Correspondence should be addressed to Sevgen Tanır Basaranoglu; sevgent@gmail.com

Academic Editor: Alexandre Rodrigues Marra

Optimal therapy for infections with carbapenem resistant GNB is not well established due to the weakness of data. Patients presenting with bloodstream infections caused by multidrug resistant *Klebsiella pneumoniae* were treated with a combination treatment. Optimal therapy for infections with carbapenem resistant Gram-negative bacteria is a serious problem in pediatric patients. We presented three cases who were successfully treated with addition of ertapenem to the combination treatment for bacteremia with multidrug resistant *Klebsiella pneumoniae*. Dual carbapenem treatment approach is a new approach for these infections and requires more data in children.

1. Introduction

The emergence of multidrug resistant (MDR) Gram-negative bacteria (GNB) poses a significant threat for global public health because of the limited therapeutic options for treatment. Optimal therapy for infections with carbapenem resistant GNB is not well established [1], while increasing amount of evidence suggests that combination therapy is more effective than monotherapy. In addition, promising novel agents are under development for MDR-GNB, such as ceftazidime-avibactam. This paper presents three pediatric cases of MDR-GNB infection successfully treated with dual carbapenem for bacteremia caused by MDR-GNB.

2. Case 1

A three-month-old male was admitted with chronic diarrhea and a diagnosis of infantile hemochromatosis. He was hospitalized for investigational studies for the underlying condition. In the follow-up, he exhibited fever, as well as signs and symptoms of sepsis. He had to be transferred to the pediatric intensive care unit (PICU). A blood culture performed at the beginning of the fever revealed MDR *Klebsiella pneumoniae* (*K. pneumoniae*) (Table 1). Because the bacteria displayed a multidrug resistant profile, meropenem and ciprofloxacin were commenced (Figure 1). On the following day, tigecycline was added. On the fourth day of treatment, when the control blood culture was still positive for *K. pneumoniae*, ertapenem was added to the combination. The blood culture was negative on the 11th day of ertapenem treatment, and the patient clinically improved. All treatment was ceased on the 22nd day of ertapenem treatment (Figure 1).

3. Case 2

The second case was a three-year-old female patient who had been followed up in the PICU after corrective cardiac surgery for tetralogy of Fallot. She was on mechanical ventilation with a central venous catheter. She had been on meropenem, ciprofloxacin, and vancomycin treatment for systemic inflammatory response syndrome postoperatively when MDR *K. pneumoniae* resulted in both peripheral and catheter-driven blood cultures (Table 1). Her central venous catheter was removed, and a new one was placed into another location. Since the microorganism displayed colistin susceptibility, colistin was added on the fourth day due to

Table 1: Demographic characteristics of patients and features of resistant microorganisms.

	Age	Underlying diagnosis	Clinical syndrome	Site of cultivation	Microorganism	Antibiotic sensitivity profile				
						MPM/MIC	ERT/MIC	AMK/MIC	CPR/MIC	TGC/MIC
Case 1	3 moa	Infantile hemochromatosis	Bacteremia	Blood culture	*Klebsiella pneumoniae*	R/>6	R/>8	IR/16	R/>2	S/1
Case 2	3 yoa	Operated tetralogy of Fallot	Bacteremia	Blood culture	*Klebsiella pneumoniae*	R/>32	R/>32	R/>64	R/>4	R/>2
Case 3	8 moa	Primary hemophagocytic syndrome (after bone marrow transplantation)	Bacteremia	Blood culture	*Klebsiella pneumoniae*	R/>32	R/>32	R/>64	R/>4	S/2

MPM: meropenem; ERT: ertapenem; AMK: amikacin; TGC: tigecycline; CPR: ciprofloxacin; R: resistant; S: sensitive; IR: intermediate resistance; MIC: minimum inhibitory concentration (mg/L); yoa: years of age; moa: months of age.

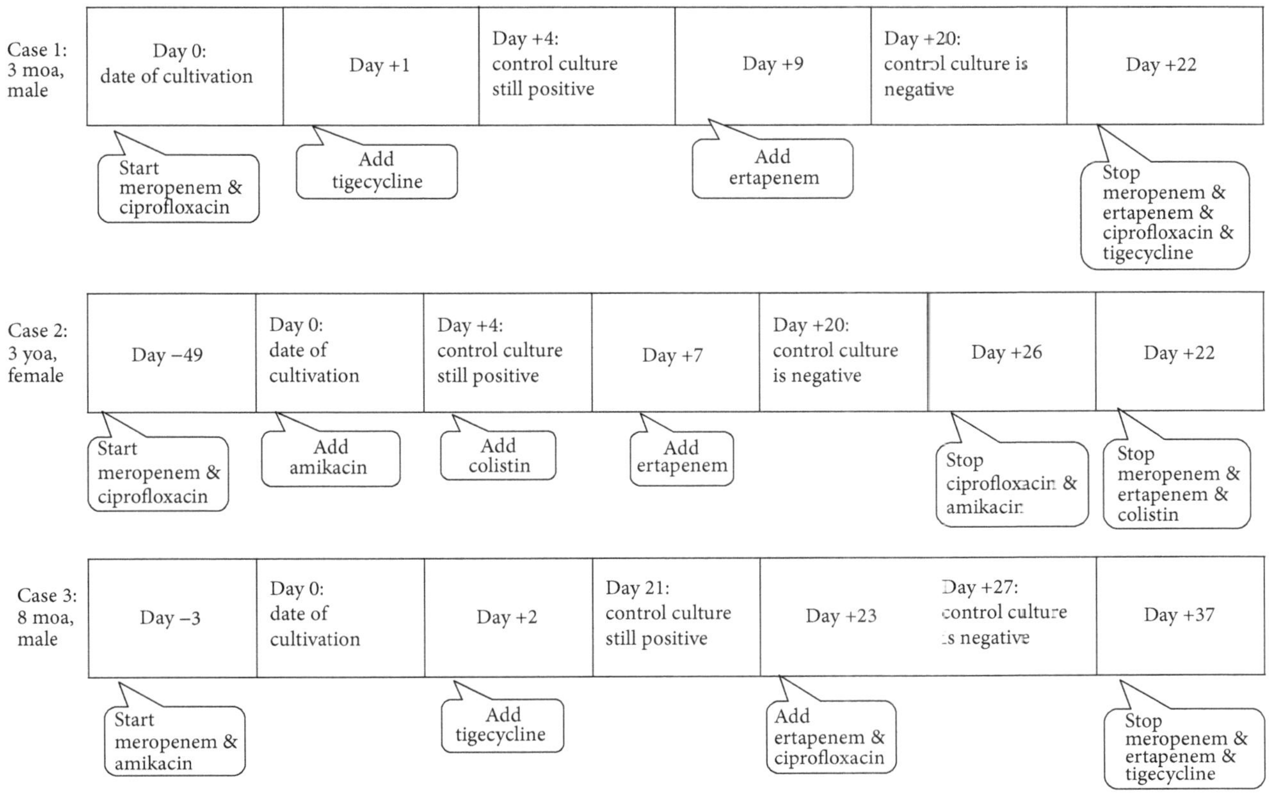

FIGURE 1: Timeline of treatment for Gram-negative bacteria and follow-up. *Dosages of Drugs.* Meropenem: 20–40 mg/kg every 8 hours; ciprofloxacin: 6–8 mg/kg every 8 hours; tigecycline: 1–1.5 mg/kg every 12 hours; ertapenem: 15 mg/kg every 12 hours; amikacin: 15 mg/kg every 24 hours; colistin: 2.5–5 mg/kg/day in 3 divided doses.

ongoing positive blood culture (Figure 1). On the seventh day, the patient was still bacteremic; therefore, ertapenem was commenced in addition to meropenem, ciprofloxacin, amikacin, and colistin. A control blood culture was negative on the fourth day of the dual carbapenem regimen. Complete recovery from infection was achieved on the 25th day of ertapenem treatment.

4. Case 3

An eight-month-old male was diagnosed with primary hemophagocytic lymphohistiocytosis, and he had undergone bone marrow transplantation after chemotherapeutics. In the first month of transplantation, while he was waiting for bone marrow recovery and was on the third day of meropenem and amikacin treatments because of the suspicion of catheter-associated bloodstream infection (CRBSI), he developed a fever. MDR *K. pneumoniae* was isolated both from a culture of peripheral blood and from a culture of blood from the central venous catheter (Table 1). His central venous catheter was removed, and a new one was placed into another central vein. Although tigecycline was added based on the patient's susceptibility profile in light of the CRBSI, blood culture was still positive for the microorganism on the 21st day. Ertapenem was started on the 23rd day of cultivation. On the fourth day of dual treatment, a negative blood culture was achieved. Treatment against GNB was successfully stopped on the 37th day (Figure 1).

5. Discussion

To the best of our knowledge, these are the first reported pediatric cases with bacteremia caused by carbapenemase-producing *K. pneumoniae* and successfully treated with a double-carbapenem regimen. GNBs are becoming increasingly nonsusceptible to carbapenems, due to the acquisition of new resistance mechanisms, usually accompanied by resistance to all β-lactam agents and often to many other classes, such as quinolones and aminoglycosides. Furthermore, treatment options for these microorganisms are extremely limited, and no consensus has been established for their management [1, 2]. In the context of infections with these microorganisms—especially those resistant to carbapenems—the role of double-carbapenem regimens containing ertapenem has been previously reviewed [3–5]. Ertapenem is used as an indicator of the expression of carbapenemases, resulting from the ease of hydrolysis compared to other members of the group. Because carbapenemases have an increased affinity for ertapenem, it is believed to be the least active agent against carbapenemase-producing *K.*

pneumoniae, and it behaves like a suicide substrate [6–8]. This belief is the rationale for the use of combination carbapenem therapy.

The mainstay of therapy for patients with bacteremia remains antimicrobial therapy, together with optimal management of the consequences, including treatment of shock and surgical treatment of infection sites, such as drainage of abscesses and removal of intravascular devices. In our cases, in addition to arrangement of combinations of antimicrobial agents, replacement of central venous catheters into other veins may have contributed to the successful results.

Our institution cares for clinically high-risk patient groups, including those suffering from primary immunodeficiencies, hematologic/oncologic malignancies, and many chronic conditions requiring long hospital stays. The possibility of encountering MDR-GNB in these patients is ever-increasing, and the situation necessitates new therapy options. For the present pediatric cases, a combination of ertapenem with meropenem, despite individual resistance to both, was a successful choice. However, larger studies are required in order to lighten the consequences of this therapy.

References

[1] R. R. Watkins and S. Deresinski, "Is combination therapy for carbapenem-resistant Klebsiella pneumoniae the new standard of care?" *Expert Review of Anti-Infective Therapy*, vol. 13, no. 4, pp. 405–407, 2015.

[2] H. W. Boucher, G. H. Talbot, J. S. Bradley et al., "Bad bugs, no drugs: no ESKAPE! An update from the Infectious Diseases Society of America," *Clinical Infectious Diseases*, vol. 48, no. 1, pp. 1–12, 2009.

[3] G. Ceccarelli, M. Falcone, A. Giordano et al., "Successful ertapenem-doripenem combination treatment of bacteremic ventilator-associated pneumonia due to colistin-resistant KPC-producing Klebsiella pneumoniae," *Antimicrobial Agents and Chemotherapy*, vol. 57, no. 6, pp. 2900-2901, 2013.

[4] G. L. Daikos and A. Markogiannakis, "Carbapenemase-producing Klebsiella pneumoniae: (When) might we still consider treating with carbapenems?" *Clinical Microbiology and Infection*, vol. 17, no. 8, pp. 1135–1141, 2011.

[5] Z. A. Qureshi, D. L. Paterson, B. A. Potoski et al., "Treatment outcome of bacteremia due to KPC-producing *Klebsiella pneumoniae*: superiority of combination antimicrobial regimens," *Antimicrobial Agents and Chemotherapy*, vol. 56, no. 4, pp. 2108–2113, 2012.

[6] C. C. Bulik and D. P. Nicolau, "Double-carbapenem therapy for carbapenemase-producing Klebsiella pneumoniae," *Antimicrobial Agents and Chemotherapy*, vol. 55, no. 6, pp. 3002–3004, 2011.

[7] A. Oliva, A. D'Abramo, C. D'Agostino et al., "Synergistic activity and effectiveness of a double-carbapenem regimen in pandrug-resistant Klebsiella pneumoniae bloodstream infections," *Journal of Antimicrobial Chemotherapy*, vol. 69, no. 6, pp. 1718–1720, 2014.

[8] K. S. Thomson, "Double-carbapenem therapy not proven to be more active than carbapenem monotherapy against KPC-positive Klebsiella pneumoniae," *Antimicrobial Agents and Chemotherapy*, vol. 56, no. 7, p. 4037, 2012.

40

Massive Haemoptysis due to Obscure Aetiology: Perils and Management Dilemmas

A. Shreenivasa,[1] K. A. Vishak,[2] K. Sindhu,[1] Kauslya Sahu,[3] and G. V. Chaithra[4]

[1]*Senior Resident, Department of Pulmonary Medicine, KMC Mangalore, MAHE University, Udupi, India*
[2]*Professor, Department of Pulmonary Medicine, KMC Mangalore, MAHE University, Udupi, India*
[3]*Professor, Department of Pathology, KMC Mangalore, MAHE University, Udupi, India*
[4]*Assistant Professor, Department of Pathology, KMC Mangalore, MAHE University, Udupi, India*

Correspondence should be addressed to A. Shreenivasa; shreenivasa.a@manipal.edu

Academic Editor: Tomoyuki Shibata

Pulmonary actinomycosis is an important differential diagnosis in patients with long-standing pulmonary infiltrates related to poor oral hygiene or compromised immune function. Up to a quarter of cases of thoracic actinomycosis are misdiagnosed as lung malignancy. Here, we report a 56-year-old man with a hypodense lesion in the left lower lobe presenting with recurrent massive haemoptysis for about one year. He underwent left lower lobe lobectomy due to intractable haemoptysis. Histopathological examination demonstrated actinomycosis infiltrating the left lower lobe. Rarity of the case was the presence of actinomycosis in an immunocompetent individual and without underlying preexisting lung disease. Also, intractable massive haemoptysis necessitating surgical excision which proved to be both diagnostic and curative due to actinomycosis is an unusual occurrence.

1. Background

Actinomycosis is an uncommon, chronic, and slowly progressive bacterial infection caused by *Gram-positive anaerobic bacteria*, belonging to the family Actinomycetaceae [1]. In humans, actinomycosis is associated with suppurative and granulomatous inflammation characterized by swelling, sinus tract formation, and purulent discharge containing yellowish sulfur granules [2]. Pulmonary actinomycosis accounts for 15–20% total incidence of actinomycosis [3]. Actinomyces are thought to colonize devitalized tissues; thus, higher incidence of pulmonary actinomycosis has been reported in patients with underlying lung disorders, such as emphysema, chronic bronchitis, and bronchiectasis [4].

Pulmonary actinomycosis is caused by aspiration of oropharyngeal or gastrointestinal secretions into the respiratory tract. Pulmonary actinomycosis usually presents with chest pain, productive cough, and dyspnea [5]. Pulmonary actinomycosis is rarely included in the differential diagnosis of a patient with pulmonary infiltrates [6], with most patients being investigated for other possible diseases, before the final diagnosis is made.

2. Case Report

A 53-year-old male, smoker (20 pack-years), occasional alcoholic, presented with complaints of blood expectoration of 400 ml in one episode followed by 100–150 ml for 2–3 days. He had 3 episodes of similar history which required hospitalizations and emergency care since 9 months. He denied history of fever, chest pain, and loss of appetite. He underwent cholecystectomy 3 years ago. There was no history of systemic immune suppression like diabetes. He had undergone bronchial artery embolization for massive haemoptysis; however, his haemoptysis persisted and diagnosis remained elusive after evaluation with sputum studies and CT-guided aspiration cytology, biopsy, and bronchoscopic lavage. He was treated for LRTI with multiple courses of antibiotics for more than 9 months.

On examination, vitals were normal with no respiratory distress. Oral hygiene was poor with dental caries. Respiratory examination revealed scattered crackles in the left lower lobe area. Chest X-ray showed an inhomogeneous opacity in the left lower zone with raised left diaphragm (Figure 1), and CECT (contrast-enhanced computer tomogram) chest showed a hypodense lesion with irregular margins in the anterior segment of the left lower lobe adjacent to the descending aorta and associated subcarinal lymphadenopathy (Figures 2 and 3). Image-guided transthoracic biopsy showed type 2 alveolar cell hyperplasia with negative immunohistochemistry. Bronchoscopy confirmed left lower lobe bleed with any endoluminal lesion. Bronchial wash was negative for microbiological and cytological studies including AFB stain, geneXpert for MTB complex, and pyogenic culture. Patient's symptoms of haemoptysis persisted; hence, CT angiogram was performed, which showed dilated vascular channels within the lesion without any obvious extravasations of contrast and no aortic abnormality.

Probable diagnosis of the left intrapulmonary vascular lesion was made and hence the patient underwent left lower lobe lobectomy. Intraoperatively, the left lower lobe was adherent posterolaterally to the aorta and diaphragm. Multiple prominent blood vessels in areas of adhesion were seen. Histopathology was suggestive of chronic inflammatory cells with focal aggregates of lymphocytes with positive GMS staining for actinomycosis (Figure 4). Postoperatively, the patient received parenteral benzylpenicillin 20 lakh units 6th hourly for 3 months. The patient was in regular follow-up, and no further episodes of haemoptysis and no recent respiratory complaints are reported.

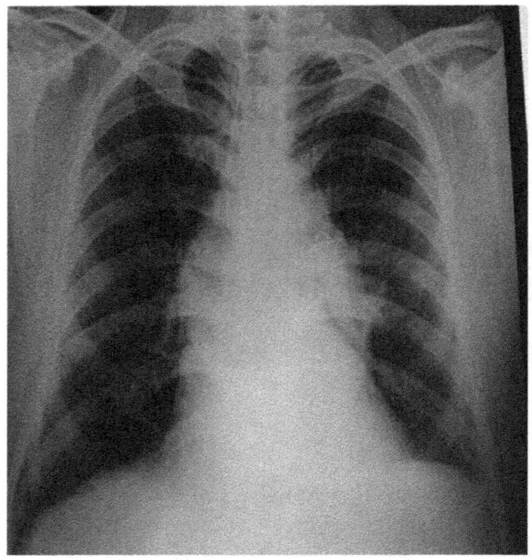

FIGURE 1: Chest X-ray revealed raised left hemidiaphragm and left midzone opacity, creating a positive silhouette sign with the left cardiac border.

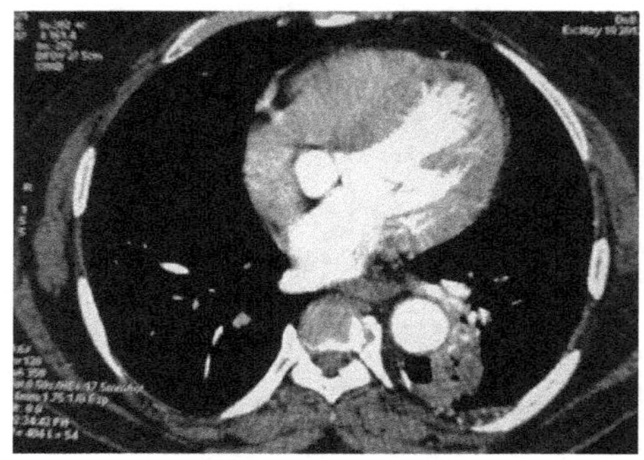

FIGURE 2: Irregular margin air space consolidation with cavitations seen in the left anterior segment adjacent to descending aorta.

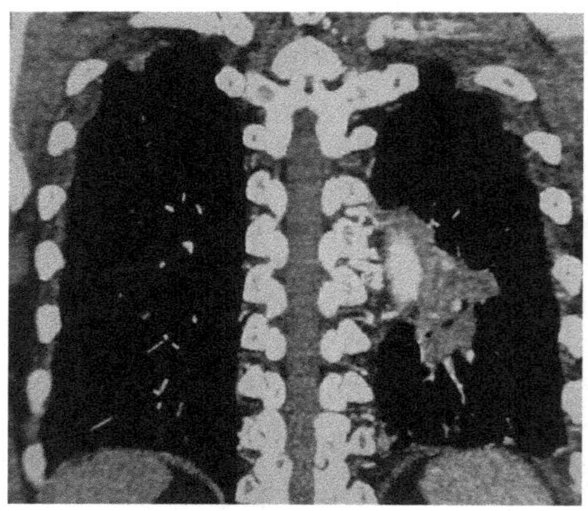

FIGURE 3: An irregular mass is seen on the left lower lobe adjacent to aorta with pleural involvement.

3. Discussion

Pulmonary actinomycosis is seen at all ages, commonly in adults and peak incidence described in the 4th and 5th decades [7]. In recent years, with the improvement in oral hygiene and early use of antibiotics, the presentation of pulmonary actinomycosis has changed from aggressive to less aggressive, making diagnosis more difficult [8]. Clinical manifestations of pulmonary actinomycosis are variable although cough and sputum are the most common symptoms [9]. Haemoptysis, although not common, has been reported often in pulmonary actinomycosis [2] and may be explained by the underlying structural diseases such as bronchiectasis. The disease usually affects the lower lobe [10], probably reflecting the role of aspiration in its pathogenesis. Pulmonary actinomycosis is usually characterized by a fibrotic lesion that is slowly progressive through the anatomical barriers which is often confused with malignancy [1].

Pulmonary actinomycosis shares many similar clinical features with chronic suppurative lung infections such as tuberculosis, fungal infections, and lung abscesses and also lung malignancy with which it is frequently confused [4]. Culture of bacteria from the sputum or bronchoalveolar secretions is technically difficult [11], and sometimes it also represents colonization of nonpathological microorganisms [12]. To confirm the diagnosis of pulmonary actinomycosis, lung biopsy is usually required [10].

Pulmonary actinomycosis may present as masses, nodules, patchy infiltrates, and solitary lesions [8]. A CT chest or ultrasound-guided biopsy is usually recommended

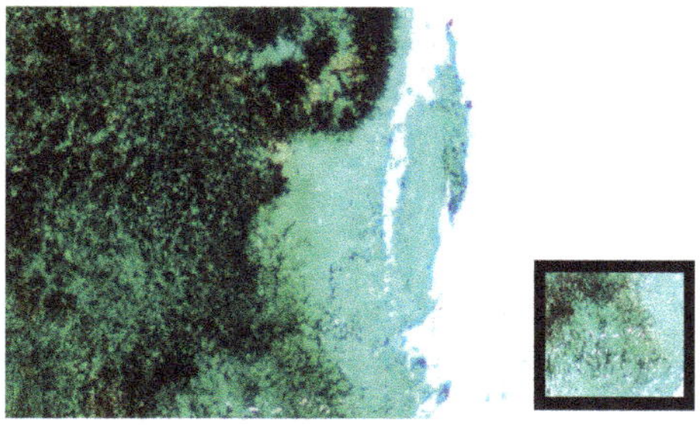

FIGURE 4: GMS stain highlighting delicate branched filaments.

prior to the surgical biopsy. However, the CT-guided biopsies may not be diagnostic as reported in our case. There could also be a case for percutaneous aspirated abscess to be sent for cultures routinely along with cytology to improve diagnostic accuracy. Thus, the gold standard for diagnosis of thoracic actinomycosis is a histological confirmation on lung biopsy.

Most cases of pulmonary actinomycosis have been diagnosed from postsurgical specimens taken on suspicion of lung cancer [1] as done in our case. Inadvertent use of antibiotics and nonspecific clinical presentations make pulmonary actinomycosis difficult to be diagnosed and often lead to misdiagnosis as malignancy rather than an infective disease [13]. Coexistence of lung cancer with pulmonary actinomycosis results in diagnostic challenge [14]. Reduction of alcohol abuse and improvement of dental hygiene may limit the occurrence of pulmonary actinomycosis [1] and require prolonged high-dose antimicrobial therapy with beta-lactam antibiotics for about 6–12 months [1].

In conclusion, this case is remarkable not only for the development of pulmonary actinomycosis in an immunocompetent patient but also for associated recurrent massive haemoptysis which eluded diagnosis and finally resection surgery confirmed the diagnosis and was also curative.

References

[1] F. Valour, A. Sénéchal, C. Dupieux et al., "Actinomycosis: etiology, clinical features, diagnosis, treatment and management," *Infection and Drug Resistance*, vol. 7, pp. 183–197, 2014.

[2] S. R. Kim, L. Y. Jung, I. J. Oh et al., "Pulmonary actinomycosis during the first decade of 21st century: cases of 94 patients," *BMC Infectious Diseases*, vol. 13, no. 1, p. 216, 2013.

[3] V. K. Wong, T. D. Turmezei, and V. C. Weston, "Actinomycosis," *BMJ*, vol. 343, article d6099, 2011.

[4] G. F. Mabeza and J. Macfarlane, "Pulmonary actinomycosis," *European Respiratory Journal*, vol. 21, no. 3, pp. 545–551, 2003.

[5] T. S. Kim, J. Han, W. J. Koh et al., "Thoracic actinomycosis: CT features with histopathologic correlation," *American Journal of Roentgenology*, vol. 186, no. 1, pp. 225–231, 2006.

[6] T. M. Alfaro, J. Bernardo, and H. Garcia, "Organizing pneumonia due to actinomycosis: an undescribed association," *Respiration*, vol. 81, no. 5, pp. 433–436, 2011.

[7] J. E. Heffner, "Pleuropulmonary manifestations of actinomycosis and nocardiosis," *Seminars in Respiratory Infections*, vol. 3, no. 4, pp. 352–361, 1988.

[8] X.-F. Sun, P. Wang, H.-R. Liu, and Ju-H. Shi, "A retrospective study of pulmonary actinomycosis in a single institution in China," *Chinese Medical Journal*, vol. 128, no. 12, 2015.

[9] J. S. Kwong, N. L. Muller, J. D. Godwin, D. Aberle, and M. R. Grymaloski, "Thoracic actinomycosis: CT findings in eight patients," *Radiology*, vol. 183, no. 1, pp. 189–192, 1992.

[10] F. Ahmed, R. Teoh, J. Kastelik, A. Campbell, and D. McGivern, "Case series of thoracic actinomycosis presenting as a diagnostic challenge," *Respiratory Medicine CME*, vol. 2, no. 1, pp. 47–50, 2009.

[11] R. H. Wong, A. D. Sihoe, K. H. Thung, I. Y. Wan, M. B. Ip, and A. P. Yim, "Actinomycosis: an often forgotten diagnosis," *Asian Cardiovascular and Thoracic Annals*, vol. 12, no. 2, pp. 165–7, 2004.

[12] I. Ariel, R. Breuer, N. S. Kamal, I. Ben-Dov, and P. Mogel, "RosenmannE Endobronchialactinomycosis simulating bronchogenic carcinoma. Diagnosis by bronchial biopsy," *Chest*, vol. 99, no. 2, pp. 493–495, 1991.

[13] L. Qiu, L. Lan, Y. Feng, Z. Huang, and Y. Chen, "Pulmonary actinomycosis imitating lung cancer on ^{18}F-FDG PET/CT: a case report and literature review," *Korean Journal of Radiology*, vol. 16, no. 6, pp. 1262–1265, 2015.

[14] F. Charif, A. Harb, M. Alfano et al., "Bronchial carcinoma and actinomycosis: a dangerous trap," *Revue des Maladies Respiratoires*, vol. 26, no. 9, pp. 1003–1006, 2009.

41

Presentation of Ocular Syphilis in a HIV-Positive Patient with False-Negative Serologic Screening

Mahsaw N. Motlagh [1] **and Cameron G. Javid** [2]

[1] *University of Arizona College of Medicine, Tucson, AZ, USA*
[2] *Department of Ophthalmology, University of Arizona College of Medicine, Tucson, AZ, USA*

Correspondence should be addressed to Mahsaw N. Motlagh; motlaghm@email.arizona.edu

Academic Editor: Paola Di Carlo

Purpose. The ocular sequelae of syphilis are devastating and may cause blindness. The ambiguous nature of its ocular manifestations makes syphilis difficult to detect. Though uncommon, the rise of syphilis in the United States requires a renewed understanding of its ophthalmic presentation to prevent devastating outcomes. We present this case to raise awareness for the increasing prevalence of ocular syphilis and appropriate serologic testing. *Observations.* We describe a 65-year-old HIV-positive male with worsening retinitis, uveitis, and rapid visual loss. Initial lab results showed a nonreactive rapid plasma reagin (RPR) for syphilis. However, subsequent *Treponema pallidum* antibody testing was positive 48 hours after initial false-negative serologic screening. The patient had a rapid and successful recovery following treatment with penicillin. *Conclusions and Importance.* The incidence of syphilis is on the rise once again, and patients living with HIV are at increased risk. Ocular syphilis should be considered in susceptible populations in the clinical setting of retinitis, uveitis, and worsening visual loss with unknown cause. In addition, retesting for syphilis will decrease the prevalence of false-negative results, especially in patients with high clinical suspicion.

1. Introduction

Syphilis has a notorious reputation as the great masquerader. Caused by the spirochete bacterium *Treponema pallidum*, syphilis has a myriad of typical and atypical presentations. With syphilis rates on the rise in the United States, it is important to be aware of ocular symptoms [1]. In this case, described below, a 65-year-old HIV-positive male presents with worsening visual loss and a negative RPR. Furthermore, the repeated testing for treponemal antibodies was positive, promoting the importance of repeat testing in patients with high clinical suspicion.

2. Case Report

A 65-year-old male with a past medical history positive for HIV was referred for ophthalmic consultation for new onset flashes and floaters in the left eye. The patient also reported decreased and blurry vision in the left eye. At the initial time of presentation, the visual acuity test revealed 20/20 in the right eye and 20/50 in the left eye. Optical coherence tomography (OCT) findings were unremarkable (Figure 1(a)). Fluorescein angiography (FA) revealed focal hyperfluorescence in the right eye and vasculitis in the left eye (Figure 1(b)). Fundus photography was unremarkable for the right eye but revealed peripheral retinitis, slight disc edema, and 2+ vitritis in the left eye (Figure 1(c)). The patient's CD4 count was >600 cells/mm^3, and viral load was undetectable. At this point, the clinical presentation suggested acute retinal necrosis (ARN), and a sample of anterior fluid was sent to be analyzed for varicella-zoster virus (VZV), herpes simplex virus (HSV), and cytomegalovirus (CMV). The patient was started on prophylactic valacyclovir and requested for follow-up in 2 days.

Forty-eight hours later, the patient's visual acuity had decreased to 20/60 in the left eye, but no changes were noted

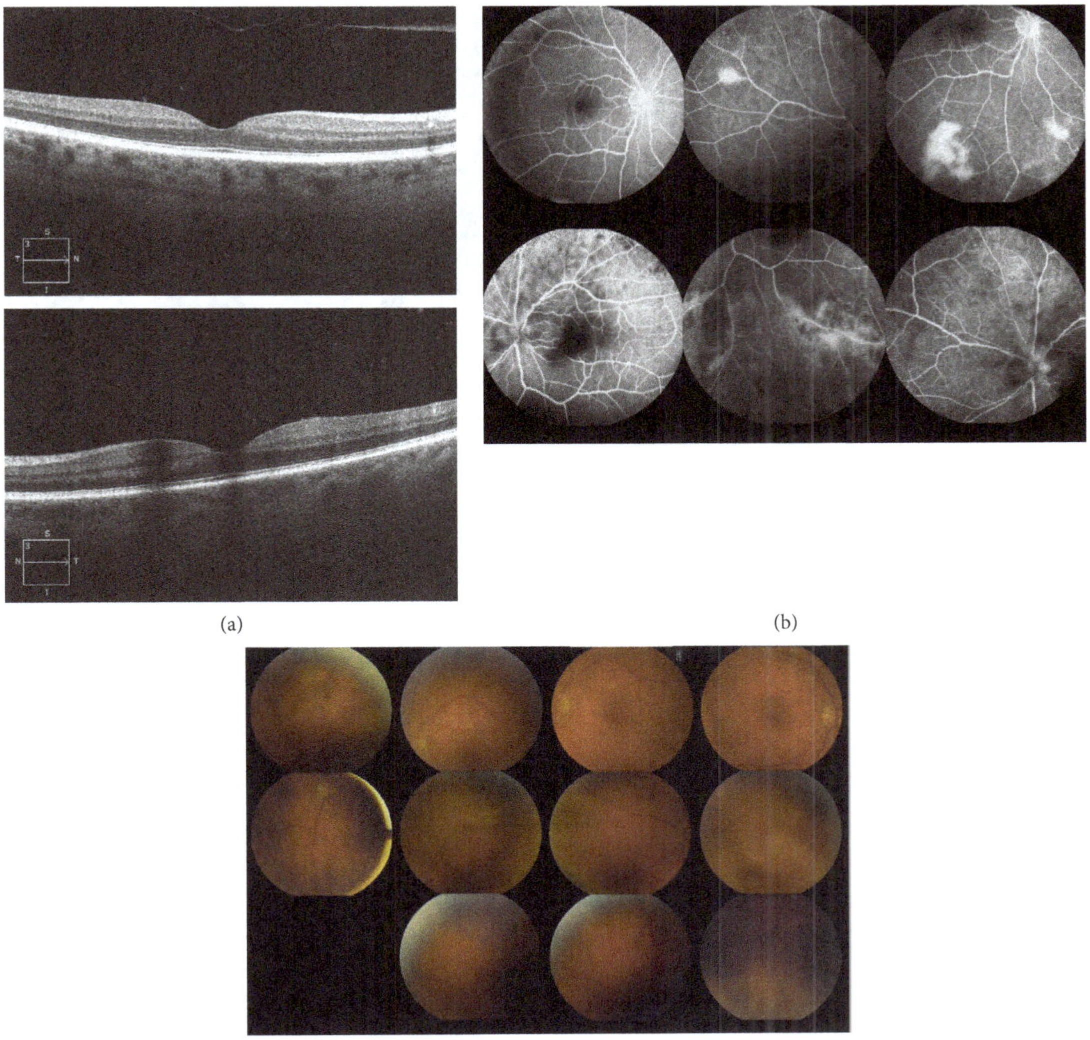

(a) (b) (c)

FIGURE 1: Baseline imaging results. (a) Optical coherence tomography upon initial presentation was unremarkable. (b) Fluorescein angiography at the first visit revealed focal hyperfluorescence inferior to the optic nerve in the right eye (*top*) and vasculitis of the inferotemporal vessels in the left eye (*bottom*). (c) Fundus photos upon initial presentation. Normal retinal vessels in the right eye. Peripheral retinitis with white yellow necrotic retina and slight disc edema in the left eye.

in the right eye. The remainder of the physical exam was unremarkable, and the patient was again scheduled for follow-up one week later.

The following week, just 8 days after initial presentation, the patient presented with dramatically worsened vision. His acuity was still preserved in the right eye at 20/25 but had decreased to 20/200 in the left eye. The concern grew stronger as the PCR results returned negative for HSV-1, HSV-2, VZV, and CMV. Despite worsened visual acuity on exam, the patient's vitritis and retinitis improved, further complicating the case. Given this clinical picture, the patient was started on 30 mg prednisone daily in addition to the previously prescribed valacyclovir. The patient was then requested for follow-up appointment in 2 weeks.

At the next follow-up visit, 20 days after initial presentation, it was apparent that the patient's ophthalmologic condition was progressively worsening. Visual acuity in the right eye was now decreased to 20/150. In the left eye, the patient could only recognize hand motion. Expectedly, OCT, FA, and fundus views were all limited in the left eye due to worsening of the vitreous debris (Figure 2). From limited views, physical exam revealed 1+ vitritis in the right eye and 4+ vitritis in the left eye (Figure 2(c)). FA of the right eye showed retinitis superiorly and inferiorly, which extended into the macula (Figure 2(b)). Both eyes were affected by posterior uveitis. Despite the worsening condition of the patient, serum testing obtained by the referring infectious disease specialist was all unremarkable. This included a nonreactive RPR screen with reflex titer for syphilis. At this point, it was discussed with the patient that visual prognosis was considered extremely poor. Even with the negative screening results from the referring physician, there was still

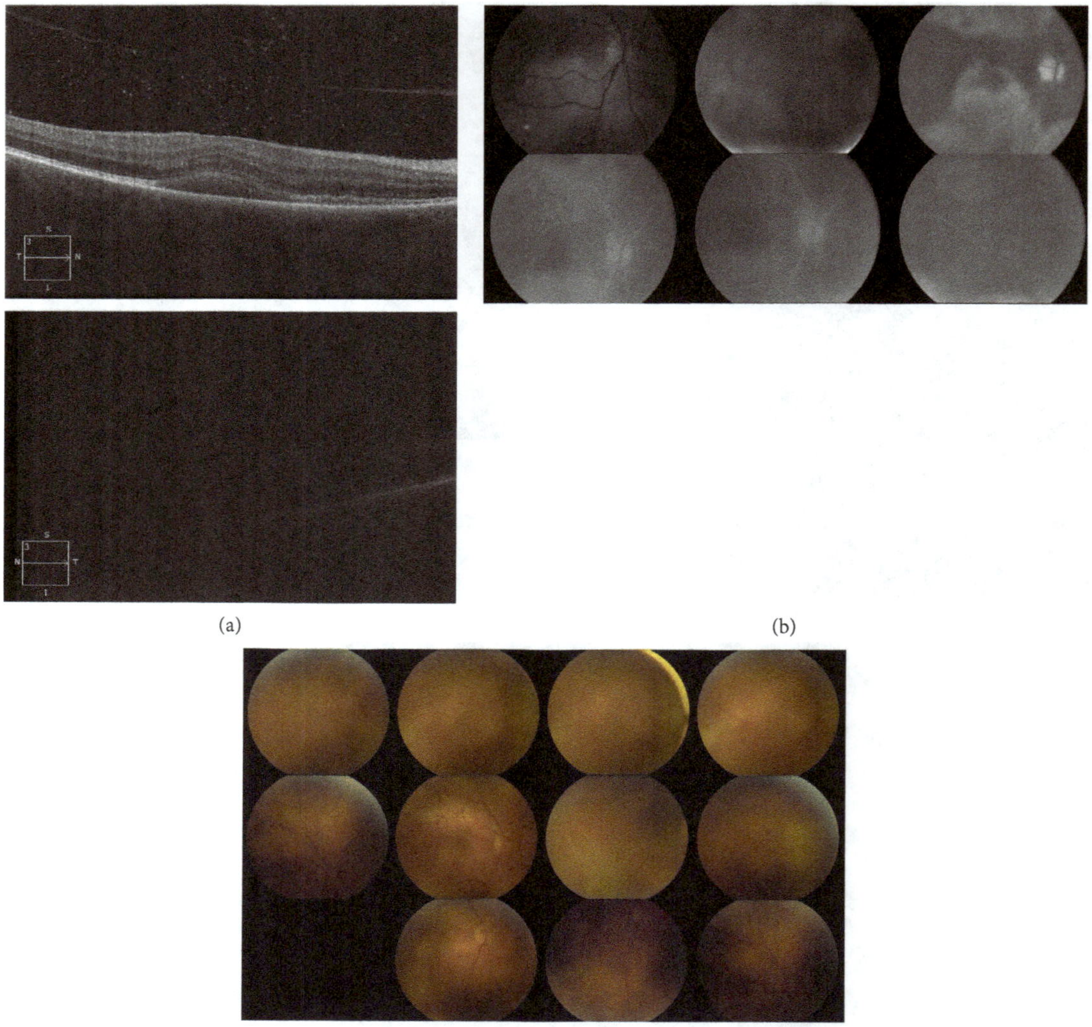

(a) (b) (c)

Figure 2: Imaging results 21 days after initial presentation. (a) Optical coherence tomography of the right eye (*top*) showed vitreous debris with no evidence of subretinal fluid. The view of the left eye (*bottom*) was limited due to heavy vitreous debris. (b) Fluorescein angiography following visual decline. There are marked retinitis and vitreous debris in the right eye (*top*) and limited views due to heavy vitreous debris in the left eye (*bottom*). (c) Fundus photos revealed vitreous debris with 1+ vitritis and peripheral retinitis in the right eye. Heavy vitreous debris with 4+ vitritis causing limited views in the left eye.

suspicion for syphilis as the patient was at considerable risk. It is well known that a nonreactive RPR test does not rule out syphilis infection; therefore, it was decided to repeat serologic testing. However, this time, the patient was tested using the alternative serologic screening algorithm for syphilis, which tests directly for treponemal antibodies (Figure 3) [2, 3].

Follow-up testing with the alternative method was reactive. Additionally, the RPR titer was now high, confirming the diagnosis of syphilis (Table 1). The patient was admitted on the same day for treatment with IV penicillin. The patient's vision dramatically improved, and he was discharged the following day on a 14-day course of penicillin. At one-week after treatment, the patient's acuity had progressed to 20/40 with pinhole improvement to 20/30 in the right eye and 20/50 with pinhole improvement to 20/30 in the left eye. A summary of the patient's visual acuity decline and subsequent improvement following treatment are found in Table 2. The repeat RPR testing promoted the significance of understanding the available serologic tests for syphilis. Had an antibody test been ordered initially, it likely would have yielded positive results. In addition, if repeat testing was not conducted for RPR, the diagnosis for this patient with extremely poor prognosis would have been delayed, potentially resulting in blindness. The aggressive nature of ocular syphilis is unforgiving, but with a quick and accurate diagnostic tool, simple treatment with IV penicillin yields excellent outcomes (Table 2).

3. Discussion

Syphilitic uveitis remains a rare condition in the United States [5]. However, in conjunction with the continued

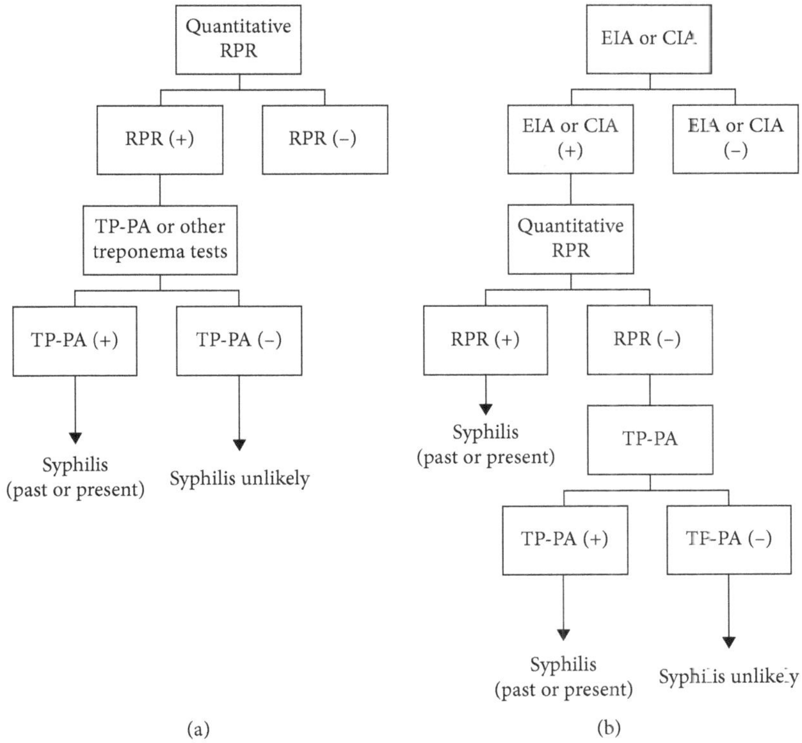

FIGURE 3: Syphilis screening algorithms. Traditional serologic screening (a) compared to reverse sequence serologic screening (b). Screening algorithms adopted from CDC recommendations [3, 4]. RPR, rapid plasma reagin; TP-PA, *Treponema pallidum* particle agglutination; EIA, enzyme immunoassay; CIA, chemiluminescence immunoassay.

TABLE 1: Serologic screening results. Upon initial presentation, the traditional testing algorithm was utilized. However, at the time of follow-up (secondary results), the alternative testing algorithm was followed.

Serologic test	Initial test results	Secondary test results (48 hours later)	Reference ranges
RPR screen	Nonreactive	Reactive	Nonreactive
RPR titer	Nonreactive	1 : 512	Nonreactive
Syphilis antibody total	N/A	6.8	≤0.8
Syphilis antibody result	N/A	Reactive	Nonreactive
Treponema pallidum antibody	N/A	Reactive	Nonreactive

RPR, rapid plasma reagin.

TABLE 2: Summary of visual acuity decline.

Date	OD	OS
Initial consult (day = 0)	20/20	20/50
Follow-up 1 (day = 2)	20/20	20/60
Follow-up 2 (day = 8)	20/25	20/200
Follow-up 3 (day = 20)	20/25	20/400
Follow-up 4 (day = 21)	20/150	20/400
Follow-up 5 (day = 41)	20/40 PH 20/30	20/50 PH 20/30

increase in prevalence, it is imperative to remain aware of the ophthalmic diseases associated with syphilis [1, 6]. Uveitis is the most common ophthalmologic presentation of syphilis and can appear at any course of the disease [7, 8]. The diagnosis of ocular syphilis should be considered in any patient with unexplained uveitis or vision loss, especially in patients with comorbid risk factors such as HIV and men who have sex with men [9]. The prognosis of this rare complication of syphilis, if left untreated, is extremely poor and can lead to complete vision loss [10, 11]. Thus, in consideration of the above, we recommend setting a low threshold for considering syphilitic uveitis in high-risk populations.

More notably, this case in particular promotes the importance of considering a false-negative screening result. For a patient with high clinical suspicion of syphilis, retesting is warranted. Though long-held practice recommends serologic screening with a nontreponemal test, most commonly RPR or Venereal Diseases Research Laboratory (VRDL) test, followed by confirmatory treponemal testing, it may be time to consider an alternative screening algorithm as the standard of care. In fact, many laboratories have begun adopting a reverse sequence of screening, in which a treponemal enzyme and chemiluminescence immunoassay (EIA/CIA) is used first, followed by a nontreponemal test for confirmation (Figure 3) [3]. This would gradually eliminate the need for repeat testing, as the treponemal antibody testing has no false-negative results [3]. This paradigm shift requires better understanding from the clinician of the serologic screening that is available.

The RPR test does not measure the bacterium directly, but instead measures antibodies to lipoidal material released from damaged host cells [12]. Therefore, the possibility of false-negative results remains plausible during any period within the course of the disease. Moreover, a reactive nontreponemal test does not confirm *Treponema pallidum* infection [12]. This discrepancy, in the context of acute ocular syphilis, warrants the use of an alternate algorithm that seeks the most accurate and precise serologic testing first [3, 13].

4. Summary Statement

A 65-year-old man with HIV developed rapid visual loss with unknown cause. Serologic testing with traditional rapid plasma regain was negative. However, subsequent testing with treponemal antibody testing was positive, indicating initially false-negative results.

Consent

Written consent from this patient was obtained for the publication of this case report.

Disclosure

All authors attest that they meet the current ICMJE criteria for authorship.

References

[1] Centers for Disease Control and Prevention, *Sexually Transmitted Disease Surveillance, 2015*, U.S. Department of Health and Human Services, Atlanta, GA, USA, 2016.

[2] Centers for Disease Control and Prevention, *Sexually Transmitted Diseases Treatment Guidelines, 2015*, U.S. Department of Health and Human Services, Atlanta, GA, USA, 2016.

[3] Centers for Disease, "Control and Prevention, U.S. Department of Health and Human Services, Discordant results from reverse sequence syphilis screening—five laboratories, United States, 2006–2010," *Morbidity and Mortality Weekly Report*, vol. 60, pp. 133–137, 2011.

[4] K Hoover, I Park, and Centers for Disease Control and Prevention, "Reverse sequence syphilis screening: an overview by CDC," July 2017, https://www.cdc.gov/std/syphilis/syphilis-webinar-slides.pdf.

[5] T. Albini, N. F. Callaway, S. Pershing, S. K. Wang, A. A. Moshfeghi, and D. M. Moshfeghi, "Trends in hospitalization and incidence rate for syphilitic uveitis in the United States from 1998 to 2009," *American Journal of Ophthalmology*, vol. 180, pp. 133–141, 2017.

[6] J. R. Chao, R. N. Khurana, A. A. Fawzi, H. S. Reddy, and N. A. Rao, "Syphilis: reemergence of an old adversary," *Ophthalmology*, vol. 113, no. 11, pp. 2074–2079, 2006.

[7] A. J. Aldave, J. A. King, and E. T. Cunningham Jr., "Ocular syphilis," *Current Opinion in Ophthalmology*, vol. 12, no. 6, pp. 433–441, 2001.

[8] R. R. Tamesis and C. S. Foster, "Ocular syphilis," *Ophthalmology*, vol. 97, no. 10, pp. 1281–1287, 1990.

[9] W. E. Abara, K. L. Hess, R. Neblett Fanfair, K. T. Bernstein, and G. Paz-Bailey, "Syphilis trends among men who have sex with men in the United States and western Europe: a systematic review of trend studies published between 2004 and 2015," *PLoS One*, vol. 11, no. 7, Article ID e0159309, 2016.

[10] M. Oette, J. Hemker, T. Feldt, A. Sagir, J. Best, and D. Häussinger, "Case report: acute syphilitic blindness in an HIV-positive patient," *AIDS Patient Care and STDs*, vol. 19, no. 4, pp. 209–211, 2005.

[11] B. C. Amaratunge, J. E. Camuglia, and A. J. Hall, "Syphilitic uveitis: a review of clinical manifestations and treatment outcomes of syphilitic uveitis in human immunodeficiency virus-positive and negative patients," *Clinical & Experimental Ophthalmology*, vol. 38, no. 1, pp. 68–74, 2010.

[12] Centers for Disease Control and Prevention, "Rapid plasma reagin (RPR) 18-mm circle card test," in *Manual of Tests for Syphilis*, U.S. Department of Health and Human Services, Atlanta, GA, USA, 9th edition, 1998.

[13] A. C. Seña, B. L. White, and P. F. Sparling, "NovelTreponema pallidumSerologic tests: a paradigm shift in syphilis screening for the 21st century," *Clinical Infectious Diseases*, vol. 51, no. 6, pp. 700–708, 2010.

Successful Management of Biliary Ascariasis in a High-Endemic Zone and Low-Resource Setting in Ethiopia

Yonathan Aliye Asfaw,[1] Girum Tesfaye Asrat,[1] Tesfanew Bekele Uddo,[2] Bethlehem Aliye Asfaw,[1] Ayush Anand,[3] Helen Huang,[4] Eden Demessie Firew,[5] and NagaSpurthy Reddy Anugu[6]

[1]*University of Gondar Collage of Medicine and Health Sciences, Gondar, Ethiopia*
[2]*Addis Ababa University, Addis Ababa, Ethiopia*
[3]*B.P. Koirala Institute of Health Sciences, Dharan, Nepal*
[4]*Royal Collage of Surgeons in Ireland, Dublin, Ireland*
[5]*Mekelle University, Mek'ele, Ethiopia*
[6]*Mediciti Institute of Medical Sciences, Hyderabad, India*

Correspondence should be addressed to Yonathan Aliye Asfaw; dreaminglatee@gmail.com

Academic Editor: Mohamed A. Dkhil

Ascariasis lumbricoides is a roundworm that causes one of the most common soil-transmitted helminth infections worldwide. Ascariasis is typically found in the jejunum and transmitted through the intake of *Ascaris lumbricoides* eggs through food and water. Initially, ascariasis can cause pulmonary symptoms during the first 6–8 weeks of ingestion and can progress to serious complications of intestinal obstruction and hepatobiliary manifestations. Biliary ascariasis is a complication of ascariasis migration from the jejunum to the hepatobiliary tree and can present with a variety of symptoms ranging from biliary colic to more serious features such as acute cholangitis. Though the mortality rate is low, limited resources for management can make it challenging to manage.

1. Introduction

Approximately one-fourth of the world's population is infected by soil-transmitted helminths (STH) [1], caused by various parasites such as roundworms, whipworms, and hookworms [2]. These infections are widespread in economically poorer regions such as sub-Saharan Africa and south-east Asia [1–3], with Ethiopia alone accounting for approximately 29 million cases of STH among children in the year 2020 [1], which can be attributed to inadequate water sanitation, poor personal hygiene, and socioeconomic disparities [4]. Ascariasis is one of the commonly occurring STH infections [5] caused by *Ascaris lumbricoides* (roundworm), most commonly found in the jejunum [2, 6]. According to the Global Burden of Disease 2019 data, the estimated global prevalence of ascariasis was 594 per 100,000 people, with 2090 deaths and 754000 disability-adjusted life years [7]. It is transmitted through the intake of food and water contaminated with infectious *Ascaris lumbricoides* eggs [8]. Most patients are symptomatic, and the early phase pulmonary manifestations of Loeffler syndrome are uncommon in high endemic zones [3, 8]. Usually, the symptoms occur after 6–8 weeks of egg ingestion, which are often nonspecific [8] and can lead to complications such as intestinal obstruction [9], hepatobiliary and pancreatic involvement [10, 11].

Biliary ascariasis is one of the complications caused due to migration of *Ascaris* from jejunum to duodenum and through ampulla of Vater to the biliary tree [12], and is more common in women and children [10]. It can present as biliary colic, acute cholecystitis, and acute cholangitis [3, 10], and can be diagnosed based on clinical evaluation, stool

Table 1: Laboratory investigations of the patient.

Investigation	Result	Reference range
Hb (g/dl)	13.4	11.0–17.5
MCV (fl)	83.9	79–94.8
MCH (pg)	30.4	25.6–32.2
MCHC (g/dl)	36.2	32.2–36.5
RBC ($\times 10^6/\mu l$)	4.41	3.93–6.08
WBC ($\times 10^3/\mu l$)	16.31	3.98–10.04
DLC (%)	N 89 L 7.4	N 34–71.1 L 19.3–53.1
Platelet ($\times 10^3/\mu l$)	231	150–450
Liver function test		
Total serum bilirubin (mg/dl)	5.1	0.3–1.3
Direct bilirubin (mg/dl)	0.46	0.1–0.4
AST (IU/l)	92	12–38
ALT (IU/l)	106	7–41
ALP (IU/l)	57	44–147
AST/ALT	0.87	

Hb = hemoglobin concentration; MCV = mean corpuscular volume; MCH = mean corpuscular hemoglobin, MCHC = mean corpuscular hemoglobin concentration; RBC = red blood cell; WBC = white blood cell; DLC = differential leucocyte count; AST = aspartate transferase; ALT = alanine transaminase; ALP = alkaline phosphatase.

examination, and imaging modalities such as plain X-ray, barium swallow, ultrasonography, endoscopy, and a computed tomography scan [13]. This condition can be treated by conservative management of clinical syndromes, administration of antihelminthic drugs, and endoscopy or surgical approaches if subsequent medical therapy fails [13, 14].

Though the mortality associated with ascariasis is low [15], the limited resources available for its management, coupled with its high endemicity in low-income countries, can make it challenging to manage. Herein, we report a rare case of obstructive jaundice secondary to biliary ascariasis in the high-endemic region of Ethiopia.

2. Case Report

A 35-year-old woman presented to our hospital, Dilla University Referral Hospital, located in Dilla, southern Ethiopia, with abdominal pain of one-day duration. The pain was in the right upper abdomen, intermittent, colicky, and nonradiating, with no aggravating or relieving factors, and accompanied by anorexia and nausea. She denied any history of fever or vomiting. On physical examination, her vitals were normal, and icteric sclera was noted. Her abdominal examination revealed tenderness in the right hypochondriac region. Her laboratory investigations (Table 1) revealed neutrophilic leucocytosis, conjugated hyperbilirubinemia, and elevated alanine transaminase. On stool examination, ova of *Ascaris lumbricoides* were seen. Furthermore, ultrasonography (USG) of the abdomen revealed worms in the distal common bile duct with partial obstruction, a dilated gallbladder, and dilated right and left hepatic ducts (Figures 1 and 2).

Based on the high endemicity of ascariasis that is limited to the gastrointestinal tract in Ethiopia, the patients' history, clinical evaluation, stool examination, and USG report,

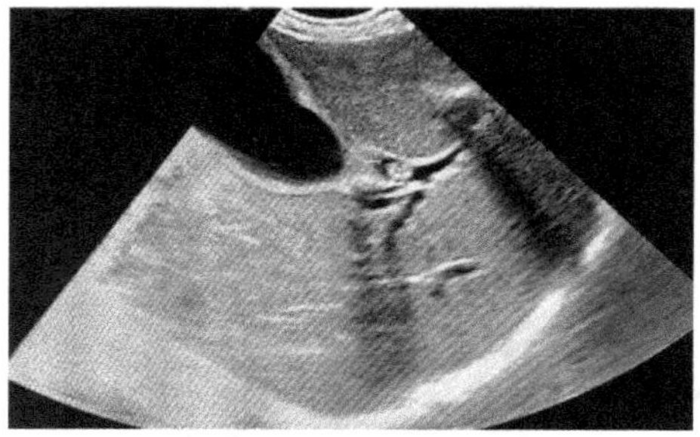

Figure 1: Ultrasound image of ascaris worm in the common bile duct, transverse section.

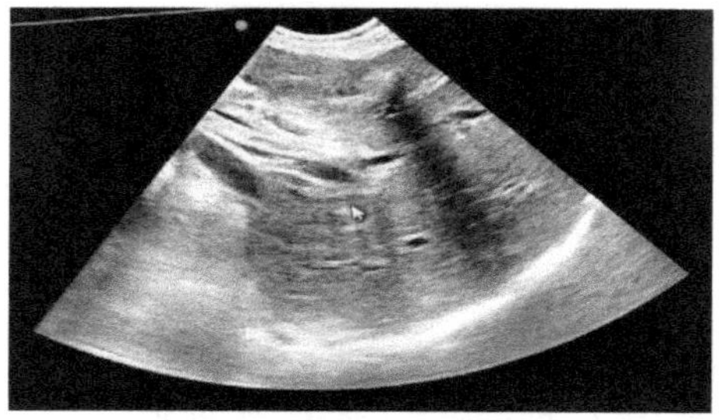

Figure 2: Ultrasound image of ascaris worm in the common bile duct, vertical section.

a diagnosis of obstructive jaundice secondary to biliary ascariasis was made. To the best of our knowledge, this is the first case report in Ethiopia about biliary ascariasis, although it is quite common to see ascariasis cause disease manifestations limited to the small and large bowel. The management was done by administering intravenous normal saline, intravenous ceftriaxone 1 g bid, intravenous metronidazole 500 mg bid, intravenous hyoscine butyl bromide, and a single dose of 200 mg oral albendazole. A follow-up USG after 2 days did not reveal any worm in the common bile duct (Figure 3). The bile duct also didn't show any sign of dilation or stenosis after the worm exit. But it was not possible to check if the bile duct had developed any complications later on as the patient didn't show up for a follow-up USG scan. The hematologic profile of the patient returned to normal values (the total bilirubin came down to 1.2 mg/dl and the direct bilirubin decreased to 0.2 mg/dl) after the worm exit. After three days of hospital stay, the patient showed complete recovery and was discharged with a prescription for oral amoxicillin-clavulanate and metronidazole for one week.

3. Discussion

Biliary ascariasis is more prevalent in high-endemic zones and shows a female preponderance, with patients usually presenting in their mid-thirties [10]. There have been cases of ascariasis presenting as colic abdominal pain [16] and leading to obstructive jaundice [10]. Similarly, the patient was a female in her mid-thirties belonging to a high-endemic region of Ethiopia [1]. Her symptoms of colicky abdominal pain and conjugated bilirubinemia, coupled with elevated ALT and AST, most likely indicate obstructive jaundice due

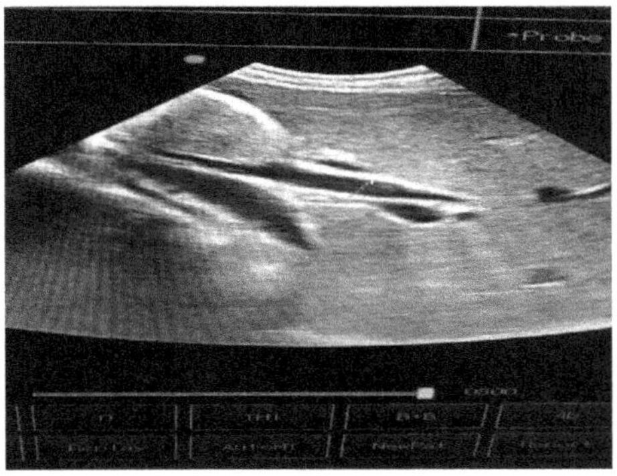

Figure 3: Ultrasound image showing normal common bile duct after worm exit.

to acquired causes. Usually, we would expect a significant rise in ALP level in cases of obstructive jaundice, but this may not always be the case across all patients [17, 18].

Imaging of the biliary tree is indicated in patients presenting with right upper abdominal pain or jaundice [19–21]. Various imaging modalities, such as plain X-ray, barium swallow, ultrasonography, endoscopy, and computed tomography scanning can be used for imaging [13]. A plain X-ray of the abdomen may reveal a collection of worms contrasting against the bowel, known as the whirlpool effect, and a barium swallow can reveal elongated filling defects in the small intestine [22]. In addition, endoscopic retrograde cholangiopancreatography (ERCP) may be indicated in these patients as a diagnostic tool to determine the presence of worms in the CBD and can also act as a therapeutic modality with a high success rate [23]. Often, these patients are initially investigated with sonography, which can help detect various congenital and acquired abnormalities in the biliary tree [19–21]. Various studies and case reports have supported the use of USG in the diagnosis of biliary diseases [24–27]. In clinical guidelines, USG is already an established imaging modality for diagnosing biliary ascariasis and is crucial in low-resource settings due to its cost-effectiveness [28–31]. In our case, the patient was evaluated with USG, which suggested the presence of worms obstructing the CBD. In addition, stool examination revealed the presence of *Ascaris* eggs. Hence, a diagnosis of obstructive jaundice secondary to biliary ascariasis was made.

The management of biliary ascariasis can be done by conservative, endoscopic, and surgical approach [6]. These patients are hospitalized and treated with intravenous fluids, antispasmodic, and broad-spectrum antibiotics [10, 32, 33]. Antihelminthic drugs such as Albendazole, Mebendazole, and Pyrantel pamoate can be used to treat ascariasis [6]. A recent obervational study by Djune-Yemeli et al. concluded that a single dose of albendazole was insufficient to eliminate STH in high endemic regions [34]. However, a meta-analysis by Conterno et al. in 2020 revealed the cure rate of ascariasis by single-dose Albendazole and multiple-dose Albendazole as 93.2% and 94.3%, respectively [35]. Albendazole has also been concluded to have high efficacy and high safety profile for children and adults, making this treatment a viable option for patients [35]. Luckily, most patients recover with conservative management within 3 days and tend to be the best course of treatment for patients with milder symptoms [6, 10]. Nevertheless, for patients who are acutely sick or failed to respond to conservative management, ERCP or open exploration is the subsequent management option [6]. An endoscopic or surgical approach was not required in our case, as conservative management improved the patient's condition and resulted in the exit of worms from the common bile duct.

Biliary ascariasis will remain as a public health concern in high endemic and low-resource settings. Clinicians should approach biliary ascariasis with a high index of suspicion, as symptoms of abdominal pain and jaundice creates a wide variety of differentials that often cause the misdiagnosis of biliary ascariasis with other hepatobiliary pathologies, such as hepatocellular carcinoma or gallbladder stones. Though the development of efficient diagnostic tools have aided in the timely management of biliary ascariasis, it is common for tertiary hospitals to not have readily available tools such as an ERCP. Future research is warranted to determine the most efficacious diagnostic modality that is feasible for low-resource settings in the case of biliary ascariasis. Moreover, studies should investigate the sensitivity of biliary markers such as ALP, AST, and ALT in determining the presence of obstructive jaundice with biliary ascariasis to better guide informed clinical decisions.

There were several limitations to the case. We did not obtain GGT levels which would have further aided in the diagnosis of obstructive jaundice.

4. Conclusion

We report a case of a female patient in her mid-thirties presenting with right upper quadrant pain. She was diagnosed with obstructive jaundice secondary to biliary ascariasis based on endemicity, clinical evaluation, USG, and stool examination. This case highlights that biliary ascariasis should be suspected in patients presenting with symptoms of right upper abdominal pain in endemic areas. Also, abdominal ultrasonography can be a rapid, safe, noninvasive, and reasonably affordable imaging modality for diagnosing biliary ascariasis. Moreover, adequate conservative management with intravenous fluids, antispasmodics, broad-spectrum antibiotics, and antihelminthic treatment results in the successful management of these patients.

References

[1] "Soil-transmitted helminthiases. WHO," 2020, https://apps.who.int/neglected_diseases/ntddata/sth/sth.html.

[2] "Soil-transmitted helminth infections. World health organization," 2022, https://www.who.int/news-room/fact-sheets/detail/soil-transmitted-helminth-infections Accessed.

[3] P. M. Jourdan, P. H. L. Lamberton, A. Fenwick, and D. G. Addiss, "Soil-transmitted helminth infections," *The Lancet*, vol. 391, no. 10117, pp. 252–265, 2018.

[4] A. K. C. Leung, A. A. M. Leung, A. H. C. Wong, and K. L. Hon, "Human ascariasis: an updated review," *Recent Patents on*

Inflammation & Allergy Drug Discovery, vol. 14, no. 2, pp. 133–145, 2021.

[5] R. L. Pullan, J. L. Smith, R. Jasrasaria, and S. J. Brooker, "Global numbers of infection and disease burden of soil transmitted helminth infections in 2010," *Parasites & Vectors*, vol. 7, no. 1, p. 37, 2014.

[6] O. J. Shah, S. A. Zargar, and I. Robbani, "Biliary ascariasis: a review," *World Journal of Surgery*, vol. 30, no. 8, pp. 1500–1506, 2006.

[7] "Global burden of disease," *Ascariasis — Level 4 Cause*, Institute for Health Metrics and Evaluation, 2019, https://www.healthdata.org/results/gbd_summaries/2019/ascariasis-level-4-cause.

[8] K. Leder, F. Weller, N. Reddy, Ascariasis - UpToDate, T. Ryan, and L. Baron, Eds., 2022,https://www.uptodate.com/contents/ascariasis?search=ascariasis&source=search_result&selectedTitle=1%7E46&usage_type=default&display_rank=1.

[9] N. R. de Silva, H. L. Guyatt, and D. A. P. Bundy, "Morbidity and mortality due to Ascaris-induced intestinal obstruction," *Transactions of the Royal Society of Tropical Medicine and Hygiene*, vol. 91, no. 1, pp. 31–36, 1997.

[10] M. S. Khuroo, S. A. Zargar, and R. Mahajan, "Hepatobiliary and pancreatic ascariasis in India," *The Lancet*, vol. 335, no. 8704, pp. 1503–1506, 1990.

[11] M. S. Khuroo, A. A. Rather, N. S. Khuroo, and M. S. Khuroo, "Hepatobiliary and pancreatic ascariasis," *World Journal of Gastroenterology*, vol. 22, no. 33, p. 7507, 2016.

[12] J. Shah and A. Shahidullah, "<b><i>*Ascaris lumbricoides*</i></b>: a Startling Discovery during Screening Colonoscopy," *Case Rep Gastroenterol*, vol. 12, no. 2, pp. 224–229, 2018.

[13] A. K. Das, "Hepatic and biliary ascariasis," *Journal of Global Infectious Diseases*, vol. 6, no. 2, p. 65, 2014.

[14] U. Jethwani, G. J. Singh, P. Sarangi, and V. Kandwal, "Laproscopic management of wandering biliary ascariasis," *Case Reports in Surgery*, vol. 2012, pp. 1–4, 2012.

[15] M. S. Khuroo, S. A. Zargar, G. N. Yattoo et al., "Ascaris-induced acute pancreatitis," *British Journal of Surgery*, vol. 79, no. 12, pp. 1335–1338, 2005.

[16] Y. Hassan, S. A. Rather, A. A. Rather, and M. K. Banday, "*Ascaris lumbricoides* and the surgical complications: our experience from Medical College Hospital," *Irish Journal of Medical Science*, vol. 191, no. 4, pp. 1815–1821, 2021, Published online October 7, 2021.

[17] S. Gowda, P. B. Desai, V. v. Hull, A. A. K. Math, S. N. Vernekar, and S. S. Kulkarni, "A review on laboratory liver function tests," *Pan Afr Med J*, vol. 3, p. 17, 2009.

[18] J. O. Hayat, C. J. Loew, K. N. Asrress, A. S. McIntyre, and D. A. Gorard, "Contrasting liver function test patterns in obstructive jaundice due to biliary structures and stones," *QJM: International Journal of Medicine*, vol. 98, no. 1, pp. 35–40, 2005.

[19] S. D. Yarmenitis, "Ultrasound of the gallbladder and the biliary tree," *European Radiology*, vol. 12, no. 2, pp. 270–282, 2002.

[20] D. J. Rubens, "Ultrasound imaging of the biliary tract," *Ultrasound Clinics*, vol. 2, no. 3, pp. 391–413, 2007.

[21] W. D. Foley and F. A. Quiroz, "The role of sonography in imaging of the biliary tract," *Ultrasound Quarterly*, vol. 23, no. 2, pp. 123–135, 2007.

[22] M. M. Reeder, "The radiological and ultrasound evaluation of ascariasis of the gastrointestinal, biliary, and respiratory tracts," *Seminars in Roentgenology*, vol. 33, no. 1, pp. 57–78, 1998.

[23] P. S. Patra, A. Das, S. M. Ahmed, S. Mitra, and G. K. Dhali, "Treatment response and long-term outcomes in biliary ascariasis: a prospective study," *Arab Journal of Gastroenterology*, vol. 22, no. 2, pp. 164–169, 2021.

[24] A. Pinto, A. Reginelli, L. Cagini et al., "Accuracy of ultrasonography in the diagnosis of acute calculous cholecystitis: review of the literature," *Critical Ultrasound Journal*, vol. 5, no. S1, pp. S11–S14, 2013.

[25] J. R. Wertz, J. M. Lopez, D. Olson, and W. M. Thompson, "Comparing the diagnostic accuracy of ultrasound and CT in evaluating acute cholecystitis," *American Journal of Roentgenology*, vol. 211, no. 2, pp. W92–W97, 2018.

[26] L. H. Blackbourne, R. C. Earnhardt, C. L. Sistrom, P. Abbitt, and R. S. Jones, "The sensitivity and role of ultrasound in the evaluation of biliary obstruction," *The American Surgeon*, vol. 60, no. 9, pp. 683–690, 1994, https://pubmed.ncbi.nlm.nih.gov/8060040/.

[27] G. Ghimire, B. Lohani, and S. Pradhan, "Accuracy of ultrasonography in evaluation of level and cause of biliary obstruction: a prospective study - PubMed," *Kathmandu University Medical Journal*, vol. 3, no. 1, pp. 17–521, 2005, https://pubmed.ncbi.nlm.nih.gov/16401938/.

[28] M. Absi, A. M. Qais, M. al Katta, M. Gafour, and A. H. Al-Wadan, "Biliary ascariasis: the value of ultrasound in the diagnosis and management," *Annals of Saudi Medicine*, vol. 27, no. 3, pp. 161–165, 2007.

[29] M. S. Khuroo, S. A. Zargar, R. Mahajan, R. L. Bhat, and G. Javid, "Sonographic appearances in biliary ascariasis," *Gastroenterology*, vol. 93, no. 2, pp. 267–272, 1987.

[30] N. A. Gomez, C. J. Leon, and O. Ortiz, "Ultrasound in the diagnosis of roundworms in gallbladder and common bile duct. Report of four cases," *Surgical Endoscopy*, vol. 7, no. 4, pp. 339–342, 1993.

[31] B. Lentz, T. Fong, R. Rhyne, and N. Risko, "A systematic review of the cost-effectiveness of ultrasound in emergency care settings," *The Ultrasound Journal*, vol. 13, no. 1, p. 16, 2021.

[32] M. S. Khuroo and S. A. Zargar, "Biliary ascariasis," *Gastroenterology*, vol. 88, no. 2, pp. 418–423, 1985, https://pubmed.ncbi.nlm.nih.gov/3965331/.

[33] M. Sultan Khuroo, S. Ali Zargar, G. Nabi Yattoo et al., "Worm extraction and biliary drainage in hepatobiliary and pancreatic ascariasis," *Gastrointestinal Endoscopy*, vol. 39, no. 5, pp. 680–685, 1993.

[34] L. Djune-Yemeli, H. C. Nana-Djeunga, C. G. Lenou-Nanga et al., "Serious limitations of the current strategy to control Soil-Transmitted Helminths and added value of Ivermectin/Albendazole mass administration: a population-based observational study in Cameroon," *PLoS Neglected Tropical Diseases*, vol. 14, no. 11, Article ID e0008794, 2020.

[35] L. O. Conterno, M. D. Turchi, I. Corrêa, and R. A. Monteiro de Barros Almeida, "Anthelmintic drugs for treating ascariasis," *Cochrane Database of Systematic Reviews*, vol. 4, no. 4, 2020.

Emergence of Lassa Fever Disease in Northern Togo: Report of Two Cases in Oti District in 2016

Akouda Akessiwe Patassi,[1,2] Dadja Essoya Landoh,[3] Agballa Mebiny-Essoh Tchalla,[4] Wemboo Afiwa Halatoko,[2,5] Hamadi Assane,[6] Bayaki Saka,[7] Mouchedou Abdoukarim Naba,[8] Issifou Yaya,[9] Kossi Atsissinta Edou,[10] Tsidi Agbeko Tamekloe,[2,11] Abiba Kere Banla,[2,5] Kokou Mawule Davi,[3] Magloire Manga,[12] Yao Kassankogno,[2] and Dominique Salmon-Ceron[13]

[1]*Service des Maladies Infectieuses, CHU Sylvanus Olympio, Lomé, Togo*
[2]*Comité national de lutte contre les Urgences, Lomé, Togo*
[3]*Organisation Mondiale de la Santé, Lomé, Togo*
[4]*Direction Préfectorale de la santé de Sotouboua, Sotouboua, Togo*
[5]*Institut National d'Hygiène-Laboratoire, Lomé, Togo*
[6]*Direction Préfectorale de la santé de Tchamba, Tchamba, Togo*
[7]*Service de Dermatologie CHU Sylvanus Olympio, Lomé, Togo*
[8]*Direction Préfectorale de la santé de Doufelgou, Niamtougou, Togo*
[9]*Aix Marseille Université, INSERM, IRD, SESSTIM, Sciences Economiques & Sociales de la Santé & Traitement de l'Information Médicale, Marseille, France*
[10]*Direction Préfectorale de la santé de Oti, Mango, Togo*
[11]*Division de l'Epidémiologie du Ministère de la Santé, Lomé, Togo*
[12]*Université de Casamance, Ziguinchor, Senegal*
[13]*Service de Maladies Infectieuses, Hôpital Cochin, Paris, France*

Correspondence should be addressed to Dadja Essoya Landoh; mlandoh@yahoo.fr

Academic Editor: Tomoyuki Shibata

Background. Lassa fever belongs to the group of potentially fatal hemorrhagic fevers, never reported in Togo. The aim of this paper is to report the first two cases of Lassa fever infection in Togo. *Case Presentation.* The two first Lassa fever cases occurred in two expatriate's health professionals working in Togo for more than two years. The symptoms appeared among two health professionals of a clinic located in Oti district in the north of the country. The absence of clinical improvement after antimalarial treatment and the worsening of clinical symptoms led to the medical evacuation. The delayed diagnosis of the first case led to a fatal outcome. The second case recovered under ribavirin treatment. *Conclusion.* The emergence of this hemorrhagic fever confirms the existence of Lassa fever virus in Togo. After a period of intensive Ebola virus transmission from 2013 to 2015, this is an additional call for the establishment and enhancement of infection prevention and control measures in the health care setting in West Africa.

1. Background

Lassa fever is an old hemorrhagic fever discovered for the first time in West Africa in Nigeria in 1969. The single-stranded RNA virus was isolated for the 1st time from the town of Lassa in Nigeria [1–3]. The animal reservoir of the virus is the multimammate mouse (*Mastomys natalensis*). The virus is transmitted to humans via contact of human food with urine or feces of an infected animal living in the house or in the bush [2, 4]. Person-to-person infections and laboratory transmission

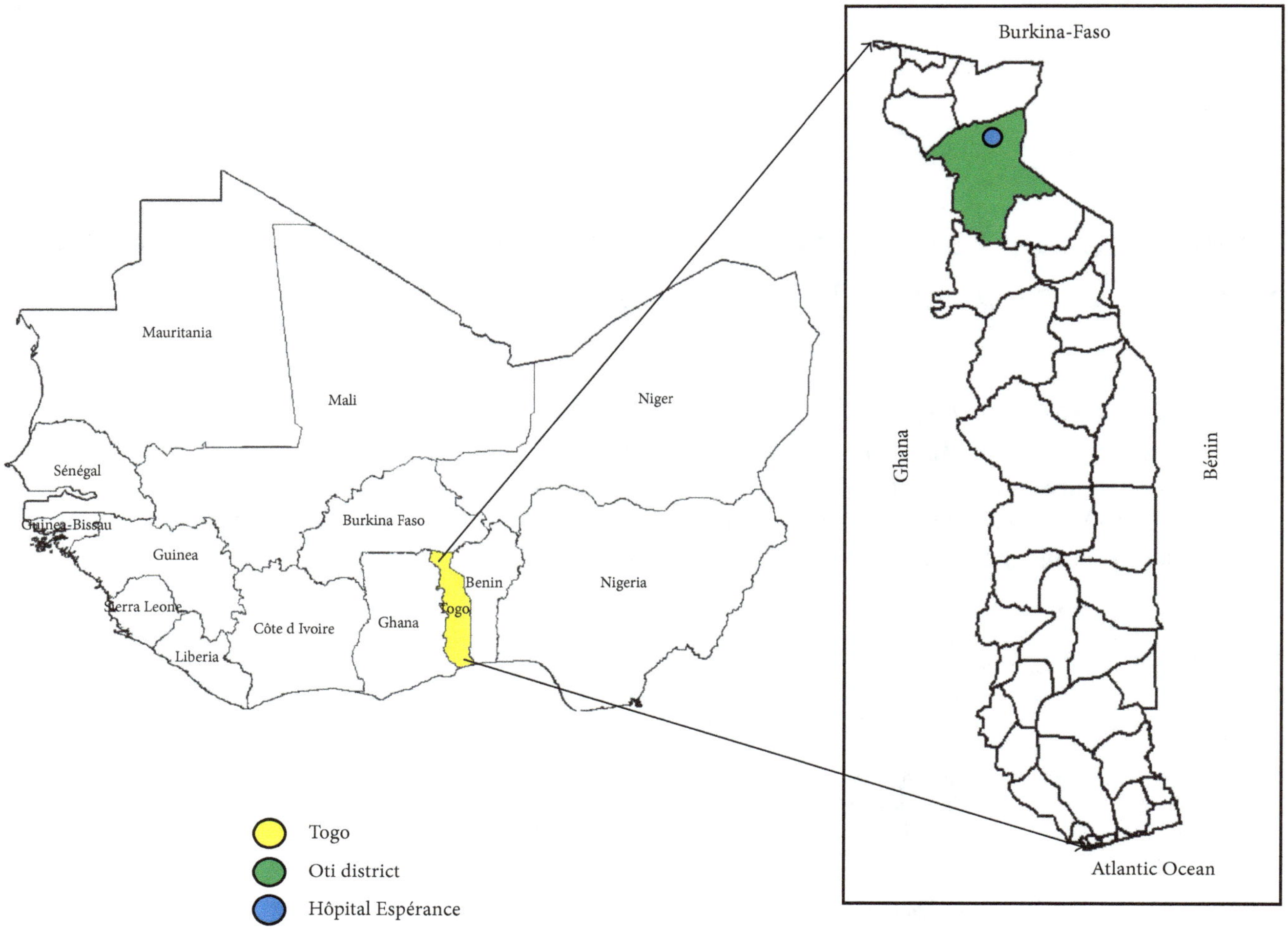

FIGURE 1: Geographical location of Oti district where "Hôpital de l'Espérance" is located.

are also possible, particularly in the absence of adequate infection control measures in the health care environment. Sexual transmission has been described in humans [3]. All humans can develop the disease after infection [1, 3, 4]. The incubation period varies from 3 to 21 days after contact with a Lassa fever patient or contaminated food or water. In 80% of the cases, the infection is asymptomatic or a mild illness with mild fever, malaise, vomiting, or muscle pain. In 20% of the cases, the clinical presentation is severe with externalized bleeding from the mouth or gastrointestinal tract. Digestive, respiratory, and neurological disorders (convulsive seizures, hearing deficit, meningitis, and encephalitis) have been described [1, 3–5]. The reported actual illness-to-infection ratio in endemic areas is presumably 20% [5, 6]. Approximately, 15–20% of patients hospitalized for Lassa fever die from the illness. The case fatality rate may reach 50% in hospitalized patients during occasional Lassa fever epidemics [2, 4]. In 2014, Shaffer et al. reported a case fatality rate of 69% in Sierra Leone [7]. Ribavirin administered early during the first six days of symptoms significantly reduces the fatality rate from 55 to 5%. In endemic areas, 300,000 to 500,000 cases of Lassa fever are estimated to occur yearly, leading to 5,000 to 10,000 deaths in West African countries such as Nigeria, Liberia, Sierra Leone, Guinea, and Mali. Neighboring countries have also declared the presence of the rodent vector of Lassa virus and the occurrence of epidemics in this region [5, 8–12]. Togo, a West African country (Figure 1), had so far reported no Lassa fever cases on its soil. The prediction of the occurrence of Lassa virus in various geographical regions, compatible with the ecology of the rodent reservoir, showed that the emergence of clinical Lassa fever is not unexpected in some West African countries including Togo [12].

In a context of providing health care workers in Togo with a working tool to combat Ebola disease, are the preparedness and alert measures implemented in the Savanes health region enough to detect timely hemorrhagic fever diseases?

The suspicion of recent Lassa fever led to take preventive and infection control measures around the environment of these cases according to WHO guidelines.

2. Case Presentation

A 47-year-old man, surgeon in "Hôpital de l'Espérance," a private hospital in the north of Togo about 550 km from Lomé, the capital [13], consulted in the same hospital on February 12, 2016, for fever. He was vaccinated against yellow fever. The thick smear performed was positive for malaria and received artemether/lumefantrine without any favorable clinical course after six days. Due to the persistence of high-grade fever and a generalized weakness, he was hospitalized in a private room and a nurse was designated for his care. On day 6 after consultation, he complained of fever, chills, malaise, headaches, pharyngitis hypoacusis, and diffuse abdominal pain. Laboratory tests showed leukopenia (1,100 cells/mm^3) and thrombocytopenia (65,000/mm^3). His epigastric pain gradually exacerbated. Based on syndromic abdominal pain with febrile illness, an exploratory laparotomy was conducted, which was followed by a bleeding on the operative wound. He was thus air-lifted using an air ambulance from Togo to Cologne, Germany, on day 13. Before the evacuation, the patient was transfused with two units of packaged red blood cells in the airport as his hemoglobin dropped to 6.8 g/dL with evidence of hemolysis symptoms. Despite intensive medical care in Germany, the patient's condition deteriorated rapidly on the second day of admission, and he died on day 14. A postmortem diagnosis of Lassa fever was confirmed by polymerase chain reaction (PCR) in Germany [13].

On March 5, 2016, the 33-year-old health care professional who took care of the surgeon presented with fever, headaches, chills, and body aches. He then had abdominal pain, generalized fatigue and myalgia, and diarrhea. The rest of the clinical status was normal. He was vaccinated against yellow fever. A thick smear was performed, and the patient received antimalarial treatment (artemether/lumefantrine) without success. Laboratory results showed a hemoglobin level of 7 g/d, a white cell count of 3300 × 109/L, and a platelet count of 30 × 109/L. The sedimentation rate was 17 mm at the 1st hour. The patient's renal function was impaired with urea increase to 27.5 mmol/L and creatinine increase to 637 mmol/L. The liver function tests were also impaired with a total bilirubin level of 50 µmol/L and aspartate aminotransferase (AST) and alanine transaminase (ALT) levels of 1321 IU/L and 1060 IU/L, respectively.

Based on the clinical presentation, and the fact that both were health workers in the same hospital, the hypothesis of a viral hemorrhagic fever (Lassa fever) was suggested, and the blood sample of this second patient was taken and sent to Accra at Noguchi Memorial Institute for Medical Research (Ghana) and at "Centre National de Recherche des Fièvres hémorragiques de l'Institut Pasteur" of Lyon (France). A reverse transcriptase polymerase chain reaction (RT-PCR) assay was performed on the blood sample on day 5 after onset, which confirmed the presence of Lassa fever virus. The same day, intravenous (IV) ribavirin regimen was initiated with a loading dose of 30 mg/kg IV (maximum, 2 g) followed by 17 mg/kg IV (maximum, 1 g/dose) every 6 hours for 4 days, and then 8 mg/kg IV (maximum, 500 mg/dose) every 8 hours for 6 days in addition to other supportive treatment. On day 7, the patient was evacuated to Atlanta aboard an air ambulance. The patient gradually regained his strength and completed 10 days of ribavirin with supportive treatment and appropriate nutrition. He was discharged in May 2016 with hearing disorders. These disorders persisted during the first six months after leaving the hospital.

2.1. Contact Tracing. This tracing was done on two axes: (i) the tracing of the so-called primary cases and (ii) the follow-up of the contacts around the two cases described above.

Primary cases were suspected to be the source of the contamination of these two cases. The search of these primary cases was done through the review of the medical records of all patients who consulted in the health facilities of the region from January 1 to April 4, 2016. Death tracing in the villages of the area was performed from December 1, 2015 to March 23, 2016.

Among patients who went through the operating room from January 14 to February 2, 2016, three patients were suspected to be primary cases from a total of 78 patients operated on by the same surgeon.

> *Case 1.* A 7-month-old child, who resided in Sadori (north Togo, Oti district), presented with a persistent fever and a cervical tumefaction. He was operated on February 8; he presented with bleeding of operative wounds and died 3 days later.
>
> *Case 2.* An 8-year-old child residing in Kankandou, Oti district, presented with a fever, swelling of the face, and hematuria.
>
> *Case 3.* A 31-year-old woman residing in Gando, Oti district, presented with a suspicion of abortion; but after analyzing her history, the case of abortion due to Lassa fever was rejected.

Blood samples for confirmation were taken from the 8-year-old child. Samples were taken also from the mother of the 7-month-old child because of the close contact between them. The search for anti-Lassa IgM and IgG using an enzyme-linked immunosorbent assay (ELISA) technique was negative for this 8-year-old child residing in Kankandou. For the mother of Case 1, the IgG was positive. These tests were performed at Noguchi Memorial Institute for Medical Research (Ghana). The surgeon was consulted for medical advice in outpatient clinics and hospitalizations. Of the 2,051 files reviewed, 36 cases with febrile diseases were selected. Five (05) of the 36 files were cases with arguments in favor of suspect cases.

In public health centers of the region, 19,074 patients were seen of whom 7319 cases were consulted for fever. None of the 7319 cases met the case definition of Lassa fever. There were 21 cases of spontaneous abortions recorded without any context of fever.

After the occurrence of the two Lassa fever cases, 110 contacts were identified and followed up for 21 days. There were 81 contacts among health workers: 80 from Hôpital de l'Espérance and one ambulance driver from Mango military camp. In the community, 29 contacts were followed up by the nurses in health facilities and community health workers. None of the 110 contacts developed symptoms.

3. Discussion

This first Lassa fever outbreak was reported in Togo in a context of the epidemiological transition of malaria in Africa. Indeed, following the large mobilization of funding to support malaria control strategies in low- and middle-income countries, a decrease in morbidity and mortality due to malaria in most of the African countries has been noted since a few years [14, 15]. However, malaria remains a major cause of consultation and hospitalization in sub-Saharan African countries including Togo. Therefore, malaria is the first diagnosis suspected by health workers and community health workers, in case of fever in children, pregnant women, travelers, and adults [14, 16, 17]. In this context, it is difficult to diagnose nonmalarial fevers from the first consultation. The two patients in our study were foreigners, one more reason to think first about malaria. This led to a delayed diagnosis and a worsening of the patient's clinical conditions. It is well known that the delay in the diagnosis of hemorrhagic fevers is the starter of most outbreaks reported, increases the rate of human-to-human transmission, and finally, makes it difficult to stop the dissemination of the disease [16, 18]. It becomes urgent to explain to the patients and convince health workers that there are many causes of fever. Fever is a major symptom of hemorrhagic diseases transmitted (i) from human to human in the hospital, (ii) by diurnal mosquitoes, (iii) by ticks or fleas, and (iv) by animals (domestic and game). Some hemorrhagic fevers are lethal without treatment but less frequent. Fever during malaria is more often severe [16, 19, 20]. Our first reported case began with fever. The positive result of the thick smear and the duration of malaria treatment by artemether were the factors that delayed the true diagnosis of Lassa fever and led to a fatal outcome.

3.1. Prevention and Response Measures. Once the hypothesis of Lassa fever was established, measures were taken to limit the dissemination of the virus and regain the eventual sources of contamination within the hospital. This outbreak of Lassa fever occurred in a dual context of Ebola disease in the West African subregion and of a Lassa fever outbreak in Benin and Nigeria. Nigeria experienced an Ebola epidemic in 2014 and a reemergence of Lassa fever in 2016. The epidemic of Lassa fever reappeared in Benin in 2015 and 2016. This is evident that arenaviruses are reemerging in African countries due to climatic or ecological changes and sometimes resulting in case fatalities.

The primary transmission occurs from the natural reservoir to the human. Once the first case appears, the transmission becomes human to human and the family or the health care workers are at risk. This explains the occurrence of the second case of nosocomial Lassa fever in Oti district. This second case was a health care professional who took care of the first Lassa fever case. At the onset of symptoms, the patient was isolated at home. The good level of hygiene in this hospital has limited the transmission although this first fatal case was operated upon in the same hospital. The other factor at risk of expansion of the infection was the long delay for diagnostic confirmation, a delay of 3 weeks which was too long due to the need to send the samples for diagnosis confirmation in Ghana and France [4]. This shows the importance of having locally the means of rapid diagnosis and qualified person for hemorrhagic fever diagnosis. The diagnosis of the first case was post mortem, but the country started preparing since 2014 for the fight against Ebola declared in Guinea while human cases of Lassa fever were already present in the neighboring countries Benin and Nigeria. Moreover, despite these risks, the country did not have ribavirin in any public or private health centres. Fortunately, the second case has received an intravenous ribavirin regimen.

Several measures have been rapidly implemented locally to stop the transmission: sorting of patients in the regional hospitals of the region on the basis of their clinical signs and country of origin (Benin, Nigeria, and Burkina Faso). Hospital hygiene measures were also enhanced (implementation of handwashing devices; decontamination and disinfection of medical equipment after use; provision of personal protective equipment; sorting, collection, storage, and destruction of biomedical waste; disinfection of the surgeon's home (index case); installation of a tent at Hôpital de l'Espérance, to serve as an isolation room for suspected cases; follow-up of contact cases by recording body temperature twice daily; and briefing of laboratory staff on sampling, processing, and infection control measures).

Hôpital de l'Espérance opened its doors in 2015 by an American Baptist mission. It has a medical service, a general surgery ward, an obstetric gynecology ward, a general laboratory, and an administrative block. More than a dozen African nationalities seek health care in this hospital.

Public sensitization was conducted through communication and social mobilization in public places and the production of health messages on the media. The Emergency Management Committee Meeting conducted training for health personnel of the district on Lassa fever, and urgent measures were taken for prevention and control of the disease. A district response plan and supervision of health sites plan on the implementation of guidelines for prevention and control measures were developed. Radio programs translated into local languages on the two radio channels of the district were broadcast. Sensitization sessions were organized in schools, mosques, churches, and at the border (Gando).

4. Conclusion

Togo experienced its first Lassa fever outbreak in the health district of Oti, North Togo. The source of the infection of the first case remained inconclusive: the serological research in the indigenous population and the animal reservoir remain a determinant element to guide preventive measures. Health workers in the region should keep in mind the existence of Lassa fever infection in the differential diagnosis of various fevers during consultations.

Additional Points

The data sets supporting the conclusions of this article are included within the manuscript and its supporting material.

Consent

The Department of Infectious Diseases of CHU of Lomé, University of Lomé, authorized the publication of this manuscript.

Authors' Contributions

Akouda Akessiwe Patassi, Agballa Mebiny-Essoh Tchalla, Wemboo Afiwa Halatoko, Hamadi Assane, Mouchedou Abdoukarim Naba, Kossi Atsissinta Edou, Tsidi Agbeko Tamekloe, Abiba Kere Banla, and Kokou Mawule Davi participated in the protocol design, in case investigation, and in data collection and wrote the manuscript. Dadja Essoya Landoh, Bayaki Saka, Issifou Yaya, Magloire Manga, Yao Kassankogno, and Dominique Salmon-Ceron have revised and finalized the manuscript. All the authors had read and approved the final manuscript to be submitted for publication.

Acknowledgments

The authors would like to thank health workers from the Hôpital de l'Esperance for their collaboration during the Lassa fever outbreak response. They also thank Mr. Diamenu Stanley, public health specialist at WHO in Ghana, for his help in revising the manuscript.

References

[1] World Health Organization, *WHO Lassa Fever Fact Sheet No. 179*, WHO, Geneva, Switzerland, 2000.

[2] N. N. A. Kyei, M. M. Abilba, F. K. Kwawu et al., "Imported Lassa fever: a report of 2 cases in Ghana," *BMC Infectious Diseases*, vol. 15, p. 217, 2015.

[3] O. Ogbu, E. Ajuluchukwu, and C. J. Uneke, "Lassa fever in West African sub-region: an overview," *Journal of Vector Borne Diseases*, vol. 44, no. 1, pp. 1–11, 2007.

[4] S. Wolff, T. Schultze, S. K. Fehling et al., "Genome sequence of Lassa virus isolated from the first domestically acquired case in Germany," *Genome Announcements*, vol. 4, no. 5, p. e00938-16, 2016.

[5] J. K. Richmond and D. J. Baglole, "Lassa fever: epidemiology, clinical features, and social consequences," *BMJ*, vol. 327, no. 7426, pp. 1271–1275, 2003.

[6] D. G. Bausch, A. H. Demby, M. Coulibaly et al., "Lassa fever in Guinea: I. Epidemiology of human disease and clinical observations," *Vector Borne and Zoonotic Diseases*, vol. 1, no. 4, pp. 269–281, 2001.

[7] J. G. Shaffer, D. S. Grant, J. S. Schieffelin et al., "Lassa fever in post-conflict sierra leone," *PLoS Neglected Tropical Diseases*, vol. 8, no. 3, p. e2748, 2014.

[8] Y. H. Kingbêwé, *Urgent: La fièvre Lassa refait surface au Bénin*, La Nouvelle Tribune, Cotonou, Benin, 2016.

[9] N. Bond, J. S. Schieffelin, L. M. Moses, A. J. Bennett, and D. G. Bausch, "A historical look at the first reported cases of Lassa fever: IgG antibodies 40 years after acute infection," *American Journal of Tropical Medicine and Hygiene*, vol. 88, no. 2, pp. 241–244, 2013.

[10] J. B. McCormick, I. J. King, P. A. Webb et al., "A case-control study of the clinical diagnosis and course of Lassa fever," *Journal of Infectious Diseases*, vol. 155, no. 3, pp. 445–455, 1987.

[11] J. B. McCormick, "Epidemiology and control of Lassa fever," *Current Topics in Microbiology and Immunology*, vol. 134, pp. 69–78, 1987.

[12] E. Fichet-Calvet and D. J Rogers, "Risk maps of Lassa fever in West Africa," *PLoS Neglected Tropical Diseases*, vol. 3, no. 3, p. e388, 2009.

[13] World Health Organization, "Lassa fever–Togo," in *Disease Outbreak News*, WHO, Geneva, Switzerland, 2016.

[14] S. Bhatt, D. J. Weiss, E. Cameron et al., "The effect of malaria control on *Plasmodium falciparum* in Africa between 2000 and 2015," *Nature*, vol 526, no. 7572, pp. 207–211, 2015.

[15] E. D. Landoh, P. Tchamdja, B. Saka et al., "Morbidity and mortality due to malaria in Est Mono district, Togo, from 2005 to 2010: a times series analysis," *Malaria Journal*, vol. 11, no. 1, p. 389, 2012.

[16] J. T. Hertz, O. M. Munishi, J. P. Sharp, E. A. Reddy, and J. A. Crump, "Comparing actual and perceived causes of fever among community members in a low malaria transmission setting in northern Tanzania," *Tropical Medicine and International Health*, vol 18, no. 11, pp. 1406–1415, 2013.

[17] V. D'Acremont, M. Kilowoko, E. Kyungu et al., "Beyond malaria—causes of fever in outpatient Tanzanian children," *New England Journal of Medicine*, vol. 370, no. 9, pp. 809–817, 2014.

[18] A. Olayemi, D. Cadar, N. Magassouba et al., "New hosts of the Lassa virus," *Scientific Reports*, vol. 6, no. 1, Article ID 25280, 2016.

[19] E. Lecompte, E. Fichet-Calvet, S. Daffis et al., "*Mastomys natalensis* and Lassa fever, West Africa," *Emerging Infectious Diseases*, vol. 12, no. 12, pp. 1971–1974, 2006.

[20] S. P. Fisher-Hoch, O. Tomori, A. Nasidi et al., "Review of cases of nosocomial Lassa fever in Nigeria: the high price of poor medical practice," *BMJ*, vol. 311, no. 7009, pp. 857–859, 1995.

44

Severe Presentation of Nontypeable *Haemophilus influenzae* (NTHi) Infection in a Previously Healthy Toddler

Eiman Al Bouloushi,[1] Abdulla Al Amri,[2] Ghassan Ghatasheh,[3] and Huda Al Dhanhani[3]

[1]*Academic Affair Department, Tawam Hospital, Al Ain, UAE*
[2]*General Pediatrics Department, Tawam Hospital, Al Ain, UAE*
[3]*Pediatrics Infectious Disease Department, Tawam Hospital, Al Ain, UAE*

Correspondence should be addressed to Huda Al Dhanhani; dr.hdhanhani@gmail.com

Academic Editor: Tomoyuki Shibata

Background. Cellulitis is the inflammation of the skin and subcutaneous tissue. It is usually caused by Gram-positive organisms such as *Staphylococcus and Streptococcus pyogenes* infection. Nontypeable *Haemophilus influenzae* (NTHi) is an uncommon cause of cellulitis. Hence, we report on this case. *Case Presentation.* A previously healthy 19-month-old girl presented with a fever and two-day history of progressive right leg swelling and redness. Her physical examination revealed significant induration and swelling of her right lower leg but no obvious signs of abscess formation. Given the clinical picture, she was admitted as a case of cellulitis. Parenteral clindamycin was started empirically, as the blood culture preliminary report showed Gram-negative rods. Ceftriaxone was added to broaden the coverage. Final blood culture grew NTHi. Despite the use of proper antibiotics (amoxicillin clavulanic acid), the clinical course was complicated with abscess formation that required surgical intervention. *Conclusions.* We are reporting a previously healthy child who developed NTHi cellulitis of the lower leg. To the best of our knowledge, there have been no formal reports pertaining to leg cellulitis following infection by NTHi, yet published in UAE, and reports of HIB cellulitis of the extremities still appear to be rare; hence, we report on this case.

1. Introduction

Haemophilus influenzae is a Gram-negative coccobacillus bacterium. There are two major types of *Haemophilus* species, the typeable *Haemophilus influenzae* and nontypeable *Haemophilus influenzae* (NTHi), which were classified according to the availability of the polysaccharide layer in its capsule [1]. *Haemophilus influenzae* can cause multiple infectious diseases such as meningitis, pneumonia, septicemia, epiglottitis, septic arthritis, osteomyelitis, cellulitis, and peritonitis, and it is also one of the HACEK organisms which contribute to infective endocarditis (HACEK: *Haemophilus*, *Actinobacillus*, *Cardiobacterium*, *Eikenella*, and *Kingella*) [2]. Cellulitis due to *Haemophilus* species is very rare to be encountered in the clinical practice.

We are reporting a case of severe presentation of nontypeable *Haemophilus influenzae* skin and soft tissue infection in a previously healthy toddler, an unusual clinical presentation with diagnostic and treatment challenges.

2. Case Summary

A previously healthy 19-month-old girl presented with a two-day history of right-leg progressive edema and erythema associated with high fever, irritability, and reduced appetite. She was limping and unable to bear weight due to pain. The patient had a recent history of insect bites in multiple areas of her body including both legs. She was fully immunized including HIB (*Haemophilus influenza* type B) vaccination as per the United Arab Emirates childhood vaccination schedule. The family history was unremarkable.

Her 3 siblings were well, and there was no family history of consanguinity or immunodeficiency.

On examination, the patient had numerous marks of insect bites all over the body, particularly the exposed skin areas. There was significant induration and swelling of her right lower leg but no obvious signs of abscess formation. Otherwise, she looked systemically stable with normal vital signs, and her cardiovascular and respiratory examinations were normal. She had no hepatosplenomegaly.

Given the clinical picture, the girl was admitted with a provisional diagnosis of cellulitis. She underwent a partial septic screen, which showed an increased total white cell count (WCC 20.2×10^9/L), significantly elevated C-reactive protein (CRP 348.5 mg/L), and anemia for age (Hb 106 g/L). Her platelet count was 348×10^9/L. Blood cultures were obtained, and she was started on parenteral clindamycin. The blood culture was reported to be positive in one bottle for Gram-negative rods after 18 hours of incubation; therefore, a third generation cephalosporin (ceftriaxone) was added to broaden antimicrobial cover. Final identification revealed nontypeable *Haemophilus influenzae* bacteria where serotype was not performed, as it is not available. Despite the broad-spectrum antibiotics, the girl continued to suffer high-grade fever and progressive swelling in her right leg, despite repeatedly negative blood cultures. Furthermore, she developed bilateral purulent conjunctivitis, which was thought to be caused by NTHi. She underwent MRI imaging (Figure 1) and an ultrasound scan to exclude deep tissue collection or bone/joint involvement. The imaging showed evidence of soft tissue edema and signs of inflammation with free fluid between the muscles but no signs of osteomyelitis or septic arthritis.

The possibility of staphylococcal infection (MSSA, methicillin-sensitive *S. aureus*) was also suspected; therefore, ceftriaxone was switched to Augmentin (amoxicillin and clavulanate). The patient made clinical improvement; however, after 8 days, she developed localized erythema and swelling (Figure 2). The repeated ultrasound scan at this point showed a significant fluid collection (5 cm × 10 cm) requiring incision and drainage. During the procedure, she was noted to have marked fat tissue necrosis, which raised the possibility of necrotizing fasciitis. On the other hand, the histological examination of the collected specimens showed findings consistent with abscess formation with no evidence of acute necrotizing fasciitis with negative culture. Following the surgical intervention, the patient improved dramatically with no further fevers and settling inflammatory markers, and she was able to walk again with normal gait. She had a repeated MRI scan, which showed no evidence of osteomyelitis. Given the severity of complicated cellulitis caused by the unusual organism, the girl underwent immunological assessment and investigations including lymphocyte subsets and complement studies, which were completely normal.

3. Discussion

The patient described above suffered from invasive skin and soft tissue infection due to *Haemophilus influenzae* which is a Gram-negative coccobacillus discovered in 1889. The bacterium is described to be a nonmotile, non-spore-forming organism and has the ability to grow in different environmental conditions (aerobically and anaerobically). There are multiple serotypes of typeable strains which were further classified according to polysaccharides in their capsule into A, B, C, D, and F, while *Haemophilus influenzae* type B (HIB) is the most common strain isolated from infections in the clinical practice [1]. The dramatic decline in the invasive disease due to HIB since the introduction of HIB conjugate vaccines has been well documented [3, 4]. In our case with invasive NTHi disease, the most striking observation is the young age. This observation is supported by the studies from the United Kingdom. Falla et al. identified 24 children in Oxford, England, with serious NTHi disease during the period from 1985 to 1991 and found that 83% of these children were less than 3 years old [5], and it was also reported by CDC that the global incidence of invasive infections related to NTHi was 1.3 per 100,000 in children younger than 5 years [6]. The predominance of disease among young children may reflect the high prevalence of nasopharyngeal colonization with NTHi and the high incidence of viral respiratory infection (and therefore increased mucosal inflammation and the potential for bacterial invasion) in this age group [7]. It has also been reported that levels of immunoglobulin (IgG, IgM, and IgA) antibodies to NTHi are relatively low until 2 years of age, reaching adult levels by 4 years of age [8]. In contrary to other reported risk factors for developing invasive NTHi [9, 10], our patient did not have underlying medical problems, but it might be related to high virulence strain of *Haemophilus* as the bacteria has multiple virulence factors, such as the ability to produce specific enzymes that can cleave protective immunoglobulin A (IgA) that protects the mucosal layer, which is called the bacterial IgA protease enzyme. A recent study by Vitovski et al. revealed that invasive isolates of NTHi exhibit increased IgA1 protease activity compared to isolates from asymptomatic carriers [11]. The level of IgA1 protease activity was not assayed in our case, but it may be one factor that contributes to the patients with NTHi

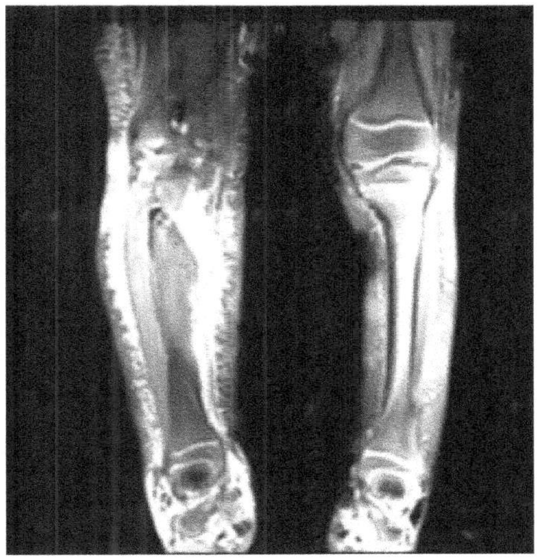

Figure 1: MRI scab showing the deep tissue inflammation and soft tissue edema.

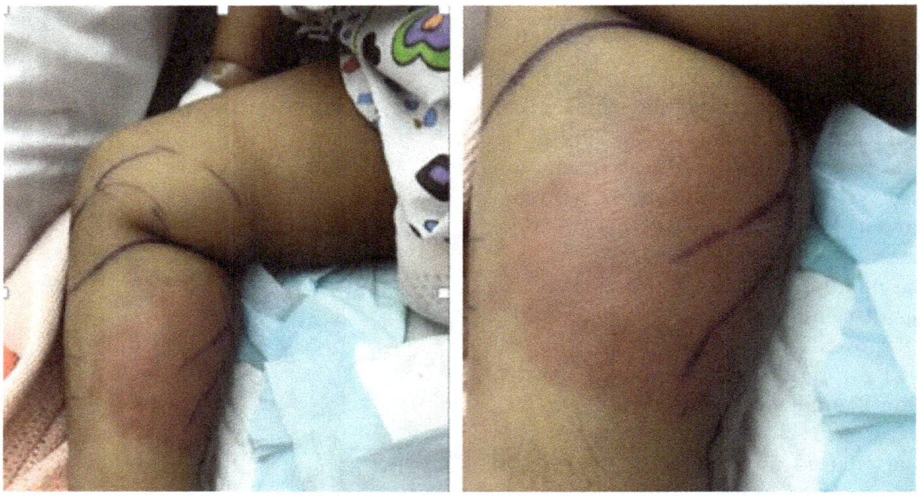

FIGURE 2: Right leg swelling and redness.

invasive disease. Moreover, the *Haemophilus* bacterium can also survive in the respiratory epithelial cells which is called intracellular sequestration, which might explain not only its colonization in the respiratory tract epithelium but also that it can migrate below the cells through transmural migration to the subepithelial area and get access to the vascular system, resulting in severe invasive infections like bacteremia and meningitis [4]. Another factor described by Arnold et al. is the ability of NTHi to form microcolonies on its mucosal surfaces which can inhibit the function of the secreted bacteriostatic products such as lactoferrin and lysozymes and to some potential can inhibit the antibody production [12].

It is known in the literature that the protection against invasive *H. influenzae* requires both innate and acquired humoral immunity. Similar to other infections, maternal antibodies against HIB were noticed to protect newborns against this strain, but they are still prone to infections with nontypeable strains. Furthermore, breastfeeding provides some protection against *H. influenzae* [13]. Although the associated clinical manifestations in NTHi infections make it a target for vaccine development, there are some challenges, e.g., the lack of the capsular polysaccharides and the described high rate of heterogeneity among the isolates from the same infection site [14]. In our patient, we thought about the possibility of primary immune deficiency contributing to the severe presentation since the patient was previously immunized, but no immune defect was identified as she had normal complete blood count, normal immunoglobulin level, and lymphocyte subset.

In conclusion, skin and soft tissue infection due to nontypeable *Haemophilus influenzae* species is quite rare, and there are few case reports in the literature; therefore, we suggest keeping it in consideration in patients with immune deficiency and those who responds slowly to the empirical antimicrobials with limited coverage. Moreover, we described in our patient slow response to the nonsurgical approach, and therefore, we encourage early surgical intervention in cases of complicated *Haemophilus influenzae* cellulitis with collections. On the other hand, more research is needed to understand risk factors for such invasive infection.

References

[1] W. Joseph, S. Geme III, and K. A. Rempe, *Principles and Practice of Pediatric Infectious Diseases (Chapter 172)*, S. S. Long, L. K. Pickering, and C. G. Prober, Eds., Elsevier, Amsterdam, Netherlands, 3rd edition, 2009.

[2] K. Oikonomou, B. Alhaddad, K. Kelly, R. Rajmane, and A. George, "*Haemophilus influenzae* serotype f endocarditis and septic arthritis," *IDCases*, vol. 9, pp. 79–81, 2017.

[3] M. P. E. Slack, "The evidence for non-typeable *Haemophilus influenzae* as a causative agent of childhood pneumonia," *Pneumonia*, vol. 9, no. 9, 2017.

[4] M. S. Reddy, J. M. Bernstein, T. F. Murphy, and H. S. Faden, "Binding between outer membrane proteins of nontypeable *Haemophilus influenzae* and human nasopharyngeal mucin," *Infection and Immunity*, vol. 64, no. 4, pp. 1477–1479, 1996.

[5] T. J. Falla, D. W. M. Crook, W. A. G. Kraak et al., "Population-based study of non-typable *Haemophilus influenzae* invasive disease in children and neonates," *The Lancet*, vol. 341, no. 8849, pp. 851–854, 1993.

[6] K. van Wessel, G. D. Rodenburg, R. H. Veenhoven et al., "Nontypeable *Haemophilus influenzae* invasive disease in the Netherlands: a retrospective surveillance study 2001–2008," *Clinical Infectious Diseases*, vol. 53, no. 1, pp. e1–e7, 2011.

[7] H. Faden, L. Duffy, A. Williams, D. A. Krystofik, and J. Wolf, "Epidemiology of nasopharyngeal colonization with non-typeable *Haemophilus influenzae* in the first 2 years of life," *Journal of Infectious Diseases*, vol. 172, no. 1, pp. 132–135, 1995.

[8] D. A. Krystofik, L. Brodsky, H. Faden et al., "Immune response to nontypeable *Haemophilus influenzae* in the general population and among children with otitis media with effusion," *Annals of Otology, Rhinology & Laryngology*, vol. 97, no. 3, pp. 34–36, 1988.

[9] J. R. Gilsdorf, "*Haemophilus influenzae* non-type b infections in children," *American Journal of Diseases of Children*, vol. 141, no. 10, pp. 1063–1065, 1987.

[10] P. T. Heath, R. Booy, H. J. Azzopardi et al., "Non-type b *Haemophilus influenzae* disease: clinical and epidemiologic characteristics in the *Haemophilus influenzae* type b vaccine era," *The Pediatric Infectious Disease Journal*, vol. 20, no. 3, pp. 300–305, 2001.
[11] S. Vitovski, K. T. Dunkin, A. J. Howard, and J. R. Sayers, "Nontypeable *Haemophilus influenzae* in carriage and disease," *JAMA*, vol. 287, no. 13, pp. 1699–1705, 2002.
[12] C. J. Arnold, G. Garrigues, J. W. Geme III, and D. J. Sexton, "Necrotizing fasciitis caused by *Haemophilus influenzae* Serotype f," *Journal of Clinical Microbiology*, vol. 52, no. 9, pp. 3471–3474, 2014.
[13] B. D. Gessner, B.-M. Njanpop-Lafourcade, and M. A. Herbert, "Haemophilus influenza," 2006, http://antimicrobe.org/b67.asp.
[14] D. M. Musher, "Haemophilus Species," in *Medical Microbiology*, University of Texas Medical Branch at Galveston, Galveston, TX, USA, 4th edition, 1996.

45

A Case of Malaria Predisposing to *Salmonella* Bacteremia in a Returning Traveler from Nigeria

Robert Jakubowski,[1] Lisa L. Steed,[2] Susan E. Dorman,[1] and Camelia Marculescu[1]

[1]*Division of Infectious Diseases, Department of Medicine, Medical University of South Carolina, 135 Rutledge Avenue, MSC 752, Charleston, SC, USA*
[2]*Department of Pathology and Laboratory Medicine, Medical University of South Carolina, 171 Ashley Avenue, MSC 908, Charleston, SC, USA*

Correspondence should be addressed to Robert Jakubowski; jakubowr@musc.edu

Academic Editor: Alexandre R. Marra

We describe a febrile adult returning to the U.S. from Nigeria. Malaria was diagnosed by rapid antigen testing, but recognition of invasive nontyphoidal *Salmonella* disease was delayed. While the moniker, "typhomalaria," once used to describe an illness with features of malaria and typhoid fever, has fallen out of favor, it may nevertheless be a helpful reminder to clinicians that both infectious diseases can arise in the same patient. Blood cultures should be obtained routinely in febrile returning travelers from malaria-endemic regions, including those in whom the diagnosis of malaria has already been established.

1. Introduction

The moniker "typhomalaria" first appeared in the medical literature in 1876 when U.S. Army surgeon J. J. Woodward used it to describe a febrile illness that had been observed among U.S. Civil War soldiers and had features of typhoid as well as periodic chills and rigors [1, 2]. At that time, the parasitic etiology of malaria was only on the verge of discovery [3]. Nevertheless, Woodward correctly concluded based on postmortem examinations of intestinal ulcers and serum pigment granules that typhomalaria was caused by "two varieties of miasmata," typhoid fever and a malarial disease [4]. In 1929, Dr. George Giglioli, working in British Guiana, noticed an association between *Salmonella* paratyphi C and malaria. He observed that paratyphoid C was more prevalent and severe during malaria outbreaks [5]. Malaria was largely eradicated from the U.S. by 1949, and typhomalaria has since faded from the medical lexicon [6]. In this case report, we present a case of concomitant malaria and invasive nontyphoidal *Salmonella* infection in a returning traveler to the U.S.

2. Case Presentation

A 50-year-old female returning traveler presented to an emergency room in South Carolina for evaluation of syncope. Thirteen days prior she had returned from a 10-day trip to Lagos, Nigeria, where she visited family. While in Lagos, she felt well. Six days after returning to the U.S., she developed nausea and diarrhea. Three days later, she developed fevers and sweats that occurred multiple times daily. Twelve days after returning to the U.S., she experienced two episodes of syncope and then sought medical care. She had no headache, neck stiffness, sore throat, or respiratory symptoms. She reported that while in Lagos, she stayed in a home in an urban environment. She used mosquito repellent with N, N-diethyl-meta-toluamide (DEET), and slept indoors with closed windows but no mosquito net. She did not recall any mosquito bites. While in Lagos, she ate food prepared in the home after purchase from a local grocery store, and she drank only bottled water. She did not recall having been in contact with anyone who was sick while she was in Lagos. She reported having taken a prescription medication for malaria prevention, but we were unable to verify this. She had received oral typhoid, yellow fever, hepatitis A, TDaP, influenza, and meningococcal vaccines within the preceding year. The recent trip was her third to Nigeria; she had been well during and after her previous two trips. She was born and raised in South Carolina and had no other international travel. She had no significant past medical history and was not taking any medications at the time of presentation. She worked as a manager at a retail clothing store.

On examination at presentation, the temperature was 100.8°, pulse 117/minute and regular, blood pressure 127/78, respirations 18/minute and unlabored, and O_2 saturation was 99% breathing ambient air. She appeared comfortable, well-nourished, and not chronically ill. There was no jaundice or lymphadenopathy. Lungs were clear. Heart sounds were normal aside from tachycardia, and there was no murmur. The abdomen was not tender, and there was no hepatosplenomegaly. She was alert, and neurologic exam was unremarkable. Laboratory test results are shown in Table 1.

Table 1

Variable	Hospital day 1
White cell count	8500/μL
Hemoglobin	10.7 gm/dL
Platelet count	142,000/μL
Sodium	123 mmol/L
Potassium	3.9 mmol/L
Chloride	90 mmol/L
Bicarbonate	24 mmol/L
Blood urea nitrogen	16 mg/dL
Creatinine	1.0 mg/dL
Glucose	107 mg/dL
Calcium	7.7 mg/dL
Total protein	6.7 g/dL
Albumin	2.3 g/dL
AST	49 U/L
ALT	52 U/L
Alkaline phosphatase	111 U/L
Total bilirubin	2.4 mg/dL

There was no hemoglobin detected in the urine. Blood cultures were drawn. Thick and thin blood smears were prepared and Giemsa-stained. Microscopic examination showed a microcytic normochromic anemia, numerous erythrocytes with trophozoite rings, and rare banana gametocytes characteristic of *P. falciparum* malaria. Parasitemia was 3.5%. Rapid malaria diagnostic testing using the BinaxNOW® Malaria test (Alere Inc., Waltham Massachusetts) was positive for *P. falciparum*. An ARCHITECT HIV Ag/Ab Combo (Abbott, Wiesbaden, Germany) test was negative. Nucleic acid amplification-based testing of a stool specimen was negative for adenovirus, *Campylobacter*, *Cyclospora cayetanensis*, *Clostridium difficile*, enteroaggregative *Escherichia coli*, enteropathogenic *E. coli*, enterotoxigenic *E. coli*, Shiga-like toxin producing *E. coli*, *Shigella*, enteroinvasive *E. coli*, *Entamoeba histolytica*, *Giardia lamblia*, human astrovirus, norovirus GI/GII, *Plesiomonas shigelloides*, rotavirus A, *Salmonella*, sapovirus, *Vibrio*, *Vibrio cholera*, and *Yersinia enterocolitica* (FilmArray™ Gastrointestinal Panel, BioFire Diagnostics LLC, Salt Lake City, UT). At 48 hours of incubation, blood cultures obtained at presentation grew gram-negative rods identified as a *Salmonella* species by MALDI-TOF mass spectrometry. A triple sugar iron agar slant showed a nontyphoidal *Salmonella* phenotype. The isolate was identified as *Salmonella enterica* subspecies *enterica* serovar *stanleyville* (1,4,12,27:z4,z23:[1,2]) by the South Carolina Department of Health and Environmental Control Public Health Laboratory using serotyping with specific O and H antisera according to the Kaufman–White scheme. She was treated for uncomplicated *P. falciparum* malaria with oral doxycycline and quinidine for 7 days. Fevers resolved by day 3 at the hospital and repeat blood smear remained negative for malaria 16 days later. For nontyphoidal *Salmonella* bacteremia, she was treated with ceftriaxone for 2 weeks; diarrhea and all other signs/symptoms resolved within 10 days.

3. Discussion

We report the occurrence of concomitant *P. falciparum* malaria and nontyphoidal *Salmonella* bacteremia in a traveler returning from Nigeria. Each of these infectious diseases is a major cause of morbidity and mortality in sub-Saharan Africa. Nigeria bears the majority of the worlds' burden of malaria, accounting for 27% of cases globally—in 2016, there were an estimated 57 million malaria cases and 100,700 deaths, and over 85% of cases were due to *P. falciparum* [7, 8]. Invasive salmonellosis mostly affects young children, those with severe malnutrition, HIV, or sickle cell anemia [9, 10]. A systematic review showed that among adults in Africa, 42% of (nonmalaria) bloodstream infections were due to *Salmonella* enterica, mostly nontyphoidal *Salmonella* [11]. In Nigeria, one-quarter to one-half of all bacteremias have been shown to be due to *Salmonella enterica*, about half of which are due to nontyphoidal *Salmonella* [12, 13].

Co-infection with malaria and *Salmonella* has been recognized for some time and is expected based on the overlapping geographical distribution of these infectious diseases [14, 15]. The epidemiology of malaria-*Salmonella* co-infections is limited by a lack of good surveillance data on invasive salmonellosis in sub-Saharan Africa. Overall, there is inconsistent access to culture and molecular techniques outside of vaccination trials [16]. However, a meta-analysis of over 11,000 patients (adults and children) in Africa showed that 6.5% of patients with malaria had fungal or bacterial bloodstream co-infections [11]. Co-infection was initially attributed to the parallel rise of both organisms during the rainy season. However, a study in Tanzania controlled for precipitation by comparing two locations with similar rainy seasons and contrasting malaria prevalence [17]. In children admitted with fever, bacteremia of any etiology was about twice as common (9.2% vs. 4.3%) in the area with high malarial burden, but nontyphoidal *Salmonella* isolates were almost ten times more common (48.2% vs. 5%) in the area with high malarial burden [17]. The same parallel rise in co-infection was seen in Gambian children during the rainy season. However, stool carriage of nontyphoidal *Salmonella* did not share the seasonal pattern leading authors to conclude that malaria predisposed to invasive nontyphoidal *Salmonella* infection [14].

The immunosuppressive effects of malaria have been well documented since the early 1970s. Recent work has shed light on a pathophysiologic mechanism for malaria as a risk factor for *Salmonella* bacteremia. This is through the adaptive phenomenon of immune tolerance, which limits self harm in response to the parasite. Malaria infection impairs the production proinflammatory cytokines by dendritic cells by inducing a state of refractory TLR signaling in favor of a downregulatory T cell response [18, 19]. In addition, in 2012, Cunnington et al. showed that malaria-induced hemolysis specifically suppressed the oxidative burst capacity of neutrophils, thereby allowing for sustained *Salmonella* bacterial replication in circulating, but functionally impaired, neutrophils in addition to mononuclear phagocytes [20]. Together, these hamper what normally would be a robust response by phagocytic cells to the bacteria facilitating their dissemination.

Awareness of the association between malaria and *Salmonella* bacteremia is important for clinicians. In patients with malaria, undiagnosed *Salmonella* bacteremia may lead to morbidity due to untreated salmonellosis and/or changes in antimalarial treatment if fevers are incorrectly attributed to malaria drug resistance. Thus, the moniker "typhomalaria" might be a useful reminder for clinicians that both infectious diseases can coexist in the same patient. Blood cultures should be obtained routinely in all febrile returning travelers from malaria-endemic regions, including those in whom the diagnosis of malaria has already been established.

Acknowledgments

This work was supported in part by a grant from the National Institutes of Health to SED (K24AI104830) and to SRC (K23AI23607). We thank Dr. Scott R. Curry for his care of the patient and comments on the manuscript.

References

[1] J. Billings, *Memoir of Joseph Janvier Woodward, 1833–1884*, National Academy of Sciences, Washington, DC, USA, 1886.

[2] C. Steele, "Was it typhomalarial fever?," *Western Lancet*, vol. 9, no. 7, pp. 193–200, 1880.

[3] CDC, *Malaria-About Malaria-History-Laveran and the Discovery of the Malaria Parasite*, CDC, Atlanta, GA, USA, 2018, https://www.cdc.gov/malaria/about/history/laveran.html.

[4] D. Smith, "The rise and fall of typhomalarial fever: i. origins," *Journal of the History of Medicine and Allied Sciences*, vol. 37, no. 2, pp. 182–220, 1982.

[5] G. Giglioli, "Paratyphoid C, an endemic disease in British Guiana," *Journal of Hygiene*, vol. 29, no. 3, pp. 273–281, 1929.

[6] CDC, *Malaria-About Malaria-History-Elimination of Malaria in the United States (1947-1951)*, CDC, Atlanta, GA, USA, 2018, https://www.cdc.gov/malaria/about/history/elimination_us.html.

[7] World Health Organization, *World Malaria Report 2017*, World Health Organization, Geneva, Switzerland, 2017.

[8] CDC, *Malaria-Travelers-Malaria Information and Prophylaxis, by Country*, CDC, Atlanta, GA, USA, 2018, https://www.cdc.gov/malaria/travelers/country_table/a.html.

[9] A. Brent, J. Oundo, I. Mwangi, L. Ochola, B. Lowe, and J. Berkley, "Salmonella Bacteremia in Kenyan Children," *Pediatric Infectious Disease Journal*, vol. 25, no. 3, pp. 230–236, 2006.

[10] S. Morpeth, H. Ramadhani, and J. Crump, "Invasive non-typhisalmonelladisease in Africa," *Clinical Infectious Diseases*, vol. 49, no. 4, pp. 606–611, 2009.

[11] E. Reddy, A. Shaw, and J. Crump, "Community-acquired bloodstream infections in Africa: a systematic review and meta-analysis," *The Lancet Infectious Diseases*, vol. 10, no. 6, pp. 417–432, 2010.

[12] K. Akinyemi, B. Bamiro, and A. Coker, "Salmonellosis in Lagos, Nigeria: incidence of plasmodium falciparum-associated co-infection, patters of antimicrobial resistance, and emergence of reduced susceptibility to fluoroquinolones," *Journal of Health, Population and Nutrition*, vol. 25, no. 3, pp. 351–358, 2007.

[13] S. Obaro, F. Hassan-Hanga, and E. Olateju, "Salmonella bacteremia among children in central and northwest Nigeria, 2008-2015," *Clinical Infectious Diseases*, vol. 61, no. 4, pp. S325–S331, 2015.

[14] D. Mabey, A. Brown, and B. Greenwood, "Plasmodium falciparum malaria and salmonella infections in Gambian children," *Journal of Infectious Diseases*, vol. 155, no. 6, pp. 1319–1321, 1987.

[15] R. Bronzan, T. Taylor, J. Mwenechanya et al., "Bacteremia in Malawian children with severe malaria: prevalence, etiology, HIV coinfection, and outcome," *Journal of Infectious Diseases*, vol. 195, no. 6, pp. 895–904, 2007.

[16] N. Feasey, G. Dougan, R. Kingsley, R. Heyderman, and M. Gordon, "Invasive non-typhoidal salmonella disease: an emerging and neglected tropical disease in Africa," *The Lancet*, vol. 379, no. 9835, pp. 2489–2499, 2012.

[17] H. Biggs, R. Lester, B. Nadjm et al., "Invasive salmonella infections in areas of high and low malaria transmission intensity in Tanzania," *Clinical Infectious Diseases*, vol. 58, no. 5, pp. 638–647, 2013.

[18] J. A. Perry, C. Olver, R. Burnett, and A. Avery, "Cutting edge: the acquisition of TLR tolerance during malaria infection impacts T cell activation," *Journal of Immunology*, vol. 174, no. 10, pp. 5921–5925, 2005.

[19] C. Roux, B. Butler, J. Chau et al., "Both hemolytic anemia and malaria parasite-specific factors increase susceptibility to nontyphoidal *Salmonella enterica* serovar typhimurium infection in mice," *Infection and Immunity*, vol. 78, no. 4, pp. 1520–1527, 2010.

[20] A. Cunnington, J. de Souza, M. Walther, and E. Riley, "Malaria impairs resistance to Salmonella through heme- and heme oxygenase–dependent dysfunctional granulocyte mobilization," *Nature Medicine*, vol. 18, no. 1, pp. 120–127, 2011.

46

Plasmodium vivax Infection in Multiple Family Members in Texas, USA

Roukaya Al Hammoud, James R. Murphy, and Michael L. Chang

Department of Pediatrics, Division of Pediatric Infectious Diseases, The University of Texas Health Science Center at Houston, McGovern Medical School, Houston, TX 77030, USA

Correspondence should be addressed to Roukaya Al Hammoud; roukaya.alhammoud@uth.tmc.edu

Academic Editor: Paul Horrocks

We report a cluster of 6 pediatric residents of Houston, Texas, USA, who presented with *Plasmodium vivax* infection within an eight-week period. All had immigrated to the United States from Afghanistan within the previous year. The clustering raises the possibilities of local mosquito vectored infection and/or synchronous relapses. Molecular typing and local mosquito testing are crucial in delineating the source of similar clusters in nonendemic regions. Single-dose hypnozoite eradication treatment may be considered in emigrating children to malaria nonendemic countries.

1. Introduction

Plasmodium vivax (*P. vivax*) is the most widespread human malaria with 2.5 billion people at risk for infection [1]. In the United States (US), residents visiting Asia are at highest risk of returning with this infection. While clustering is common in endemic regions, imported *P. vivax* clustering among immigrant family members in the US has not been described. We report a cluster of six pediatric patients who were recent immigrants from Afghanistan diagnosed with vivax malaria within a 2-month period centered around 8 months after immigration. We report this cluster to remind practitioners that some strains of vivax malaria may become symptomatic (from relapse or long incubation period) many months after an immigrant has arrived to the United States. This cluster also raises the question of a potential benefit from screening or presumptive treatment of *P. vivax* in asymptomatic immigrants from endemic regions arriving to areas with transmission competent *Anopholene* mosquito vectors, similar to the current guidelines in those departing from sub-Saharan Africa [2, 3].

2. Case Presentation

A 7-year-old previously healthy girl (patient 1, family A) presented to a children's hospital in Houston, Texas, in the spring of 2017 (day 1) with symptomatic vivax malaria. On day 5, patient 2, the twin brother of patient 1, presented with symptomatic vivax malaria. Subsequently, on day 9, 15, 41, and 55, patient 3, patient 4, patient 5, and patient 6, respectively, sought medical care for the same diagnosis. Diagnoses were made via microscopic examination of blood smears in our institution's laboratories. Table 1 summarizes demographic, clinical, and laboratory characteristics of the patients. The patients belong to 2 related families (families A and B; the fathers are brothers) who live in 2 different apartment units on the same floor of the same residential complex. Both families emigrated from the temperate Jowzjan province in Northern Afghanistan, a country where vivax malaria is endemic (70–95%), even at high altitudes [4]. Patients were treated in Afghanistan for symptomatic vivax malaria with presumed chloroquine but the exact dates of their treatment could not be recalled by the parents. None of the patients received primaquine in the past. Patients arrived in Houston between 6 and 10.5 months prior to presentation with symptomatic vivax infection (Table 1). Both families reported exposure to mosquitoes in Houston. The 6 patients were initially treated by emergency physicians with atovaquone/proguanil as malaria speciation was not readily available. Patient 5 had an unusual high parasitemia (5%) and had no further confirmation of her results. All

TABLE 1: Clinical and laboratory characteristics of the patients.

	Patient 1	Patient 2	Patient 3	Patient 4*	Patient 5	Patient 6
Age (years)	7	7	11	2.8	5	6
Gender	Female	Male	Male	Male	Female	Female
Family	A	A	B	A	B	B
Relation to patient 1		Twin brother	Cousin	Sibling of patient 1 and 2	Sibling of patients 3	Sibling of patients 3 and 5
Day of presentation	Day 1	Day 5	Day 9	Day 15	Day 41	Day 55
Presenting symptoms	Fever, chills, headache, and myalgia	Fever, myalgia, and fatigue	Fever, chills, nausea, and fatigue	Fever, chills, emesis, headache, and myalgia	Fever, fatigue, emesis, and abdominal pain	Fever, nausea, emesis, headache, and cough
Organomegalies	None	None	None	None	None	Mild splenomegaly
Hemoglobin (g/dl)	9.4	11.2	13.7	11.3	11.3	11.2
Platelets (per mm$^{3)}$	51,000	87,000	152,000	99,000	108,000	69,000
Initial parasitemia (%)	0.25	0.11	1.3	2.4	5	1.2
Period between immigration to US and illness	~6 months	~6 months	~9 months	~6 months	~10 months	~10.5 months
Previous malaria history	Yes	Yes	Yes	Yes	Yes	Yes
Previous blood transfusion or travel outside Houston since immigration	No	No	No	No	No	No
Parasitemia (%); time after treatment	0.1, 3 days	Not done	Negative, 7 days	0.5, 2 days; negative, 65 days	Negative, 5 days	0.01, 25 days

*All patients are previously healthy except patient 4 (history of idiopathic thrombocytopenic purpura).

patients completely recovered after treatment and received primaquine as a hypnozoite-eradicating treatment.

3. Discussion

We report a cluster of vivax infections in 6 related children living in close proximity in a region considered free from endemic malaria transmission. While hypnozoite reactivation is the most probable explanation in these emigrating patients who had not previously received hypnozoite-eradicating treatment, the clustering did raise concerns for possible local mosquito-borne transmission of *P. vivax* mainly with the patients' reported history of recent mosquito contact. In the distant past, *P. vivax* was endemic in the Houston region. Mosquito transmission of *P. vivax* was reported in 1994, and *P. vivax*-competent *Anopheles* are endemic to Houston [5]. All 6 of our patients were reported to local health authorities. An epidemiological investigation was not initiated, and molecular typing and local mosquito testing were not feasible at our institution's clinical laboratories. There were no known secondary cases that occurred outside these 2 families per local health department authorities. Also, the cluster was recognized at its later stage, which made further testing impossible, given the unavailability of the patients' samples. The onset of illness in patients 1, 2, 3, and 4 was too close for *P. vivax* to complete its cycle in the mosquito and its incubation period in patients. Based on the limited available data, there was no evidence of local mosquito transmission. Less common sources of malaria as airport malaria and blood transfusion were excluded and unlikely to explain a cluster.

In nonendemic regions, familiarity with the different phenotypes may be limited, and vivax malaria presenting outside of endemic areas is often considered a single homogeneous species with providers failing to recognize the substantial phenotypic variation between *P. vivax* strains. [6] Tropical strains of *P. vivax* usually relapse at 3 weeks intervals if treated early with antimalarials. In contrast, temperate region "long-latency" *P. vivax*, considered prevalent in Afghanistan, has long incubation period (8–10 months) or extended period between malaria illness and first relapse (8–10 months) [6, 7]. As such, this cluster may be primary presentation for "hibernans" vivax malaria or long-latency relapse. It is likely that "preprogrammed" hypnozoites with biologic clock decide when they resume development, causing activation and relapse. It is both plausible and probable that our family members were primarily infected with the same "strain" of vivax malaria in Afghanistan, which could explain close incubation periods. Another factor that can influence incubation period is initial inoculum of sporozoites. The higher the dose of sporozoites inoculated in patients by mosquito, the shorter the latency period between malaria illness and first relapse and the more frequent relapses. [6] Immunity may also influence incubation period and latency. In our patients, unfortunately it was difficult to clarify through history taking, when the previous malaria illnesses occurred in Afghanistan. However, since they reported prior antimalarial therapy (though without primaquine), we suspect this to be a first relapse for a long-latency strain, as there were no reported malaria illnesses after their immigration to the US prior to this presentation.

Hypnozoites can remain dormant for months or even years. The exact mechanism of hypnozoite dormancy and activation is not well understood with multiple factors involved. For "long-latency" temperate vivax strains, subsequent relapses after the first are shorter, usually weeks, and for unclear reasons, subsequent relapses tend to occur periodically [6]. There are many concepts related to activation of hypnozoites and relapse. Activation of hypnozoites could also be induced by a new malarial febrile illness caused by a new plasmodium inoculation. It was also suggested that uninfected mosquito biting can induce hypnozoite activation, possibly via sensing of a mosquito protein [6, 8]. Hypnozoites can adapt to the phenology of local vectors, and activation would coincide mosquito season. For example, imported *P. vivax* reactivation cases in the United Kingdom were reported to be limited to the summer months irrespective of the time of initial infection. [9] As noted in these previous studies, our patients also presented at the onset of the rainy season and usual timing of mosquito population increases. Household clustering is common in malaria-endemic areas, likely secondary to simultaneous transmission, but few clusters of imported *P. vivax* infection have been reported in nonendemic areas [10, 11]. Imported *P. vivax* clustering among immigrant family members in the US has not been described. We present this case to remind providers in nonendemic regions that immigrants from some vivax malaria-endemic regions may have long incubation periods and long-latency periods prior to development of symptoms. Given the large population of *Anopholene* mosquitoes in our area, providers need to remember that treatment should include primaquine to eradicate hypnozoites (as in our patients) and also focus on minimizing transmission via mosquito repellent and good mosquito control in the local environment.

Finally, all malaria cases and especially those representing the unique circumstance of a cluster should be promptly reported to health departments so that the epidemiology of the disease can be identified. Optimally, molecular typing of clinical specimens and local mosquito testing for *Plasmodium* species will give more evidence delineating the origin of similar clusters. As migration, climate, and environmental factors change, immigrants, especially children, from regions of high prevalence of *P. vivax* could be screened (as immigrants from sub-Saharan Africa are for falciparum) and might be considered for single-dose 8-aminoquinoline treatment to prevent local transmission in nonendemic areas with *Anopholene* vectors [12].

References

[1] R. E. Howes, K. E. Battle, K. N. Mendis et al., "Global epidemiology of *Plasmodium vivax*," *American Journal of Tropical Medicine and Hygiene*, vol. 95, no. 6, pp. 15–34, 2016.

[2] C. E. Matisz, S. Z. Brown, S. Houston et al., "Post-arrival screening for malaria in asymptomatic refugees using real-time PCR," *American Journal of Tropical Medicine and Hygiene*, vol. 84, no. 1, pp. 161–165, 2011.

[3] *Overseas Refugee Health Guidelines: Malaria*, https://www.cdc.gov/immigrantrefugeehealth/guidelines/overseas/malaria-guidelines-overseas.html#sect2.

[4] WHO, *World Malaria Report Summary*, World Health Organization, Geneva, Switzerland, 2015.

[5] Centers for Disease Control and Prevention, "Local transmission of *Plasmodium vivax* malaria-Houston, Texas, 1994," *MMWR, Morbidity and Mortality Weekly Report*, vol. 44, no. 15, p. 295, 1995.

[6] N. J. White, "Determinants of relapse periodicity in *Plasmodium vivax* malaria," *Malaria Journal*, vol. 10, no. 1, p. 297, 2011.

[7] P. C. Garnham, R. S. Bray, L. J. Bruce-Chwatt et al., "A strain of *Plasmodium vivax* characterized by prolonged incubation: morphological and biological characteristics," *Bull World Health Organ*, vol. 52, no. 1, pp. 21–32, 1975.

[8] L. Hulden and L. Hulden, "Activation of the hypnozoite: a part of *Plasmodium vivax* life cycle and survival," *Malaria Journal*, vol. 10, p. 90, 2011.

[9] P. Venkatesan, M. Dedicoat, J. A. Innes, and C. J. Ellis, "Seasonality of presentation of imported *Plasmodium vivax* malaria in Birmingham, UK," *Transactions of the Royal Society of Tropical Medicine and Hygiene*, vol. 97, no. 5, p. 550, 2003.

[10] T. Weitzel, J. Labarca, C. P. Cortes, R. Rosas, M. E. Balcells, and C. Perret, "Cluster of imported vivax malaria in travelers returning from Peru," *Journal of Travel Medicine*, vol. 22, no. 6, pp. 415–418, 2015.

[11] A. Mavrogordato and A. M. Lever, "A cluster of *Plasmodium vivax* malaria in an expedition group to Ethiopia: prophylactic efficacy of atovaquone/proguanil on liver stages of *P. vivax*," *Journal of Infection*, vol. 65, no. 3, pp. 269–274, 2012.

[12] M. V. G. Lacerda, A. Llanos-Cuentas, S. Krudsood et al., "Single-dose tafenoquine to prevent relapse of *Plasmodium vivax* malaria," *New England Journal of Medicine*, vol. 380, no. 3, pp. 215–228, 2019.

Herpes Zoster Infection Presenting as Aseptic Meningitis and Dermatomal Rash in Immunocompetent Adult

Suyash Dawadi,[1] **Sudesh Lamsal**,[1] **and Bhupendra Shah**[2]

[1]*B.P. Koirala Institute of Health Sciences, Dharan, Nepal*
[2]*Department of Internal Medicine, B.P. Koirala Institute of Health Sciences, Dharan, Nepal*

Correspondence should be addressed to Bhupendra Shah; bhupendra.shah@bpkihs.edu

Academic Editor: Larry M. Bush

Herpes zoster is a localized, painful, and vesicular rash involving one or adjacent dermatomes caused by varicella-zoster virus reactivation. Herpes zoster presenting as aseptic meningitis is prevalent among elderly population and people with immunocompromised status. However, it is a rare phenomenon in the young immunocompetent adult; hence, we are reporting a case of a herpes zoster infection presenting as aseptic meningitis and dermatological manifestation in a 19-year-old immunocompetent male.

1. Introduction

Herpes zoster (HZ) is a localized, painful, and vesicular rash involving one or adjacent dermatomes caused by varicella-zoster virus (VZV) reactivation. The incidence of herpes zoster increases with age or immunosuppression [1]. Varicella-zoster virus-specific cell-mediated immunity (CMI) is required to halt the virus reactivation. During young adulthood, VZV-specific CMI is robust which explains the infrequent occurrence of HZ in this age group. Individuals with decreased cell-mediated immunity resulting from carcinoma, radiation therapy, chemotherapy, or human immunodeficiency virus (HIV) infection are at greater risk for reactivation of latent VZV [2]. Herpes zoster is uncommon in healthy immunocompetent individuals; hence, we report a case of herpes zoster infection presenting as aseptic meningitis and dermatomal rash in the immunocompetent adult.

2. Case Background

A 19-year-old farmer by occupation presented to the emergency room with complaints of a headache for 2 days and vesicular rashes over the right side of the chest for 1 day. The headache was acute in onset, bifrontal, continuous, and throbbing in nature. It was aggravated on the supine position and slightly relieved in the sitting position. The headache was associated with photophobia and multiple episodes of nonprojectile and nonbilious vomiting. The patient did not have any history of fever, altered mental status, altered sleep-wake cycle, loss of consciousness, or any abnormal body movement. The patient complained of painful erythematous lesions on the right side of the chest. The lesions were initially small and later on progressed to become large vesicles. The patient did not have any history of chickenpox in childhood or recent exposure to it. There was no history of any diabetes, immunocompromised status, cardiac diseases, pulmonary diseases or cancer, and immunosuppressive intake. The patient was not on any kind of long-term medication. On general physical examination, the patient was conscious, cooperative, and well oriented to time, place, and person. The patient's blood pressure was 120/80 mmHg, pulse rate was 80 beats per minute, respiratory rate was 18 cycles per minute, and temperature was 98°F. The patient had no pallor, icterus, lymph node enlargement, cyanosis, or clubbing. On systematic examination, the patient had neck stiffness and positive Kernig's sign. The rest of the CNS and systematic examinations were normal. No abnormalities were detected on other systemic examinations. All baseline laboratory parameters were normal except cerebrospinal fluid analysis which showed lymphocytic pleocytosis suggestive of meningitis as illustrated in Table 1. Computed tomography of the head was normal. We admitted the patient with the provisional diagnosis of meningitis and treated with intravenous ceftriaxone 2 gram twice daily and intravenous acyclovir 500 mg thrice daily. On the 2nd day of admission, the patient had a complaint of multiple vesicular, erythematous, and tender lesions on the right side of the chest as depicted in Figure 1. The final diagnosis of herpes zoster infection with aseptic meningitis and dermatome rash was made. We stopped ceftriaxone and continued acyclovir. There was a decrease in headache and vomiting on the 4th day of hospital admission. We discharged on acyclovir 800 mg 5 times a day orally. The patient was followed-up in 3 weeks of hospital discharge without any neurological sequelae.

TABLE 1: Baseline investigation reports of the patient.

Laboratory parameters	Value	Reference range
Haemoglobin (gm/dl)	16.9	11–16
Haemotocrit (%)	52.7	36–48
TLC (cell/mm^3)	5400	4000–11000
Platelet (cell/mm^3)	240000	150000–400000
RBS (mg/dl)	105	<140
HIV antibody	Negative	
CSF analysis		
TLC (cell/mm^3)	150	<10
Neutrophil (%)	35	
Lymphocyte (%)	65	
RBC (cell/mm^3)	130	
Glucose (mg/dl)	63	40–65
Protein (mg/dl)	16	15–45
ADA (U/litre)	5	<7.0

TLC: total leucocyte count; RBS: random blood sugar; mg/dl: milligram deciliter; HIV: human immunodeficiency virus; RBC- red blood cell; ADA: adenosine deaminase.

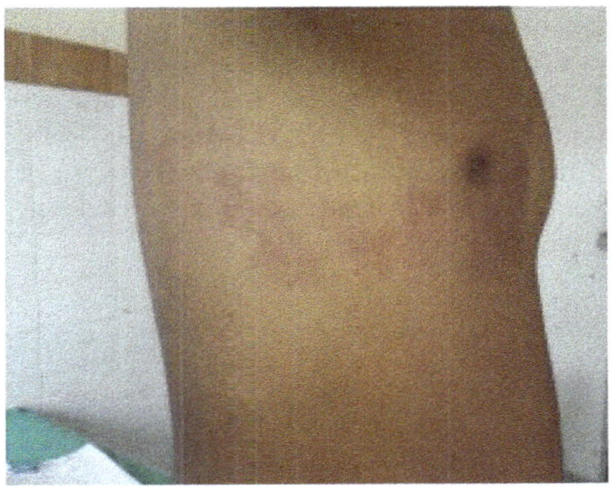

FIGURE 1: Erythematous vesicles along the right thoracic dermatome of the patient.

3. Case Discussion

We diagnosed our patient as a case of herpes zoster infection presenting as aseptic meningitis and dermatomal rash. The patient had unilateral single-thoracic dermatomal-distributed painful vesicular skin rash characteristic of herpes zoster rash. Aseptic meningitis was diagnosed as the patient had symptoms of meningeal irritation, lymphocytic pleocytosis, and culture-negative in cerebrospinal fluid and no other explainable noninfectious etiology. However, the serology test for the varicella-zoster virus was not performed due to the unavailability of the test in the hospital.

Herpes zoster is common in the elderly population; as with aging, there is a decline in cell-mediated immunity [3]. The mean age of herpes zoster reactivation was 52 years as reported by Takesima et al. [4]. However, our patient was a young adult with herpes zoster infection presenting as aseptic meningitis and dermatomal rash that make his presentation unique. A similar case report of herpes zoster in the young adult was reported by Kangath et al. [5]. Most of the patients with herpes zoster commonly occurred in the immunocompromised people as reviewed by the Bollea-Garlatti et al. [6]; however, our patient had negative workup for immunocompromised status. Only a few cases with herpes zoster presenting as aseptic meningitis in immunocompetent were reported in the medical literature [7]. Aseptic meningitis prior to vesicular eruption was notable presentation in our patient as Takeshima et al. reported only two of 11 cases had herpes zoster meningitis prior to the dermatological lesion [4]. Similar to our case, herpes zoster aseptic meningitis preceding dermatological rash was reported by Kangath et al. [5].

We treated our patient with intravenous acyclovir 500 mg thrice a day for seven days and oral acyclovir for the next two weeks. The patient had an excellent response to the treatment. Similarly, Kangath et al. reported that the patient with disseminated herpes had a good response with IV acyclovir 500 mg three times a day for seven days and transition to valacyclovir for two additional weeks [5]. We did not prescribe valacyclovir due to its unavailability in the local market. Our patient was discharged after 7 days of hospital stay and followed-up in OPD after 2 weeks and without neurological sequel. We could not perform the polymerase chain reaction of CSF to identify the virus due to the unavailability of the facility in our center.

4. Conclusion

Examining the dermatological lesion in a patient with aseptic meningitis may be helpful in diagnosing herpes zoster rarely. Even though herpes zoster infection is common in the elderly, immunecompromised, and patients with comorbidities, it is also possible in a young immunocompetent individual. Early diagnosis of herpes zoster infection in a patient with aseptic meningitis and its prompt treatment with acyclovir often have a good clinical outcome.

Acknowledgments

The authors would like to acknowledge the patient for giving them consent to publish this case report.

References

[1] R. E. HOPE-SIMPSON, "The nature of herpes zoster: a long-term study and a new hypothesis," *Proceedings of the Royal Society of Medicine*, vol. 58, no. 1, pp. 9–20, 1965.

[2] R. M. Joesoef, R. Harpaz, J. Leung, and S. R. Bialek, "Chronic medical conditions as risk factors for herpes zoster," *Mayo Clinic Proceedings*, vol. 87, no. 10, pp. 961–967, 2012.

[3] V. Mantero, L. De Toni Franceschini, N. Lillia, A. Guccione, I. Santilli, and E. Agostoni, "Varicella-zoster meningoencephaloradiculoneuropathy in an immunocompetent young woman," *Journal of Clinical Virology*, vol. 57, no. 4, pp. 361-362, 2013.

[4] S. Takeshima, Y. Shiga, T. Himeno et al., "Clinical, epidemiological and etiological studies of adult aseptic meningitis: report of 11 cases with varicella zoster virus meningitis," *Rinsho Shinkeigaku*, vol. 57, no. 9, pp. 492–498, 2017.

[5] R. V. Kangath, T. E. Lindeman, and K. Brust, "Herpes zoster as a cause of viral meningitis in immunocompetent patients," *BMJ Case Reports*, vol. 2013, Article ID bcr2012007575, 2013.

[6] M. L. Bollea-Garlatti, L. A. Bollea-Garlatti, A. S. Vacas et al., "Características clínicas y evolutivas de una población con herpes zoster diseminado: un estudio de cohorte retrospectiva," *Actas Dermo-Sifiliográficas*, vol. 108, no. 2, pp. 145–152, 2017.

[7] M. Gnoni, K. Zaheer, M. M. Vasser et al., "Varicella Zoster aseptic meningitis: report of an atypical case in an immunocompetent patient treated with oral valacyclovir," *IDCases*, vol. 13, Article ID e00446, 2018.

A Case of Bacteremia and Meningitis Associated with Piperacillin-Tazobactam Nonsusceptible, Ceftriaxone Susceptible *Escherichia coli* during *Strongyloides* Hyperinfection in an Immunocompromised Host

Santosh Dahal, Jeffrey Lederman, Jesse Berman, Marius Viseroi, and Stephen Jesmajian

Department of Internal Medicine, Albert Einstein College of Medicine, Montefiore Medical Center, New Rochelle, NY 10801, USA

Correspondence should be addressed to Santosh Dahal; sdahal@montefiore.org

Academic Editor: Alexandre R. Marra

Strongyloidiasis is an emerging parasitic infection with intriguing epidemiology, presentation, and clinical management. We report a case of hyperinfection syndrome complicated by *E. coli* bacteremia and meningitis with one of the isolates showing a unique resistance pattern recently being recognized. This report describes the aspect of invasive bacterial infections in strongyloidiasis and highlights the unique susceptibility pattern of the *E. coli* isolate and the extreme caution required during the antibiotic therapy.

1. Introduction

Invasive bacterial infections, including meningitis by enteric and other commensal bacteria, are a known complication of severe *Strongyloides* spp. infection. Mortality rates as high as 60% and 68.5% have been reported for hyperinfection syndrome and disseminated infection, respectively [1]. Furthermore, Gram-negative bacillary meningitis by itself is a serious infection with a case fatality rate between 15 and 40% [2]. Eradication of the parasite is pivotal in the management, and it can be challenging in an immunocompromised host. Appropriate antibiotic therapy is the cornerstone in the management.

2. Case Presentation

The case is a 59-year-old Hispanic female born in Mexico with a medical history of insulin-dependent type 2 diabetes and rheumatoid arthritis on methotrexate, abatacept, and prednisone. Her prednisone dose was increased because of corneal transplant two days prior to admission. The patient was seen in the emergency department multiple times over the preceding month for abdominal pain, diarrhea, and vomiting and was treated with ciprofloxacin and metronidazole a week prior. She presented with lethargy, temperature 102°F, heart rate 121 bpm, and blood pressure 102/80 mmHg. Her Glasgow Coma Scale (GCS) score was 15/15, and meningeal signs were absent. The blood leukocyte count was 16,600 cells/mcL, serum sodium was 121 mmol/L, potassium was 3.4 mmol/L, chloride was 89 mmol/L, CO_2 was 10 mmol/L, and blood sugar was 222 mg/dl. Arterial blood gas analysis showed triple acid-base disturbance with high anion gap metabolic acidosis, metabolic alkalosis, and respiratory alkalosis (pH 7.35, pCO_2 13, and HCO_3 7.1). Urine showed large ketones. CT scan of the abdomen showed possible colitis with thickening of the colon. She was started on insulin protocol after supplementing potassium. She was started on vancomycin 1.25 g every 12 hours (q12 hr) and piperacillin-tazobactam (PTZ) 3.37 g every 6 hours (q6 hr). Immunosuppressive agents were put on hold. She became more acidotic and tachypneic requiring intubation to prevent respiratory fatigue. On day 2 (D2), blood cultures grew Gram-negative bacilli (GNB). Suspicion of strongyloidiasis was high in the setting of Gram-negative bacteremia and a recent history of persistent GI symptoms in a patient from an endemic region. Single dose of ivermectin 200 micrograms/kg was given empirically. On D3, stool and

Table 1: Antibiotic sensitivity reports for *E. coli* isolates (MicroScan WalkAway, NBC44).

Test panel	*E. coli* (blood culture) MIC/KB value (specimen collected on 12/07/2016)	*E. coli* (CSF culture) MIC/KB value (specimen collected on 12/14/2016)
Ampicillin/sulbactam	Resistant $(R) > 16/8$	$R > 16/8$
Amikacin	Sensitive $(S) \leq 16$	$S \leq 16$
Ampicillin	$R > 16$	$R > 16$
Aztreonam	$S \leq 8$	$S \leq 8$
Ceftriaxone	$S \leq 8$	$S \leq 8$
Cefoxitin	$S \leq 8$	$S \leq 8$
Cefazolin	$S \leq 8$	$R > 16$
Ciprofloxacin	$R > 2$	$R > 2$
Ertapenem	$S \leq 1$	$S \leq 1$
Gentamicin	$S \leq 4$	$S \leq 4$
Imipenem	Not tested	$S \leq 4$
Piperacillin/tazobactam	$S \leq 16$	$R > 64$
Trimethoprim/sulfamethoxazole	$R > 2/38$	$R > 2/38$

sputum microscopy reported larvae of *Strongyloides* spp. GNB from blood culture was identified as *E. coli*, which was sensitive to cefazolin and piperacillin-tazobactam (PTZ) (Table 1). Hence, PTZ was continued.

She improved clinically, remained afebrile, and got extubated on D4, was started on oral diet on D5, and was moved out of ICU to regular floor on D6. Serology for *Strongyloides* was reported to be positive for immunoglobulin (Ig) A. On day 7, PTZ was switched with cephalexin 500 mg q6 hr. Early the next morning, she was found to have rapidly worsening mental status and was reintubated. Cephalexin was switched with cefepime 2 g q8 hr and ampicillin 2 g q4 hr. Lumbar puncture (LP) was done, and CSF showed GNB, WBC 330 cells/mcL with 98% granulocytes and 2% monocytes, RBC 250 cells/mcL, glucose less than 10 mg/dl, and protein 458 mg/dl. Ampicillin was stopped. Repeat stool microscopy remained positive for *Strongyloides* spp. Ivermectin dose was increased to 400 mcg/kg daily in 40% ethanol to increase absorption, and albendazole 400 mg q12 hr was also added. On D10, CSF culture reported *E. coli* resistant to PTZ and cefazolin but sensitive to ceftriaxone (CTX) (Table 1). Identification and sensitivity were done by using the MicroScan WalkAway 40 SI system with Negative combo 44 panels. Cefepime was continued. Her mental status did not improve, and the electroencephalogram was reported to be consistent with vegetative state with cerebral dysfunction. Repeat LP after 2 weeks showed WBC 82 cells/mcL with granulocytes 53%, lymphocytes, 46%, and monocytes 1%, RBC 9 cells/mcL, glucose 51 mg/dl, total protein 81 mg/dl, and LDH 192, and Gram staining and culture were negative. Repeated stool exams were negative for larvae. The patient received 14 days of ivermectin and 7 days of albendazole. She did not improve and underwent palliative extubation on D19 and died 10 days later.

3. Discussion

Strongyloidiasis is an emerging parasitic infection in developing countries of tropical and subtropical regions with small endemic areas in the temperate region. However, according to recent epidemiological studies, there is some endemicity even in developed countries, including the United States [3]. Epidemiology is complicated by international travel and migration patterns, and global data are considered inadequate [4]. In our case, the patient was born and grew up in Mexico and had a history of multiple travels to Mexico.

The life cycle of this helminthic parasite is unique and complex, with filariform larvae penetrating the skin and ending up in the gut from various routes involving connective tissue, bloodstream, and lungs. Their ability to cause autoinfection is characteristic, which is also the mechanism for hyperinfection. The clinical course is commonly chronic and symptomatically mild, but in immunosuppressed hosts, hyperinfection syndrome characterized by severe disease with high parasitic load and disseminated infection involving internal organs can occur which could be fatal [5]. Diagnosis is difficult and usually late because of variable presentation. In nonendemic settings, a very high index of suspicion is required for diagnosis. In this case, chronic GI symptoms were suggestive, and she had strong risk factors such as the use of abatacept and prednisone and diabetes [6]. No evidence could be found as to whether she was screened for *Strongyloides* spp. before she was started on immunosuppressive therapy, but the screening could have been lifesaving. History of persistent GI symptoms and Gram-negative bacteremia without other sources of infection aroused high suspicion of strongyloidiasis, so we treated her with one dose of ivermectin while waiting for stool microscopy. Our decision to start treatment prior to obtaining diagnostic evidence was based on clinical judgement, and there is no evidence regarding empirical treatment of strongyloidiasis.

Invasive bacterial infections are a well-known complication of strongyloidiasis, which is explained by bacterial translocation on the nematode's surface as it penetrates the intestinal mucosa [7]. According to one study, out of 30 patients with *S. stercoralis*, 16 had invasive infections, including sepsis, meningitis, pneumonia, peritonitis, and endocarditis caused by enteric bacteria and *Candida* spp. [8]. Although pathogenesis is still unclear, high-grade bacteremia is key to meningitis [2]. Bacterial isolates from meningitis associated with strongyloidiasis are mostly the intestinal commensals including *Escherichia coli*, *Streptococcus bovis*, *Klebsiella pneumoniae*, *Lactococcus lactis*, *Streptococcus sanguinis*, *Enterococcus faecium*, and *Staphylococcus warneri* [9–11]. We used broad-spectrum therapy with PTZ and vancomycin for our patient until blood culture reported growth of GNB.

A week after hospitalization, when the patient was moved out of ICU to regular floors and a day after switching from PTZ to cephalexin, the patient had rapid deterioration of mental status and was found to have meningitis from *E. coli* resistant to PTZ and cefazolin but susceptible to CTX. This situation could have resulted from partially treated CNS infection because of ineffective CNS concentration of PTZ, leading to selection of resistant strains or failure to control high inoculum of *E. coli* infection with seeding of the central nervous system. Clinical worsening while the patient was switched from PTZ to cephalexin which was active for less than 24 hours was most likely coincidental than contributory to worsening of the disease. It has been reported that the clinical use of β-lactam/β-lactamase inhibitor combinations results in the selection of point mutants in TEM penicillinases resistant to inhibitors, referred to as inhibitor-resistant TEMs (IRTs) which are generally susceptible to cephalosporins. Strains with complex mutant TEMs (CMTs) that combine ESBL and IRT mutations are resistant to both groups of antibiotics [12]. In this case, *E. coli* isolated from CSF was not an ESBL producer, was resistant to cefazolin, and was sensitive to CTX. A study has reported 4.1% of *E. coli* and 4.4% of *K. pneumoniae* isolates from bloodstream infections with resistance to PTZ and susceptibility to CTX. Most of these patients were hospital inpatients at infection onset and had recently received antibacterial agents, including β-lactam/β-lactamase inhibitor (BL/BLI), and gastrointestinal translocation was the most common presumed source. They have been found to be nonclonal and associated with deleted or dysfunctional porins contributing to the observed resistance pattern [13, 14].

The patient was initially started on PTZ to cover for Gram-negative infection including *Pseudomonas* spp. In a patient presenting with diabetic ketoacidosis with potential abdominal source of infection and without any meningeal signs, concern for meningitis was not significant. PTZ was switched with cephalexin as per the sensitivity report once the patient clinically improved and completed 7 days of intravenous antibiotics. Since there was no suspicion of meningitis, switching to oral therapy seemed appropriate. The optimal duration of antibiotic therapy for bloodstream infections is unknown, and shorter duration of therapy has been demonstrated to be equally effective [15]. With the view of antibiotic stewardship, there was a missed opportunity to de-escalate from PTZ to ceftriaxone once blood culture was reported. Retrospectively switching to ceftriaxone and increasing dose to the meningitic level could have altered the course of disease. When mental status worsened and meningitis was suspected, the patient was started on cefepime and ampicillin. Cefepime was continued even after the sensitivity results because we wanted to suppress the Gram-negative rods in the gut.

Meningitis could have also been caused by reinfection during the continued migration of larvae. There is a strong possibility that clinical worsening and the poor outcome were from the failure to control spread of the larvae rather than the effect of bacterial infection alone. Treatment of invasive bacterial infections is tied with parasite cure because failure in doing so poses risk for recurrent infections [11]. Ivermectin is the drug of choice, but there is no consensus regarding the dosing, and cure rates vary between 55 and 100% [16]. In our case, stool microscopy was still positive for larvae on D7 after 5 days of ivermectin 200 mcg/kg daily dose after which dosing was increased to 400 mcg/kg daily on 40% ethanol to increase absorption, and albendazole was also added.

Limitation of this report is the lack of further testing and characterization of the two *E. coli* isolates which would have provided answers as to how closely they were related and the possible mechanism of the resistance pattern. It is important for the clinical practitioners to be aware of the occurrence of such a resistance pattern and the prevalence in their practice settings. Enteric bacteria and the bowel flora can cause invasive bacterial infections including meningitis during strongyloidiasis, and there should be high suspicion of meningitis in these cases. Antibiotic therapy should be decided taking into account high rates of resistance found among enteric bacteria and the risk of reinfection until the parasitic infection is cured.

References

[1] D. Buonfrate, A. Requena-Mendez, A. Angheben et al., "Severe strongyloidiasis: a systematic review of case reports," *BMC Infectious Diseases*, vol. 13, no. 1, p. 78, 2013.

[2] K. S. Kim, "Human meningitis-associated *Escherichia coli*," *EcoSal Plus*, vol. 7, no. 1, 2016.

[3] L. A. Marcos, A. Terashima, H. L. Dupont, and E. Gotuzzo, "*Strongyloides* hyperinfection syndrome: an emerging global infectious disease," *Transactions of the Royal Society of Tropical Medicine and Hygiene*, vol. 102, no. 4, pp. 314–318, 2008.

[4] World Health Organization, *Strongyloidiasis*, WHO, Geneva, Switzerland, 2017.

[5] L. A. Marcos, A. Terashima, M. Canales, and E. Gotuzzo, "Update on strongyloidiasis in the immunocompromised host," *Current Infectious Disease Reports*, vol. 13, no. 1, pp. 35–46, 2011.

[6] S. Lim, K. Katz, S. Krajden, M. Fuksa, J. S. Keystone, and K. C. Kain, "Complicated and fatal *Strongyloides* infection in Canadians: risk factors, diagnosis and management," *Canadian Medical Association Journal*, vol. 171, no. 5, pp. 479–484, 2004.

[7] W. G. Simpson, D. C. Gerhardstein, and J. R. Thompson, "Disseminated *Strongyloides stercoralis* infection," *Southern Medical Journal*, vol. 86, no. 7, pp. 821–825, 1993.

[8] M. N. Al-Hasan, M. McCormick, and J. A. Ribes, "Invasive enteric infections in hospitalized patients with underlying strongyloidiasis," *American Journal of Clinical Pathology*, vol. 128, no. 4, pp. 622–627, 2007.

[9] T. Shimasaki, H. Chung, and S. Shiiki, "Five cases of recurrent meningitis associated with chronic strongyloidiasis," *American Journal of Tropical Medicine and Hygiene*, vol. 92, no. 3, pp. 601–604, 2015.

[10] L. Zammarchi, F. Montagnani, G. Tordini et al., "Persistent strongyloidiasis complicated by recurrent meningitis in an HTLV seropositive Peruvian migrant resettled in Italy," *American Journal of Tropical Medicine and Hygiene*, vol. 92, no. 6, pp. 1257–1260, 2015.

[11] R. N. Incani, M. Hernández, J. Cortez, M. E. E. González, and Y. D. Salazar, "*Staphylococcus warneri* meningitis in a patient with *Strongyloides stercoralis* hyperinfection and lymphoma: first report of a case," *Revista do Instituto de Medicina Tropical de Sao Paulo*, vol. 52, no. 3, pp. 169-170, 2010.

[12] J. Lee, C. E. Oh, E. H. Choi, and H. J. Lee, "The impact of the increased use of piperacillin/tazobactam on the selection of antibiotic resistance among invasive *Escherichia coli* and *Klebsiella pneumoniae* isolates," *International Journal of Infectious Diseases*, vol. 17, no. 8, pp. e638–e643, 2013.

[13] T. Baker, D. P. Calfee, L. Westblade, S. Jenkins, B. N. Kreiswirth, and M. Satlin, "Characterization of piperacillin-tazobactam-non-susceptible, but ceftriaxone-susceptible, *Escherichia coli* and *Klebsiella pneumoniae* bloodstream infections," *Open Forum Infectious Diseases*, vol. 3, no. 1, p. 2014, 2016.

[14] J. R. Mediavilla, Z. Schneider, C. Nwaigwe et al., "Molecular characterization of piperacillin-tazobactam (TZP)-resistant *Escherichia coli* susceptible to cephalosporins, monobactams, and carbapenems," *Open Forum Infectious Diseases*, vol. 2, no. 1, p. 1181, 2015.

[15] T. C. Havey, R. A. Fowler, and N. Daneman, "Duration of antibiotic therapy for bacteremia: a systematic review and meta-analysis," *Critical Care*, vol. 15, no. 6, p. R267, 2011.

[16] T. Mendes, K. Minori, M. Ueta, D. C. Miguel, and S. M. Allegretti, "Strongyloidiasis current status with emphasis in diagnosis and drug research," *Journal of Parasitology Research*, vol. 2017, Article ID 5056314, 13 pages, 2017.

Invasive *Malassezia pachydermatis* Infection in an 8-Year-Old Child on Lipid Parenteral Nutrition

Zheyi Teoh,[1] **Joel Mortensen**,[2] **and Joshua K. Schaffzin**[1,3]

[1]*Division of Pediatric Infectious Diseases, Cincinnati Children's Hospital Medical Center, Cincinnati, OH, USA*
[2]*Department of Pathology and Laboratory Medicine, Cincinnati Children's Hospital Medical Center, Cincinnati, OH, USA*
[3]*Department of Pediatrics, University of Cincinnati College of Medicine, Cincinnati, OH, USA*

Correspondence should be addressed to Zheyi Teoh; zheyi.teoh@cchmc.org and Joshua K. Schaffzin; joshua.schaffzin@cchmc.org

Academic Editor: Dawei Cui

Invasive disease due to *Malassezia pachydermatis* infection is uncommon but increasingly recognized in children, especially neonates on parenteral nutrition or immunocompromised children. We describe a case of *Malassezia pachydermatis* fungemia in a demographically distinct patient and discuss the workup and current strategies for managing this infection in the setting of a central venous catheter.

1. Introduction

The genus *Malassezia* (class Malasseziomycetes, subphylum Ustilaginomycotina, phylum Basidiomycota) comprises a group of lipid-dependent yeasts that are part of the human population skin mycobiome [1]. Though they are typically associated with common skin disorders, they are increasingly recognized as causes of invasive infections in children. Three species of *Malassezia*, *Malassezia furfur*, *Malassezia pachydermatis*, and *Malassezia sympodalis,* have been implicated in invasive infections found in humans [2].

M. pachydermatis is a zoophilic species that is part of the normal skin flora of dogs and cats [3] but has been implicated in human cases of catheter-related bloodstream infection, meningitis, and death [2, 4–6]. Pediatric cases are almost exclusively reported in premature infants on parenteral nutrition or immunocompromised children [2]. We describe an unusual case of invasive *M. pachydermatis* infection in a patient who is demographically unique compared with other pediatric cases.

2. Case Description

An 8-year-old girl with a history of short gut syndrome secondary to gastroschisis presented with fevers and fatigue. She received enteral feeds but was dependent on parenteral lipid nutrition (provided by the four-oil emulsion Smoflipid®) through a central venous catheter (CVC). She denied any new rashes, skin changes, or gastrointestinal symptoms including abdominal pain, diarrhea, or intolerance to enteral feeds. Her exposure history was notable for a 6-year-old pitbull at home.

On presentation, she was febrile to 100.6°F, but her remaining vital signs were within normal limits for her age. Her physical examination, including inspection of her CVC site, was unremarkable. The results of a complete blood count and C-reactive protein were within normal limits. Blood cultures (BacT/Alert®) obtained from the CVC subsequently flagged positive after 28 hours of incubation. A direct Gram-stained smear revealed yeast-like cells (Figure 1) that were approximately $3 \times 5\,\mu m$ with collarettes, making *Candida* species unlikely.

Slow growth was demonstrated on Sabouraud-dextrose agar (SDA) with and without long-chain fatty acid supplementation although more robust growth occurred with fatty acid supplementation over time (Figure 2).

The isolate was subsequently identified as *M. pachydermatis* using mass spectrometry time of flight (MALDI-TOF) (BioMerieuxVitek® MS) with 99.9% confidence.

The patient was started on intravenous fluconazole (12 mg/kg/day) when the Gram-stained smear was reported, and an Infectious Diseases consultation was sought upon

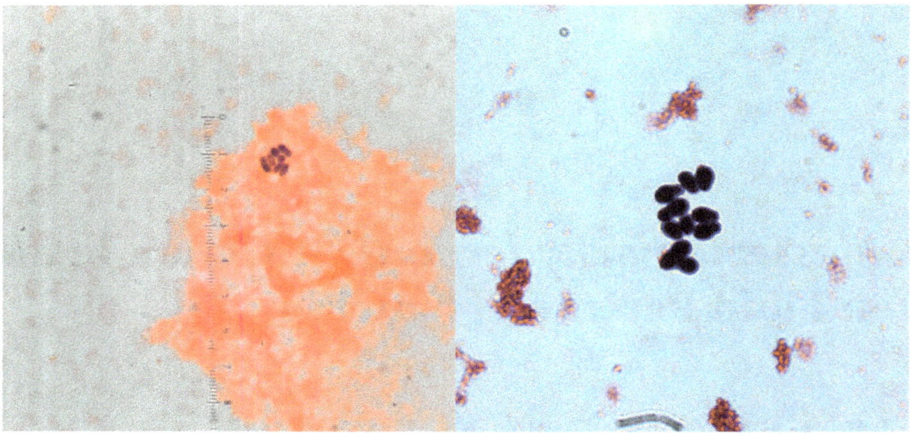

FIGURE 1: Gram-stained smear of positive blood culture revealing yeast-like cells with collarettes suspicious for a non-*Candida* organism, $40x$ and $100x$.

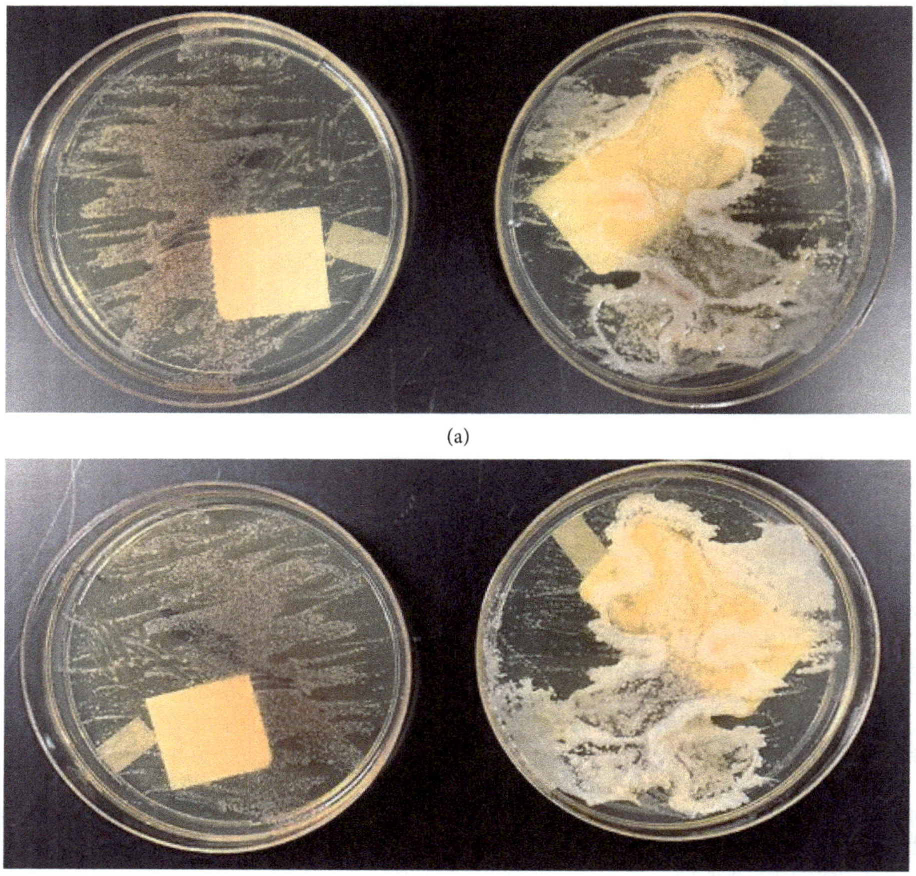

(a)

(b)

FIGURE 2: Growth on SDA vs. SDA with long-chain fatty acid supplementation, 30°C. Day 5 (a) vs. day 10 (b).

organism identification. The primary team attempted a line salvage strategy with intravenous antifungals alone as her nutritional requirements prevented discontinuation of parenteral lipid nutrition and instillation of antifungal locks. However, growth of yeast was documented on daily blood cultures obtained from the CVC for the following 5 days. Transthoracic echocardiogram and ophthalmologic funduscopic exam did not reveal evidence of cardiac or ocular involvement.

The CVC was ultimately removed and replaced with a peripherally inserted central catheter (PICC) on day 8, after which she had no further positive cultures. Results of antifungal susceptibility testing results became available on day 12, and based on these results, we decided to replace intravenous fluconazole (minimal inhibitory concentration (MIC) = 16 μg/ml) with intravenous posaconazole at 10 mg/kg daily (MIC <0.03 μg/ml). Voriconazole was another alternative option based on susceptibility testing (MIC 0.125 μg/ml). It was planned to continue therapy for 14 days, but the patient completed 18 days of antifungals before the reinsertion of a new CVC, after which she was discharged home.

3. Discussion

The majority of case reports describing invasive disease due to *M. pachydermatis* involved neonates on parenteral nutrition or immunocompromised children [2]. Our patient was demographically distinct from these children and was an unexpected case of invasive disease due to *M. pachydermatis*.

The major risk factor contributing to our patient's infection was likely the receipt of parenteral lipid nutrition and the use of a CVC. Parenteral lipid nutrition is commonly reported as a risk factor, mainly in neonatal infections, due to the lipid dependence of *Malassezia* species [2]. *M. pachydermatis* was traditionally considered the only species within the genus not to be strictly lipid dependent [1, 6]. This idea came from the observation that *M. pachydermatis* can grow on SDA without fatty acid supplementation. However, *M. pachydermatis* was recently discovered to lack the gene encoding for fatty acid synthase, as with all other *Malassezia* species. Its growth on non-supplemented SDA was explained by the discovery that commercial peptone used to prepare SDA contains small amounts of fatty acids [1]. In a completely lipid-free media, the growth of *M. pachydermatis* does not occur.

The dog exposure reported by our patient is worth discussing as *M. pachydermatis* is a known animal skin commensal with zoonotic potential given that dog owners are at increased rates of *M. pachydermatis* carriage [7]. During an outbreak investigation of 15 cases of *M. pachydermatis* in a neonatal intensive care unit, *M. pachydermatis* was also isolated from the skin of a healthcare worker and several dogs owned by different healthcare workers [4]. These isolates had similar genetic signatures based on genotyping studies, implicating dog-owning healthcare workers as potential vectors that allowed colonization of infants with *M. pachydermatis*. In our case, there were no cultures performed from the patient's dog to prove this association. Still, we suspect that the contact with the dog gave origin to the infection.

This case also illustrates the challenges with diagnosis and management of disease due to *Malassezia* species including *M. pachydermatis*. Cases of infection caused by *Malassezia* species may be underdetected because fatty acid supplementation is not routinely performed when culturing yeast on solid media. Fatty acid supplementation is also important for *M. pachydermatis* which can grow on some commercial lipid-free media, but the growth is more vigorous in the presence of fatty acids. Supplementation should be considered, especially if Gram-stain smears indicate the presence of yeast-like cells but growth is slow or lacking on solid media, as seen in our case.

Treatment of infections with *Malassezia* species is guided primarily by anecdotal experience in the absence of comparative studies and lack of standardized susceptibility testing [8, 9]. Amphotericin B or fluconazole are commonly utilized as empiric therapy [8] although in vitro resistance to fluconazole has been reported, especially for *M. pachydermatis* [10–13]. In regards to our case, we replaced fluconazole with posaconazole after susceptibility test results were made available, though at that time, the infection appeared under control. The switch to another antifungal agent was made prudentially since the very low MIC suggested a higher effectiveness of posaconazole. The apparent discrepancy between the high MIC and clinical effectiveness of fluconazole may be explained by the high dosage employed, which may have allowed reaching therapeutic blood levels. Another explanation is that the removal of the CVC contributed to the success of the fluconazole treatment.

In addition to removal of CVCs, other key aspects in managing *Malassezia* fungemia include reducing or eliminating lipid parenteral nutrition [8, 14]. Although CVC salvage may be desired, *Malassezia* species are known to form biofilms in a capacity similar to *Candida* species which may make this strategy ineffective [15, 16]. The efficacy of antifungal lock therapy for salvage of CVC-associated infections is unknown, but its successful use has been reported in one instance [17]. Not surprisingly, our patient failed catheter salvage with persistent growth of *M. pachydermatis* despite a week of antifungal therapy.

In conclusion, invasive disease due to *M. pachydermatis* is an uncommon, opportunistic infection and should also be considered for children on lipid parenteral nutrition irrespective of age or immune status. The incidence of invasive *M. pachydermatis* in older, immunocompetent children is likely underrecognized, and clear communication of a suspicion or risk of any *Malassezia* species can help the microbiology laboratory consider fatty acid supplementation of solid media culture.

References

[1] G. Wu, H. Zhao, C. Li et al., "Genus-wide comparative genomics of malassezia delineates its phylogeny, physiology, and niche adaptation on human skin," *PLoS Genetics*, vol. 11, no. 11, Article ID e1005614, 2015.

[2] W. Rhimi, B. Theelen, T. Boekhout, D. Otranto, and C. Cafarchia, "Malassezia spp. yeasts of emerging concern in fungemia," *Frontiers in Cellular and Infection Microbiology*, vol. 10, p. 370, 2020.

[3] R. Bond, D. O. Morris, J. Guillot et al., "Biology, diagnosis and treatment of malassezia dermatitis in dogs and cats clinical consensus guidelines of the world association for veterinary dermatology," *Veterinary Dermatology*, vol. 31, no. 1, pp. 28–74, 2020.

[4] H. J. Chang, H. L. Miller, N. Watkins et al., "An epidemic of malassezia pachydermatis in an intensive care nursery asso-

ciated with colonization of health care workers' pet dogs," *New England Journal of Medicine*, vol. 338, no. 11, pp. 706–711, 1998.

[5] E. Chryssanthou, U. Broberger, and B. Petrini, "Malassezia pachydermatis fungaemia in a neonatal intensive care unit," *Acta Paediatrica*, vol. 90, no. 3, pp. 323–327, 2001.

[6] A. Tragiannidis, G. Bisping, G. Koehler, and A. H. Groll, "Minireview: malassezia infections in immuno compromised patients," *Mycoses*, vol. 53, no. 3, pp. 187–195, 2010.

[7] D. O. Morris, K. O'Shea, F. S. Shofer, and S. Rankin, "Malassezia pachydermatis carriage in dog owners," *Emerging Infectious Diseases*, vol. 11, no. 1, pp. 83–88, 2005.

[8] M. C. Arendrup, T. Boekhout, M. Akova et al., "ESCMID and ECMM joint clinical guidelines for the diagnosis and management of rare invasive yeast infections," *Clinical Microbiology and Infection*, vol. 20, no. 3, pp. 76–98, 2014.

[9] A. Peano, M. Pasquetti, P. Tizzani, E. Chiavassa, J. Guillot, and E. Johnson, "Methodological issues in antifungal susceptibility testing of malassezia pachydermatis," *Journal of Fungi (Basel, Switzerland)*, vol. 3, no. 3, 2017.

[10] C. Cafarchia, L. A. Figueredo, R. Iatta, V. Colao, M. T. Montagna, and D. Otranto, "In vitro evaluation of malassezia pachydermatis susceptibility to azole compounds using E-test and CLSI microdilution methods," *Medical Mycology*, vol. 50, no. 8, pp. 795–801, 2012.

[11] K. C. Miranda, C. R. de Araujo, C. R. Costa, X. S. Passos, O. de Fátima Lisboa Fernandes, and M. do Rosário Rodrigues Silva, "Antifungal activities of azole agents against the malassezia species," *International Journal of Antimicrobial Agents*, vol. 29, no. 3, pp. 281–284, 2007.

[12] A. Peano, E. Johnson, E. Chiavassa, P. Tizzani, J. Guillot, and M. Pasquetti, "Antifungal resistance regarding malassezia pachydermatis: where are we now?" *Journal of Fungi (Basel, Switzerland)*, vol. 6, no. 2, 2020.

[13] M. Angileri, M. Pasquetti, M. De Lucia, and A. Peano, "Azole resistance of malassezia pachydermatis causing treatment failure in a dog," *Medical Mycology Case Reports*, vol. 23, pp. 58–61, 2019.

[14] L. A. Mermel, M. Allon, E. Bouza et al., "Clinical practice guidelines for the diagnosis and management of intravascular catheter-related infection: 2009 update by the infectious diseases society of America," *Clinical Infectious Diseases*, vol. 49, no. 1, pp. 1–45, 2009.

[15] L. Angiolella, C. Leone, F. Rojas, J. Mussin, M. de Los Angeles Sosa, and G. Giusiano, "Biofilm, adherence, and hydrophobicity as virulence factors in malassezia furfur," *Medical Mycology*, vol. 56, no. 1, pp. 110–116, 2018.

[16] L. A. Figueredo, C. Cafarchia, S. Desantis, and D. Otranto, "Biofilm formation of malassezia pachydermatis from dogs," *Veterinary Microbiology*, vol. 160, no. 1-2, pp. 126–131, 2012.

[17] P. M. Arnow and R. Kushner, "Malassezia furfur catheter infection cured with antibiotic lock therapy," *The American Journal of Medicine*, vol. 90, no. 1, pp. 128–130, 1991.

Permissions

All chapters in this book were first published by Hindawi Publishing Corporation; hereby published with permission under the Creative Commons Attribution License or equivalent. Every chapter published in this book has been scrutinized by our experts. Their significance has been extensively debated. The topics covered herein carry significant findings which will fuel the growth of the discipline. They may even be implemented as practical applications or may be referred to as a beginning point for another development.

The contributors of this book come from diverse backgrounds, making this book a truly international effort. This book will bring forth new frontiers with its revolutionizing research information and detailed analysis of the nascent developments around the world.

We would like to thank all the contributing authors for lending their expertise to make the book truly unique. They have played a crucial role in the development of this book. Without their invaluable contributions this book wouldn't have been possible. They have made vital efforts to compile up to date information on the varied aspects of this subject to make this book a valuable addition to the collection of many professionals and students.

This book was conceptualized with the vision of imparting up-to-date information and advanced data in this field. To ensure the same, a matchless editorial board was set up. Every individual on the board went through rigorous rounds of assessment to prove their worth. After which they invested a large part of their time researching and compiling the most relevant data for our readers.

The editorial board has been involved in producing this book since its inception. They have spent rigorous hours researching and exploring the diverse topics which have resulted in the successful publishing of this book. They have passed on their knowledge of decades through this book. To expedite this challenging task, the publisher supported the team at every step. A small team of assistant editors was also appointed to further simplify the editing procedure and attain best results for the readers.

Apart from the editorial board, the designing team has also invested a significant amount of their time in understanding the subject and creating the most relevant covers. They scrutinized every image to scout for the most suitable representation of the subject and create an appropriate cover for the book.

The publishing team has been an ardent support to the editorial, designing and production team. Their endless efforts to recruit the best for this project, has resulted in the accomplishment of this book. They are a veteran in the field of academics and their pool of knowledge is as vast as their experience in printing. Their expertise and guidance has proved useful at every step. Their uncompromising quality standards have made this book an exceptional effort. Their encouragement from time to time has been an inspiration for everyone.

The publisher and the editorial board hope that this book will prove to be a valuable piece of knowledge for researchers, students, practitioners and scholars across the globe.

List of Contributors

Linda Ponce-Rosas
Peruvian American Medical Society, Especialistas en Gestion de Salud Ocupacional, Lima, Peru

Jose Gonzales-Zamora
Department of Medicine, Division of Infectious Diseases, University of Miami Miller School of Medicine, Miami, FL, USA

Nelson Diaz-Reyes and Jorge Alave-Rosas
Peruvian Union University, Lima, Peru
Department of Internal Medicine, Good Hope Clinic, Lima, Peru

Oliver Alarco-Cadillo
Department of Internal Medicine, Good Hope Clinic, Peruvian University of Applied Sciences, Lima, Peru

Izza Mir, Sijan Basnet, David Ellsworth and Elan Mohanty
Department of Medicine, Reading Health System, 420 S. Fifth Avenue, West Reading, PA 19611, USA

Jumanah N. Algazaq
Department of Health Sciences International, e University of California, San Diego, CA, USA

Kevan Akrami, Allen McCutchan and Ajay R. Bharti
Division of Infectious Diseases, e University of California, San Diego, CA, USA

Fernando Martinez
Division of Pathology, University of Texas MD Anderson Cancer Center, Houston, TX, USA

Nosheen Nasir, Aamir Hameed Khan and Farheen Ali
Department of Medicine, Aga Khan University, Karachi, Pakistan

Kauser Jabeen, Joveria Farooqi, Binish Arif Sultan, Afia Zafar
Department of Pathology and Microbiology, Aga Khan University, Karachi, Pakistan

Muneer Amanullah
Department of Surgery, Aga Khan University, Karachi, Pakistan

Radhika Sheth and Vivek Kak
Henry Ford Allegiance Health (HFAH), Jackson, MI, USA

Ayman Battisha
University of Massachusetts Medical School-Baystate, Springfield, MA, USA

Ahmed M. Altibi
Henry Ford Allegiance Health (HFAH), Jackson, MI, USA
Harvard T. H. Chan School of Public Health, Harvard University, Boston, MA, USA

Ahmed M. Alkhunaizi
Nephrology Section, Specialty Medicine Department, Johns Hopkins Aramco Healthcare, Dhahran, Saudi Arabia

Ali M. Bazzi and Ali A. Rabaan
Department of Pathology, Johns Hopkins Aramco Healthcare, Dhahran, Saudi Arabia

Elwaleed A. Ahmed
Infectious Diseases Section, Specialty Medicine Department, Johns Hopkins Aramco Healthcare, Dhahran, Saudi Arabia

Jace Kusler
University of North Dakota School of Medicine and Health Sciences, 1301 N. Columbia Rd., Grand Forks, ND 58203, USA

Supha Arthurs
CHI St. Alexius Health, 900 E. Broadway Ave., Bismarck, ND 58503, USA

Clifford Akateh and Dathe Benissan-Messan
General and Gastrointestinal Surgery, Department of Surgery, The Ohio State University Wexner Medical Center, Columbus, OH 43210, USA

Christina A. Arnold
Department of Pathology, The Ohio State University Wexner Medical Center, Columbus, OH 43210, USA

Anthony Michaels
Division of Gastroenterology, Hepatology and Nutrition, Department of Internal Medicine, The Ohio State University Wexner Medical Center, Columbus, OH 43210, USA

Sylvester M. Black
Division of Transplant Surgery, Department of Surgery, The Ohio State University Wexner Medical Center, Columbus, OH 43210, USA

Brian L. Block and Adithya Cattamanchi
Division of Pulmonary and Critical Care Medicine, University of California, San Francisco, CA, USA

Tejas Mehta
SBKS Medical Institute and Research Centre, Gujarat, India

Gabriel M. Ortiz
Division of Hospital Medicine, Priscilla Chan and Mark Zuckerberg San Francisco General Hospital and Trauma Center, San Francisco, CA, USA

Sean P. Ferris
Division of Pathology and Laboratory Medicine, University of California, San Francisco, CA, USA

Thienkhai H. Vu
Department of Radiology and Biomedical Imaging, Priscilla Chan and Mark Zuckerberg San Francisco General Hospital and Trauma Center and University of California, San Francisco, CA, USA

Laurence Huang
Division of Pulmonary and Critical Care Medicine, University of California, San Francisco, CA, USA
HIV, Infectious Diseases, and Global Medicine Division, University of California, San Francisco, CA, USA

Akshay Khatri, Naga Sasidhar Kanaparthy, Bright Jebaraj Selvaraj and Eunna Cho
Department of Medicine, New York Medical College at Westchester Medical Center, Valhalla, NY 10595, USA

Marc Y. El Khoury
Department of Medicine, New York Medical College at Westchester Medical Center, Valhalla, NY 10595, USA
Division of Infectious Diseases, New York Medical College at Westchester Medical Center, Valhalla, NY 10595, USA

Cátia Dias, Filipa Duarte-Ribeiro, Sara Pipa and Margarida Mota
Department of Internal Medicine, Centro Hospitalar Vila Nova de Gaia/Espinho, Espinho, Portugal

Chukwunonso Chime, Charbel Ishak, Kishore Kumar, Muhammad Kamal, Srinivasan Krishna, Paul Kelly and Sridhar Chilimuri
BronxCare Health System–A Clinical Affiliate of Mount Sinai Hospital and Academic Affiliate of the Icahn School of Medicine, New York, NY, USA

Bahram Eshraghi, Alireza Ramezani-Majd and Mohsen Pourazizi
Isfahan Eye Research Center, Department of Ophthalmology, Isfahan University of Medical Sciences, Isfahan, Iran

Nastaran-Sadat Hosseini
School of Medicine, Isfahan University of Medical Sciences, Isfahan, Iran

Rasoul Mohammadi
Department of Medical Parasitology and Mycology, School of Medicine, Infectious Diseases and Tropical Medicine Research Center, Isfahan University of Medical Sciences, Isfahan, Iran

Seyed Hamid Reza Abtahi
Department of Otolaryngology, Isfahan University of Medical Sciences, Isfahan, Iran

Roya Azad
Department of Radiology, Faculty of Medicine, Isfahan University of Medical Sciences, Isfahan, Iran

Jonathan See, Kok Choon Raymond Fong and Humaira Shafi
Department of Infectious Disease, Changi General Hospital, 2 Simei Street 3, Singapore 529889

Naureen Ali and Getahun Abate
Division of Infectious Diseases, Allergy and Immunology, Saint Louis University, St. Louis, USA

Ranna Al-Dossari
University of North Texas Health Science Center, Texas College of Osteopathic Medicine, Fort Worth, TX, USA

Sana Zekri
John Peter Smith Health System, Fort Worth, TX, USA

John Gaskill and Michael Aronson
Lewis-Gale Hospital Montgomery, 3700 South Main St., Blacksburg, VA 24060, USA

Rachel Subramanian
Department of Medical Education, Santa Barbara Cottage Hospital, Santa Barbara, CA, USA

Lynn Fitzgibbons
Department of Infectious Diseases, Santa Barbara Cottage Hospital, Santa Barbara, CA, USA

Ryo Yasuhara
Tokyo Medical and Dental University Hospital Faculty of Medicine, Tokyo, Japan

Shunichi Shibazaki
Department of Emergency and General Internal Medicine, Hitachinaka General Hospital, Hitachinaka, Japan

Takayoshi Yamanouchi
Department of Cardiology, Hitachinaka General Hospital, Hitachinaka, Japan

John Ashurst and Matthew Perry
Duke Lifepoint Conemaugh Memorial Medical Center, Department of Emergency Medicine, Johnstown, PA, USA

Abdulrahman D. Algarni
Department of Orthopedic Surgery, King Saud University, Riyadh, Saudi Arabia

Berta Becerril Carral, Salvador López Cárdenas and Jesús Canueto Quintero
Unidad Clínica de Gestión de Enfermedades Infecciosas y Microbiología del Área Sanitaria del Campo de Gibraltar, Cádiz, Spain

Elvira Alarcón Manoja
Unidad Clínica de Gestión de Medicina Interna del Área Sanitaria del Campo de Gibraltar, Cádiz, Spain

Abdul Azeez Ahamed Riyaaz and Sabaratnam Sivakumaran
Department of Internal Medicine, Dr. Neville Fernando Teaching Hospital, Malabe, Sri Lanka

Vindya Perera and Nelun de Silva
Department of Microbiology, Faculty of Medicine, South Asian Institute of Technology and Medicine, Malabe, Sri Lanka

Victoria Cress
Loma Linda University School of Medicine, 11175 Campus Street Loma Linda, Loma Linda 92350, CA, USA

Michael T. Ulrich
Loma Linda University Medical Center, Department of Medicine, 1234 Anderson Street Rm. 1503 Loma Linda, Loma Linda 92354, CA, USA
Riverside University Health System, Department of Medicine, 26520 Cactus Avenue Moreno Valley, Moreno Valley 92555, CA, USA

Sue Min Sophia Kwon
Loma Linda University Medical Center, Department of Medicine, 1234 Anderson Street Rm. 1503 Loma Linda, Loma Linda 92354, CA, USA

D. Chrastek, S. Hickman, D. Sitaranjan, I. Vokshi, O. Kakisi, J. Kadlec, W. Bartosik, F. Van Tornout and V. Kouritas
Department of oracic Surgery, Norwich and Norfolk University Hospital NHS Foundation Trust, Norwich, UK

Nexhmedin Shala, Fisnik Jashari, Dren Boshnjaku, Argjend Shala and Vera Kukaj
Clinic of Neurology, University Clinical Center of Kosovo, Pristina 10000, Kosovo
Department of Neurology, Faculty of Medicine, University of Pristina "Hasan Prishtina", Pristina 10000, Kosovo

Pranvera Ibrahimi
Clinic of Cardiology, University Clinical Center of Kosovo, Pristina 10000, Kosovo
UBT College, Institute of Medical Sciences and Innovation, Pristina 10000, Kosovo

Shemsedin Dreshaj
Clinic of Infectious Disease, University Clinical Center of Kosovo, Pristina 10000, Kosovo
Department of Infectious Disease, Faculty of Medicine, University of Pristina "Hasan Prishtina", Pristina 10000, Kosovo

Syuichi Tetsuka, Tomohiro Suzuki, Tomoko Ogawa, Ritsuo Hashimoto and Hiroyuki Kato
Department of Neurology, International University of Health and Welfare Hospital, 537-3 Iguchi, Nasushiobara, Tochigi 329-2763, Japan

Deesha Bhojwani, Mohamed Zakarya and Suha Abu Khalaf
University of Missouri, One Hospital Dr DC043.00, Columbia, MO 65212, USA

Cristina Aranda Cazón, Cristina González Menchén, Zarife Daoud Pérez and José Tomás Ramos Amador
Department of Pediatrics, Hospital Clínico San Carlos, Instituto de Investigación Sanitaria del Hospital Clínico San Carlos (IdISSC), Madrid, Spain

Luis Arruza Gómez, Gloria Herranz Carrillo and José Antonio Martínez-Orgado
Division of Neonatology, Hospital Clínico San Carlos, Instituto de Investigación Sanitaria del Hospital Clínico San Carlos (IdISSC), Madrid, Spain

Jennifer Tam and Shaun K. Morris
Division of Infectious Diseases, The Hospital for Sick Children, 555 University Ave., Toronto, ON, Canada
Department of Pediatrics, Faculty of Medicine, University of Toronto, 1 King's College Circle, Room 2109, Toronto, ON, Canada

Santina J. Lee
Department of Pediatrics and Child Health, University of Manitoba, 840 Sherbrook St., Winnipeg, MB, Canada

Vibhuti Shah
Department of Paediatrics, Mount Sinai Hospital, 600 University Ave., Toronto, ON, Canada
Institute of Health Policy, Management and Evaluation, University of Toronto, 155 College Street, Suite 425, Toronto, ON, Canada

Mohsen Jari
Department of Pediatric Rheumatology, Imam HosseinChildren,s Hospital, Isfahan University of Medical Sciences, Isfahan, Iran

Gisela Borges and Maria de Jesus Silva
Internal Medicine Department, Hospital Pulido Valente, Lisbon, Portugal

Diana Neves, Inês Pintado Maury and Aida Pereira
Infectious Diseases Department, Hospital Santa Maria, Lisbon, Portugal

Purva Sharma, Mohamad Kabach, Samineh Sehatbakhsh, Rashida Tharpe, Shaun Isaac, Robert Chait and Kleper De Almeida
JFK Medical Center, University of Miami-Palm Beach Regional GME Consortium, Atlantis, FL, USA

José Leite and Diana Gonçalves
Department of Internal Medicine, Coimbra University Hospital Centre, Coimbra, Portugal

Ana Ribeiro, Luís Trindade and Victor Duque
Department of Infectious Diseases, Coimbra University Hospital Centre, Coimbra, Portugal

João Sargento-Freitas
Department of Neurology, Coimbra University Hospital Centre, Coimbra, Portugal

M. Aon
Department of Medicine, Faculty of Medicine, Cairo University, Giza, Egypt

T. Al-Enezi
Department of Medicine, Jahra Hospital, Al-Jahra, Kuwait

Ross P. Elliott
Internal Medicine Residency Program, MercyOne Medical Center and Clinics, Des Moines, IA 50314, USA

Brian P. Freeman
Mission Cancer and Blood, Des Moines, IA 50309, USA

Jeffery L. Meier
Iowa City Veterans Affairs Health Care System, Iowa City, IA 52246, USA
Division of Infectious Diseases, Department of Internal Medicine, University of Iowa Carver College of Medicine, Iowa City, IA 52242, USA

Rima ElHerte
Division of Infectious Diseases, Department of Medicine, Creighton, University School of Medicine and CHI Health, Omaha, NE 68124, USA

Nikolaos Petridis, Athanasia Apsemidou, Georgios Kalopitas, Georgios Pilianidis and Iakovos Avramidis
First Department of Internal Medicine, G. Papanikolaou General Hospital, Thessaloniki, Greece

Hazim Bukamur, Waseem Ahmed, Yazan Numan, Ibrahim Shahoub and Fuad Zeid
Department of Pulmonary Medicine, Joan C. Edwards School of Medicine, Marshall University, Huntington, WV, USA

Sevgen TanJr Basaranoglu, Yasemin Ozsurekci, Kubra Aykac, Kamile Oktay ArJkan, Ayse Buyukcam, Ali Bulent Cengiz, Mehmet Ceyhan and Ates Kara
Pediatric Infectious Disease Department, İhsan Doğramacı Children's Hospital, Hacettepe University, Ankara, Turkey

A. Shreenivasa and K. Sindhu
Senior Resident, Department of Pulmonary Medicine, KMC Mangalore, MAHE University, Udupi, India

K. A. Vishak
Professor, Department of Pulmonary Medicine, KMC Mangalore, MAHE University, Udupi, India

Kauslya Sahu
Professor, Department of Pathology, KMC Mangalore, MAHE University, Udupi, India

G. V. Chaithra
Assistant Professor, Department of Pathology, KMC Mangalore, MAHE University, Udupi, India

Mahsaw N. Motlagh
University of Arizona College of Medicine, Tucson, AZ, USA

Cameron G. Javid
Department of Ophthalmology, University of Arizona College of Medicine, Tucson, AZ, USA

Yonathan Aliye Asfaw, Girum Tesfaye Asrat and Bethlehem Aliye Asfaw
University of Gondar Collage of Medicine and Health Sciences, Gondar, Ethiopia

Tesfanew Bekele Uddo
Addis Ababa University, Addis Ababa, Ethiopia

Ayush Anand
B.P. Koirala Institute of Health Sciences, Dharan, Nepal

Helen Huang
Royal Collage of Surgeons in Ireland, Dublin, Ireland

Eden Demessie Firew
Mekelle University, Mek'ele, Ethiopia

NagaSpurthy Reddy Anugu
Mediciti Institute of Medical Sciences, Hyderabad, India

Akouda Akessiwe Patassi
Service des Maladies Infectieuses, CHU Sylvanus Olympio, Lomé, Togo
Comité national de lutte contre les Urgences, Lomé, Togo

Dadja Essoya Landoh
Organisation Mondiale de la Santé, Lomé, Togo

Agballa Mebiny-Essoh Tchalla
Direction Préfectorale de la santé de Sotouboua, Sotouboua, Togo

Hamadi Assane
Direction Préfectorale de la santé de Tchamba, Tchamba, Togo

Bayaki Saka
Service de Dermatologie CHU Sylvanus Olympio, Lomé, Togo

Mouchedou Abdoukarim Naba
Direction Préfectorale de la santé de Doufelgou, Niamtougou, Togo

Issifou Yaya
Aix Marseille Université, INSERM, IRD, SESSTIM, Sciences Economiques & Sociales de la Santé & Traitement de l'Information Médicale, Marseille, France

Kossi Atsissinta Edou
Direction Préfectorale de la santé de Oti, Mango, Togo

Magloire Manga
Université de Casamance, Ziguinchor, Senegal

Dominique Salmon-Ceron
Service de Maladies Infectieuses, Hôpital Cochin, Paris, France

Wemboo Afiwa Halatoko and Abiba Kere Banla
Comité national de lutte contre les Urgences, Lomé, Togo
Institut National d'Hygiène-Laboratoire, Lomé, Togo

Tsidi Agbeko Tamekloe
Comité national de lutte contre les Urgences, Lomé, Togo
Division de l'Epidémiologie du Ministère de la Santé, Lomé, Togo

Kokou Mawule Davi
Organisation Mondiale de la Santé, Lomé, Togo

Yao Kassankogno
Comité national de lutte contre les Urgences, Lomé, Togo

Eiman Al Boloushi
Academic Affair Department, Tawam Hospital, Al Ain, UAE

Abdulla Al Amri
General Pediatrics Department, Tawam Hospital, Al Ain, UAE

Ghassan Ghatasheh and Huda Al Dhanhani
Pediatrics Infectious Disease Department, Tawam Hospital, Al Ain, UAE

Robert Jakubowski, Susan E. Dorman and Camelia Marculescu
Division of Infectious Diseases, Department of Medicine, Medical University of South Carolina, 135 Rutledge Avenue, MSC 752, Charleston, SC, USA

Lisa L. Steed
Department of Pathology and Laboratory Medicine, Medical University of South Carolina, 171 Ashley Avenue, MSC 908, Charleston, SC, USA

Roukaya Al Hammoud, James R. Murphy and Michael L. Chang
Department of Pediatrics, Division of Pediatric Infectious Diseases, The University of Texas Health Science Center at Houston, McGovern Medical School, Houston, TX 77030, USA

Suyash Dawadi and Sudesh Lamsal
B.P. Koirala Institute of Health Sciences, Dharan, Nepal

Bhupendra Shah
Department of Internal Medicine, B.P. Koirala Institute of Health Sciences, Dharan, Nepal

Santosh Dahal, Jeffrey Lederman, Jesse Berman, Marius Viseroi and Stephen Jesmajian
Department of Internal Medicine, Albert Einstein College of Medicine, Montefiore Medical Center, New Rochelle, NY 10801, USA

Zheyi Teoh
Division of Pediatric Infectious Diseases, Cincinnati Children's Hospital Medical Center, Cincinnati, OH, USA

Joel Mortensen
Department of Pathology and Laboratory Medicine, Cincinnati Children's Hospital Medical Center, Cincinnati, OH, USA

Joshua K. Schaffzin
Division of Pediatric Infectious Diseases, Cincinnati Children's Hospital Medical Center, Cincinnati, OH, USA
Department of Pediatrics, University of Cincinnati College of Medicine, Cincinnati, OH, USA

Index

A

Aerobic Culture, 16, 20, 61-62

Anemia, 13, 60, 99-100, 125, 134, 142-143, 145-146, 148-152, 181, 185-186

Anorexia, 99, 152, 172

Antigenemia, 110-112, 114-115

Antimicrobial Therapy, 44-45, 62, 76, 96, 118, 126, 142-143, 162, 165

B

Bacteremia, 7, 42-45, 69, 74, 76-78, 80-81, 103-104, 124-125, 152-153, 159-160, 162, 182, 184-186, 193-196

Biliary Ascariasis, 171-174

Bilirubin, 20, 32, 42-43, 72, 79-80, 106, 142, 146-148, 172, 177, 185

Blood Cultures, 7, 16, 22, 43-44, 60, 64, 66, 69, 73, 79-80, 91, 99, 116, 124-125, 138, 146, 152-153, 156, 159, 181, 184-185, 197

Blood Pressure, 2, 7, 20, 37, 43, 46, 59, 76, 87, 111, 117, 127, 133, 142, 152, 185, 190, 193

Blood Urea, 79, 106, 185

C

Cell-mediated Immunity, 99, 114, 190-191

Cellulitis, 19-20, 43-44, 59, 61-63, 68-69, 180-182

Central Nervous System, 2, 15, 49, 57-59, 84, 112, 114-116, 119, 130, 132, 137, 139, 143, 195

Cerebrospinal Fluid, 49, 52, 61, 90, 111-112, 125, 130-132, 137-138, 191

Chemotherapy, 7-9, 13, 20, 23, 26-27, 44, 70, 78, 86, 89, 96, 126, 130-132, 153, 158, 162, 190

Cirrhosis, 42, 44-45, 50, 69, 77, 101

Cortex, 102-103

Cryptococcosis, 25, 49-50, 52, 59-63

Cytokines, 54, 139, 186

Cytomegalovirus, 33, 107, 110, 112, 115, 130, 132, 138, 143, 145, 150-151, 166

D

Decortication, 66, 73, 101-103, 155-157

Dermatology, 23, 58, 62-63, 105, 107, 129, 199

Diarrhea, 11, 31-34, 43, 46, 146, 159, 177, 184-185, 193, 197

Discitis, 75-77

E

Edema, 2, 11, 43, 55-56, 60, 62, 68-69, 72-73, 106-108, 127-129, 137-138, 166-167, 180-181

Empyema, 64-67, 72-73, 101-104, 155-158

Encephalopathy, 110-112, 114-115, 139

Erythema, 43, 59-60, 68-69, 83, 87, 181

F

Febrile Illness, 145, 177, 184, 189

Fluconazole, 9-10, 50-51, 53, 65-66, 157, 197, 199

Frontal Lobes, 2, 4-5, 56

Fungal Culture, 16, 39, 61-62, 112

Fungal Infections, 6, 9, 12-13, 19, 21-26, 48, 54, 57-58, 66, 121, 157-158, 164

G

Gastrointestinal Tract, 67, 145, 158, 172, 176

Gram Stain, 16, 20-21, 24-25, 61-62, 72, 77, 88, 112

H

Hematuria, 101, 142, 146, 177

Hemoglobin, 2, 7, 37, 43, 46, 49, 72, 79, 112, 117, 121, 138, 142, 172, 177, 185

Hemolysis, 143, 145-146, 148-150, 177, 186

Hepatosplenomegaly, 94, 117, 145-146, 148-149, 181

I

Immunocompetent, 19, 22, 31-34, 49-50, 52, 54, 56, 59, 64, 68, 75-78, 98-99, 110-111, 114-116, 118-119, 121, 123, 145-146, 149-151, 163, 165, 190, 192, 199

Immunodeficiency, 22-23, 33-35, 46, 48-50, 52-53, 63, 65, 69-70, 86, 110-112, 130-133, 135-136, 149, 170, 181, 190-191

Immunomodulatory Therapy, 115, 147

Immunosuppression, 3, 11, 13, 24-25, 32-34, 40, 44, 46, 59, 62-63, 102-103, 150, 190

Ischemia, 106-107, 134

L

Leukopenia, 11, 100, 127, 142-143, 145, 177

Liver Failure, 42, 101, 103

Lumbar Puncture, 29, 51, 60-62, 117, 131, 194

Lymph Nodes, 32, 72, 137

Lymphocytes, 2, 20, 28-29, 37, 94, 111-112, 121, 131, 138, 142, 146-149, 156, 164, 194

M

Macrophages, 12, 47, 117, 148-149

Malnutrition, 56, 77, 99, 185

Meningitis., 37, 52, 91, 99, 116-118

Meningoencephalitis, 111, 116, 118, 146

Mucous Membranes, 2, 80, 142

Multidrug Resistance, 76-77, 93

N

Nausea, 31, 50, 116-117, 139, 146, 155, 172, 184
Neurons, 116, 137
Neutropenia, 7-10, 19, 21, 47, 148
Neutrophils, 2, 20-21, 37, 43, 65, 76, 94, 111-112, 117, 121, 142, 146, 149, 152, 156, 186

O

Osteomyelitis, 15, 20-21, 30, 42-45, 52, 75-78, 180-181

P

Palpation, 15, 20, 46, 68, 87, 98
Parasitemia, 185, 187
Parenteral Nutrition, 124, 197, 199
Photophobia, 49, 116, 190
Posaconazole, 4, 6, 8-10, 19-23, 199
Prothrombotic Effects, 137, 139
Pulse Rate, 59, 190

R

Respiratory Rate, 2, 20, 43, 59, 64, 76, 103, 111, 117, 190

S

Salmonella, 93-97, 184-185
Sinus, 2, 4, 50, 55, 57-58, 86-88, 91, 106, 117, 134, 137-139, 141, 163
Sinusoids, 146, 148
Soft Tissue, 20, 62, 69-70, 72, 88, 180-182

T

Tonic-clonic Seizures, 110-111, 137
Tuberculosis, 38, 42, 86-89, 98-100, 112, 121, 131, 146, 152, 164

U

Ulcers, 48, 57, 59, 62, 146, 134

V

Valganciclovir, 145, 147, 150
Varicella Zoster Virus, 116, 118-119, 133, 141, 192
Vivax Infection, 187, 189
Vivax Malaria, 187, 189

www.ingramcontent.com/pod-product-compliance
Lightning Source LLC
LaVergne TN
LVHW082227200926
848484LV00008B/2315